CONTROL OF POSTURE AND LOCOMOTION

ADVANCES IN BEHAVIORAL BIOLOGY

CONTROL OF POSTURE AND LOCOMOTION

Edited by

R. B. Stein, K. G. Pearson,
R. S. Smith, and J. B. Redford

University of Alberta and University of Alberta Hospital
Edmonton, Canada

PLENUM PRESS • NEW YORK-LONDON

Library of Congress Cataloging in Publication Data

Main entry under title:

Control of posture and locomotion.

  (Advances in behavioral biology, v. 7)
  Includes bibliographies.
  1. Human locomotion—Congresses. 2. Animal locomotion—Congresses. 3. Posture—Congresses. I. Stein, R. B., 1940-   ed. II. Alberta University, Edmonton. [DNLM: 1. Locomotion—Congresses. 2. Posture—Congresses. W3 AD215 v. 7 1973 / WE103 C764 1973]
QP303.C56   591.1'852   73-19634
ISBN 0-306-37907-4

Proceedings of an International Symposium at the
University of Alberta, August 20-22, 1973

© 1973 Plenum Press, New York
A Division of Plenum Publishing Corporation
227 West 17th Street, New York, N.Y. 10011

United Kingdom edition published by Plenum Press, London
A Division of Plenum Publishing Company, Ltd.
Davis House (4th Floor), 8 Scrubs Lane, Harlesden, London, NW10 6SE, England

Printed in the United States of America

PREFACE

R. B. Stein

Department of Physiology, University of Alberta,
Edmonton, Canada

The impetus for this volume and the conference that gave
rise to it was the feeling that studies on motor control had reached
a turning point. In recent years, studies on motor units and
muscle receptors have become increasingly detailed. Attempts
to integrate these studies into quantitative models for the spinal
control of posture have appeared and preliminary attempts have
been made to include the most direct supraspinal pathways into
these models (see for example the chapters by Nashner and
Melvill Jones et al. in this volume). Thus, we felt that the time
was ripe to summarize these developments in a way which might
be useful not only to basic medical scientists, but also to clinicians
dealing with disorders of motor control, and to bioengineers
attempting to build devices to assist or replace normal control.

Over the past few years, computer methods have also made
possible increasingly detailed studies of mammalian locomotion,
and improved physiological and pharmacological studies have
appeared. There seems to be almost universal agreement now
that the patterns for locomotion are generated in the spinal cord,
and that they can be generated with little, if any, phasic sensory
information (see chapters by Grillner and Miller et al.). This
concludes a long controversy on whether chains of reflexes or
central circuits generate stepping patterns. The nature of the
pattern generators in mammals remains obscure, but invertebrate
studies on locomotion have recently made striking advances.
Several mechanisms have been demonstrated which involve spiking
interneurones (Willows et al.), non-spiking interneurones
(Pearson et al.) or coupling between motoneurones (discussion
summary by Kennedy). Again, we thought it useful to summarize

these advances and discuss their implications.

Many controversies remain. How general is the "size" principle" whereby, at least under certain conditions, increasingly large motor units are recruited to increase the force of a reflex contraction? Under what conditions is there effective compensation for variations in load and what are the relative roles of muscle properties, spinal reflexes and supraspinal pathways in this compensation? How is the coupling between the pattern generators controlling different legs mediated and how is this coupling changed during different patterns of gait?

The session chairmen in their summaries have tried to capture the flavour of the spirited discussions that developed on these points. These summaries have been supplemented with short papers submitted by discussants. These discussions and the ideas they generated should lead to improved experiments to settle these important issues. The conference ended with an impromptu and well-received reminder from Prof. C. I. J. M. Stuart of the University of Alberta that the ease of quantitative data collection does not alleviate, and may indeed make more imperative, the clear formulation of hypotheses and the careful design of experimental tests for these hypotheses. Although scientific research may be undertaken as an exciting voyage of discovery into the unknown, careful preparations are still required and a thorough analysis of existing knowledge and possible routes to be explored may be essential to the success of the voyage. We hope this volume may provide a useful summary of existing knowledge and a useful basis for planning future studies on the control of posture and locomotion.

Each part of this volume begins with a chapter which is mainly devoted to reviewing a field from the author's particular point of view. We have left it up to all the authors to organize their material in the way they thought would be most useful. Thus, except for editorial changes and the requirements of a common format (e.g. each article begins with a summary which has been indented slightly), this volume represents 44 different views of the knowledge and concepts regarding motor control, as of August, 1973.

The editors owe a particular debt of gratitude to the Faculty of Medicine, the University of Alberta, the City of Edmonton, the Muscular Dystrophy Association of Canada, and the Multiple

Sclerosis Society of Canada. Their combined generosity made
this symposium and this volume possible. We are indebted also
to the many people in the Departments of Physiology and
Continuing Medical Education who worked hard to make the
symposium such a success. We also appreciate the permission
of the many journals who have allowed reproduction of original
figures. The cover is taken from the pioneering work of
A. Vesalius in his book Icones Anatomicae. This drawing
was made at a time when dissection of human corpses represented
a substantial methodological advance. Yet Vesalius eloquently
captured the feeling of posture and locomotion under normal
physiological conditions.

TABLE OF CONTENTS

PART I: MOTOR UNITS AND MUSCLE SPINDLES

DEMAND AND ACCOMPLISHMENT IN

VOLUNTARY MOVEMENT*

R. Granit

Nobel Institute for Neurophysiology, Karolinska
Institutet, Stockholm, Sweden

A review is presented of our knowledge of the voluntary
motor act, as reflected in electrical records from man and
monkey. Thus, the electronic summation technique has revealed complex changes of cortical potentials accompanying
the act of volition and preceding execution of the willed movement. Furthermore, by monosynaptic testing with the aid of
H-reflexes, preparatory variations in the size of these reflexes have been shown to succeed a warning signal alerting
the subject to a demanded movement. Variations in size of
the H-reflex occur in a number of muscles, not only in those
taking part in the demanded movement, but even in their silent partners on the opposite side of the body. Muscle spindle
afferents in man have been recorded from in voluntary movement. Electromyography and myography have been used to
analyze the effect of varying the voluntary command and,
finally, the timing of motor events in voluntary movement has
been successfully carried out at several sites in the brain of
the awake monkey. A synthesis is attempted of the available
knowledge and the final discussion is centred on the possibilities of advancing in this field of study by considering
voluntary acts from the point of view of demand and the
checking of its accomplishment.

---

*   Being an abbreviated version of the Murlin Lecture, delivered at the University of Rochester (N.Y.) April 10, 1973.

In a recent paper, H.C. Longuet-Higgins (1972) gave an
excellent account of how I, at the close of my own experimental
career, look upon the task ahead, "In so far as the neuro-
physiologist is concerned to understand 'how the brain works',
he must equip himself with a non-physiological account of the
tasks which the brain and its peripheral organs are able to perform: only then can he form mature hypotheses as to how these
tasks are carried out by the available 'hardware' -- to borrow a
phrase from computing science" (p. 255).

Below follows an attempt at reviewing some relevant aspects
of 'hardware' research pertaining to demanded movements and
their accomplishment. Demanded movements are by definition
purposive and, when after some practice such movements become
automatic, this does not destroy their purposiveness. Auto-
matization merely relieves our consciousness of the trouble
of keeping the whole movement in permanent focus.

The new knowledge about the widespread occurrence of
anticipatory motor activity in central nuclei widely apart in the
cortex, thalamus, mesencephalon, cerebellum and the spinal
cord (see below) indicates that motor acts are operated by a
large number of subsystems of incredible complexity. Considering
with Harmon (1970) that if one has n subsystems, the number of
parameters may be still larger but even if they were n only,
there would be 2^n subsets making "complete assessment...
virtually impossible if n is large" (p. 488). Harmon, a physicist
and communications engineer, clearly realizes that we need
teleological constraints in order to narrow down the number of
possibilities in a sensible manner. My view is that demanded
movements provide natural constraints with a likewise natural
approach to the study of an instrument whose main task is to
deal with them.

REACTION TIME

Study of the simple reaction times is the·oldest example of
attempts at quantifying some aspects of a demanded movement.
Electronic summation of changes of potential over the scalp has
led to a reactivation of this approach. The technique has mostly
involved timing the act of pressing or releasing a telegraph key
in response to a stimulus signal preceded by a warning signal.
With light signals well-trained subjects (men or monkeys) have

reaction times between 160 and 180 msec (e.g. Donchin and Lindsley, 1966; Evarts, 1966; Miller and Glickstein, 1967) measured up to the electromyographic response. Hufschmidt and Hufschmidt (1954) followed by others have shown that in man inhibition of the antagonist precedes the excitatory response of the agonist by some 15-20 msec. This has also been found by Evarts (1966) in the monkey. In man, values for the efferent time vary from 30-60 msec (Miller and Glickstein, 1967; Vaughan and Costa, 1968). The latency of the evoked potential to light also varies, partly dependent on the retinal latencies which hardly could go below 15-20 msec with strong stimuli. Accepting Miller and Glickstein's value of 30-40 msec to the evoked potential in the striated area, clearly something remains to be accounted for. In his reaction time experiments, Evarts took the time to spiking of the pyramidal cells in the motor cortex of the monkey and found it to be of the order of 100 msec, as against 30 msec in the chloralosed animal. Processing of the demanded behavioural act thus added 70 msec.

In reaction time experiments a non-demanded electromyographic response may slip through the system at a faster rate than the behavioural reaction. Thus, Luschei et al. (1967, with references to earlier papers), studying the reaction time both to clicks and to visual stimuli, found an early electromyographic response after 30-50 msec. The demanded response to a click would otherwise be of the order of 80 msec. The early electromyogram definitely correlated with the stimulus, visual or acoustic, but not with the behavioural reaction. When the latter was delayed by differential reinforcement, the early response stayed put in its time-dependent relationship to the stimulus while the behavioural reaction slowed down in obedience to the new demand imposed. Training to react 'as fast as possible' does not seem to lead the reaction into pathways responsible for early electromyograms.

As is well known, the evoked potential to light is a long-lasting affair comprising several components. A late wave N_2, at 250 msec latency with visual signals, was found by Bostock and Jarvis (1970) to relate very strongly, both within and across subjects, to the speed of the reaction. This component was interpreted as an index of the moment-to-moment level of arousal. Karlin et al. (1971) found the length of the reaction time correlated with several of the evoked potential wavelets. While there is a considerable literature to show that the form and magnitude

of the evoked potential varies with the level of alertness, it is
worth emphasizing that the latency to the peaks or troughs of
the various waves has no relationship to the length of the reaction
time (Davis and Yoshie, 1963; Morell and Morell, 1966, using
visual stimulation). It is the processing within the instrument
that is decisive for the speed of the response. Of this the configuration of the evoked potential seems to be an index.

VOLUNTARY MOVEMENT

The electronic summation technique in the hands of many
recent workers (e.g. Kornhuber and Deecke, 1964; Gilden et al.,
1966; Vaughan and Costa, 1968, Deecke et al., 1969) has demonstrated the existence of a drawn-out cortical process in man and
monkey engaged in performing voluntary movements. There are
complex changes of potential preceding such acts (Deecke et al.,
1969) which I do not intend to review in their entirety with attention to details. These still belong to the frontline of research.
Voluntary movement is preceded by a slow negative bilateral
change of potential. It may begin as early as 850 msec before
the mechanogram (readiness potentials). Such changes of
potential during the time between a warning signal and the signal
to react are being eagerly studied today. The experiments need
not necessarily be completed with a motor act. Other purposive
responses may serve just as well (Donchin et al., 1971). However,
about 50-150 msec prior to contraction there appears a more
decisive and brisk unilateral change in the same direction, the
so-called motor potential, closely related in time to the spike
activity described by Evarts (1966, 1967) in the pyramidal
neurones of the monkey. The motor potential in man is unilateral and somatotopically located over the specific region in
the motor area that is engaged in the motor act. It may precede
movement of the hand by 30-40 msec. Deecke et al. (1969) find
a latency of 56 msec to the electromyogram of the index finger.

Of particular interest seems to me a paper by Vaughan et al.
(1970) in which they describe work on monkeys trained to perform
wrist extension at regular intervals. The motor potential and the
electromyogram were recorded <u>before</u> and <u>after</u> de-afferentation
of the limb. The negative motor potential was followed by a
positive deflection that had been regarded as a response to proprioceptive feedback because of its similarity to the recordable
effect of joint movements. However, it was seen also in the de-

afferented state and so, if really caused by a feedback mechanism, must have been fed back from elsewhere in the cerebrum, cerebellum or spinal cord. There had been a fresh
training period of 4 weeks interpolated between deafferentation
and the resumption of the experiments. This would give ample
time for the establishment of vicarious feedback in aid of accomplishment of the movement.

I have selected this, rather than any other of the many experiments in this field because it convincingly demonstrates a
retardment and prolongation of the cortical process itself after
deafferentation. In their work normal values for the delay between the cortical motor potential and its electromyographic
counterpart were of the order of 100 msec, never below 80
msec, occasionally as late as 250 msec. After deafferentation
the lag regularly was between 200 and 250 msec. The peripheral
motor response lasted 200-300 msec in the normal monkey,
after deafferentation 500 msec. The experiment shows that the
afferent apparatus of a limb is needed for efficient motor performance. Afferent messages must have reached the cortical
organization in advance of the motor potential, at the
time when the brain was still engaged in processing the voluntary motor act. Thus, in an animal at the monkey's level of
encephalization, the cortex must be cognizant of the peripheral
requirements conditioning execution of a demanded movement.
Except for the retardation, the cortical process itself, in terms
of potentials, was not very different before and after deafferentation. The act of processing the demand was merely slowed
down and delayed.

While papers over a period of a hundred years have shown
that deafferentation produces motor deficits, the discovery and
analysis of the cortical motor potential adds the demonstration
that, in advance of movement, the cortex itself has recorded
and made use of available information required for rapid and
efficient execution of what is being demanded. How does it
inform itself? Along what channels? The solution of this problem seems to be within reach of experimentation and one day
we shall have the answer.

While considering the subject of simple reaction times and
motor potentials, one should perhaps give a thought to the great
variations of estimates of time in this field of work. Any figure
can be doubled or even trebled, as we have seen in the papers

dealing with human subjects. Levels of arousal are known to be
very important for the outcome of experiments on reaction time
(e.g. Garcia-Austt et al., 1964), but variations are likely to depend also on temporal summation of the kind that have been illustrated so well at the spinal level by Phillips and Porter (1964)
studying the motoneurones of the baboon excited from the motor
area. Porter and Muir (1971) found the motoneurones extremely
sensitive to small variations of frequency. In studying this variable in the motoneurones of the m. abductor pollicis they found a
range of latencies from 17.6 -66.5 msec. There may be other
sites at which similar temporal summations could be equally
effective. Both non-specific and specific afferent impulses
may be responsible for such variations in levels of depolarization
as would be capable of explaining the large span of latencies
observed in experiments on reaction times.

'GHOST MOVEMENTS'

There is a considerable literature making use of monosynaptic
testing by H-reflexes and tendon jerks in man to investigate the
excitability of the motoneurones during the warning period that
alerts a subject to the signal in reaction time experiments.
During this time the cortical changes of potential indicate processing of the demanded act and the question raised is whether
anything measurable also can be recorded at the spinal level.
Some recent experiments by Requin (1969), Requin and Paillard
(1969) and Coquery and Coulmance (1971) will serve to illustrate
what is meant.

Thus, for instance, an experiment was arranged so as to
measure the size of the tendon reflex of the two soleus muscles.
The warning signal was a click, the signal to react was a light
and the response was an extension of the right foot. The monosynaptic testing reflexes were elicited by a bilateral percussion
of the two Achilles tendons and recorded by electrodes on the
soleus muscles. The right soleus alone was involved in the instruction to react, but both solei exhibited a facilitation after
the warning signal. In the muscle engaged in the demanded response the facilitation was gradually replaced by an inhibition of
unknown origin. In the motoneurones not involved the 'ghost'
movement gradually disappeared.

This experiment has been modified in several ways. In one

case the demand was elaborated as a choice-reaction-time experiment. When the warning signal was followed by a light signal on the left, the subject extended the left foot; when it was given on the right, he was requested not to respond. Random equiprobable signals were used for the two choices. Testing was by H-reflexes elicited from the popliteal fossa. Duration of the preparatory period from warning click to stimulus signal was varied from 100 to 700 msec. During this period there was a facilitation of the monosynaptic indicator reflex that again was seen on both sides and rose more slowly with the extended delay. These experiments provided more examples of the intricate changes of motoneurone excitability caused by a variation of the demand. The expectation raised by the different lengths of the preparatory period may also be regarded as a further variation of what was demanded of the subject: be attentive for a short or a long interval before the signal to react is given. It turned out that processing of the response from the very beginning was adjusted to these instructions.

Timing, localization, the relative significance of alpha and gamma motoneurones (Brunia, 1971), etc., enter into experiments making use of demand as a variable. At the Second International Symposium on Motor Control, in Varna, Bulgaria (1972), Zalkind presented a variety of 'ghost movements' by monosynaptic testing, demonstrating the intimate manner in which the cortex takes part in and prepares for movement down to the spinal level. It would be interesting to have spindle records from subjects responding with 'ghost' movements.

DEMAND AND ACCOMPLISHMENT

One of the earliest neurophysiological experiments to demonstrate the significance of varying demands was carried out by Hammond (1954, 1956), and interpreted by Hammond et al. (1956). The subject carried a steel tape wristlet connected to a stretching device. The experiments were conducted at an initial tension of 3.06 kg. Tension to pull and the biceps electromyogram were recorded. The demanded acts were: (i) respond to a tendon tap by the strongest possible contraction; (ii) when the wristlet is pulled away without warning, resist the pull; (iii) or do not resist, but let go (this will not be considered below).

Ten superimposed responses were used in each case. To (i)

the tendon tap produced a monosynaptic reflex jerk with a latency of 15-20 msec. This was succeeded by silence in the EMG
for some 50 msec. At a latency of about 80 msec followed the
subject's response. The whole experiment is thus a study of
proprioceptive reaction time.

Knowing now that in such measurements of reaction time the
afferent signal reaches the cortex to be somehow processed with
respect to the demand for a specific movement (strong biceps
contraction in this case), let us consider what could be the minimal, theoretical latency of the behavioural response, if the
fastest possible pathways were in operation. There are precise
measurements of afferent and efferent times from the work of
Phillips and his colleagues on the baboon's hand and arm muscles
and their cortical connections. Impulses in the fast primary
spindle afferents reach the cortical area 3a after a mean time
of 4.2 msec, counted from the dorsal root entry (Phillips et al.,
1971). The fast monosynaptic path from the motor cortex to the
motoneurones requires a minimum of 2.3 msec (Kernell and Wu,
1967a, b) to 2.5 msec (Landgren et al., 1962).

The additional time required to and from the biceps electrodes
can hardly account for more than a few msec. This is on the
assumption that the motoneurones are optimally depolarized in
advance by (i) the cortical paths to their interneurones and (ii)
by the maintained stretch of the arm muscles keeping the spindles
active. Adding a generous estimate of 15-20 msec a minimal
reaction time would be something of the order of 45-50 msec.
Such theoretical times probably presuppose employment of the
fast primary spindle afferents and the monosynaptic cortical
efferents. The cortical afferent latencies of spindle secondaries
are of the order of 20 msec in the baboon (Wiesendanger, 1973).
There seems to be no obvious reason why use of the fast pathways should be prohibited, provided that the subject is attentive
and well enough trained. Polysynaptic segmental excitation induced from the cortex is present in all animals and is likely
always to be engaged.

Brief reaction times are of considerable interest because
Evarts (1973) has recently carried out experiments on the monkey suggesting that in a well-trained animal these can be very
brief indeed. In this work the monkey grasped the handle of the
apparatus to trigger the rapid movement required for reward.
It responded by opposing the triggered pull. Records were taken

from pyramidal tract neurones which began to discharge 25 msec after the proprioceptive stimulus. The electromyographic response came at a total reaction time of 35 msec, so that the efferent time would have been 10 msec. The initial monosynaptic jerk at a latency of 15 msec was followed by a pause in the EMG. The reward put a premium on speed of performance, and speed, indeed, was what the monkey delivered. It was noted that the brief reaction times required attention. If the animal let his attention wander, the response time was prolonged.

Here then we have evidence proving that the cortex actually was engaged in very rapid performance. A direct connection of area 3a of the primary spindle projections to the motor area of the baboon has not been found by Phillips and his co-workers (Phillips et al., 1971; Wiesendanger, 1973), but their experiments were carried out in light anaesthesia and we have seen that brief reaction times require full attention on the part of the animal, or of man, for that matter. One would not therefore expect them to have found the key to the lock closing the path. This is tied to a definite demand. However, there are also other meeting places 'en route', for instance, in the thalamus where the actual integrative work may take place. Cerebellar impulses destined for the cortex likewise take this way. Activity in neurones of the thalamic nucleus VL has been shown to precede movement with latencies approximating those of the fastest cortical cells (Evarts, 1970). There is no information available on cortical motor potentials in those experiments. It would be desirable to have some.

I have taken up Evarts' experiment in such detail because we have a pendant to it in Hammond's second type of experiment. This shows up other aspects of the interpretation of brief reaction times.

To (ii): in this case Hammond introduced an unexpected pull on the wristlet and the instruction was to resist it when it came. Again the first effect of stretch was the monosynaptic reflex jerk at 15-20 msec, followed by a pause shortened to 35 msec. The command to resist took effect after a reaction time of about 50 msec. Evarts' results suggest that in Hammond's very similar experiment the cortex was informed and had time to act upon this information. Evarts and Hammond both used a fully awake aroused preparation, monkey or man.

At the time one could only postulate (Hammond et al., 1956) that the alpha and gamma motoneurones would be co-activated but we have since had the evidence of Hagbarth and Vallbo (1968, 1969) and of Vallbo (1970, 1971) by direct recording from spindle afferents in man that voluntary movement is executed in alpha-gamma linkage, leading to co-activation of the direct and indirect motor systems.

In Hammond's first type of experiment there would have been voluntary activation of the spindles involved in the requirement for a maximal response to a tendon tap. Assuming that in both cases the sensory message from the stimulus itself reached the cortex and was reflected back to the muscle in alpha-gamma linkage, why was the time shortened when the subject was requested to resist the pull? Very likely the effect was caused by the spindles' increased firing in load compensation to the more isometric mode of contraction implied in the instruction to resist stretching. Considering that the cortical monosynaptic path to the motoneurones operates within a span of 18-67 msec at the motoneurone, this may provide a sufficient margin for the variations of delay observed in the cases compared. (It might be remarked that there are monosynaptic corticomotoneuronal paths also to the gamma motoneurones, at least in the baboon (Clough et al., 1971). There may well be more of them in man.)

Finally, what can we say about the period of silence after the monosynaptic jerk of constant brief latency in man and monkey? This clearly precedes and, for a moment, curtails load compensations on the part of the spindles. Is it merely caused by an after-hyperpolarization of motoneurones synchronously engaged in delivering the jerk, supported by recurrent inhibition? I am inclined to be skeptical. It may well be caused by Golgi tendon organs and, in places, by spindle secondaries. However, knowing as we do that antagonist inhibitions have shorter reaction times than agonist excitation, we cannot exclude that it may be one of the properties of motor processing to sweep a path clean by a cortically generated inhibition before action. The corticomotoneuronal inhibitory path in the baboon is as fast as its excitatory counterpart and a single intercalated synapse only adds a negligible time of the order of a millisecond. More work should now be done on the inhibitions in the antagonists and their extremely brief latencies.

CHECKING ACCOMPLISHMENT

Knowing that pyramidal and extrapyramidal motor paths branch off to several nuclei on their way to the motoneurones, we have to reckon with means of internal feedback of information at many sites. Another matter is how to attack such problems in terms of 'hardware' and in their precise relation to specific motor acts. In this situation my standpoint is that one should begin with the muscle spindles and the tendon organs. These structures are situated in the contracting muscles and are accessible indicators of both force and length, of the first derivatives of these quantities and, in the case of spindles, also of the misalignment between them and the main muscle. If we cannot solve such problems, what chance is there of solving the obscure ones of internal feedback? There is little likelihood that an organ like the spindle, which is co-activated from virtually all sites capable of initiating movements (Granit and Kaada, 1953) and which returns information to both the cerebrum and the cerebellum, ever could be neglected in trying to formulate ideas on accomplishment as checked by feedback. Vallbo's (1971) recent work on afferent spindle responses from the human hand shows that even brief isometric twitch-like wrist movements are carried out in alpha-gamma linkage.

It has now become necessary for further progress to entertain some precise ideas about the structural nature of the link between the alphas and gammas that is responsible for their co-activation. I have recently (Granit, 1973) put forth a simple model which could serve as a guide in such endeavours. Its postulates should not be too difficult to test by experimentation.

Though I now have emphasised the role of the spindles in feeding back information on accomplishment, I do not think of this problem in as simple terms (Granit, 1972). There are receptors from the joints and the skin to be considered in addition to the muscular receptors. Recently Marsden et al. (1972) have studied the responses to loading and unloading of the flexor of the top joint of the thumb. By producing anaesthesia of the hand with the aid of a wrist cuff, the muscle belly (containing the spindles) has been left above the affected region and so the thumb has remained flexible. In this situation Marsden et al. found the compensatory responses to loading disappear showing that, acutely at least, spindles and tendon organs by themselves cannot operate the system. The nature of the contribution from other end organs is unknown, but it may well be in aid of maintaining the necessary level of depolarization at one or several sites along the passage to the cortex. Marsden et al. (1973) have also been led to the view that a cortical 'reflex' may be caused by stretching a muscle.

In thinking of sensory information and what it may achieve it is necessary to rid our argumentation of the unjustified assumption that isolation of a sensory input necessarily is the most informative way of studying it (Granit, 1972). This assumption is true only for the basic elementary question of conduction, convergence, divergence, etc., relating to sensory projections. Many sense organs, and particularly those concerned with movement, reveal their true significance only when allowed to cooperate in active motor acts with other input channels.

OPERATIVE USE OF 'DEMAND'

Returning finally to the original question of making demands, analyzable in terms of 'hardware' and of the need for teleological constraints, I have chosen my examples to indicate possible means of advancing. Electrodes implanted into different sites can tell us a great deal, provided that we can impose a constraint of variable purpose upon the experiments, as in those mentioned here. Explanations may not always be as plausible and testable as in those discussed above, but, on the other hand, if one merely persists in demonstrating that site a inhibits or excites site b, c or d, neglecting the teleological questions of what purpose all of it serves and how it responds to variations of 'demand', then, in the end one will be in possession of a body of knowledge, to be sure, but knowledge likely to become merely an amorphous conglomerate of well-documented facts.

Let us not underrate the difficulties. We have seen in this exposé that there is widespread cortical activity in voluntary movement, that it moulds both alpha and gamma activity according to demand, as was well illustrated by the increased spindle activity in response to a demand for greater force. We have also seen that measurable acts of preparation for a movement take place as far down as at the level of the spinal motoneurones. Evarts (1966, 1967) and those that have employed his microelectrode technique of studying wrist flexion and extension in the awake monkey, have demonstrated how widely a movement is

reflected in the brain; thalamic neurones have been mentioned
above, the pallidum is informed (DeLong, 1971) and so is the
cerebellum (Thach, 1970a, b). It seems likely that the pontine
nuclei and the dorsal column nuclei could be added to the list.
In the motor area Evarts found both pyramidal tract neurones
and non-pyramidal ones participating and also post-central
neurones in the sensorimotor cortex, the latter some 60-80
msec delayed. Humphrey et al. (1970) repeated the experiment
on the motor cortex with five tungsten microelectrodes inserted
into an area 2x3 cm centred on the forearm region. They
studied the temporal distribution of the discharges. Clearly,
in the motor area alone thousands of cells must be activated in
these simple wrist movements. The cortical neurones according
to Evarts are concerned with force and velocity of contraction.
Such discharges precede muscular contraction also in the thalamus and the dentate nucleus of the cerebellum, but there the
cells in addition fire during and after contractions. This suggests
that, like the post-central neurones, they respond to feedback
messages. For further reference to these results, see Evarts
(1973).

In view of all these findings, is it at all sensible to expect
us to understand coding in this immense 'computer' without considering that it has been moulded in the course of phylogenesis
to deliver purposive reactions in response to demands. These
were originally set by the environment, and, after development
of a cortex and cortico-subcortical interaction, also by invoking
conscious mentation of movements, remembered or created ad
libitum for some purpose.

REFERENCES

Bostock, H., and Jarvis, M.J., 1970. Changes in the form of the
    cerebral evoked response related to the speed of simple
    reaction time. Electroenceph. Clin. Neurophysiol. 29, 137-145.
Brunia, C.H.M., 1971. The influence of a task on the Achilles
    tendon and Hoffmann reflex. Physiol. Behav. 6, 367-373.
Clough, J.F.M., Phillips, C.G., and Sheridan, J.D., 1971.
    The short-latency projection from the baboon's motor cortex
    to fusimotor neurones of the forearm and hand. J. Physiol.,
    216, 257-279.
Coquery, J.M., and Coulmance, M., 1971. Variations d'amplitude
    des réflexes monosynaptiques avant un mouvement volontaire.
    Physiol. Behav. 6, 65-69.

Davis, H., and Yoshie, N., 1963. Human evoked cortical responses to auditory stimuli. Physiologist 6, 164.

Deecke, L., Scheid, P., and Kornhuber, H.H., 1969. Distribution of readiness potential, pre-motion positivity, and motor potential of the human cerebral cortex preceding voluntary finger movements. Exp. Brain Res. 7, 158-168.

DeLong, M.R., 1971. Activity of pallidal neurons during movement. J. Neurophysiol. 34, 414-427.

Donchin, E., and Lindsley, D.B., 1966. Average evoked potentials and reaction times to visual stimuli. Electroenceph. Clin. Neurophysiol. 20, 217-233.

Donchin, E., Otto, D., Gerbrandt, L.K., and Pribram, K.H., 1971. While a monkey waits: electrocortical events recorded during the foreperiod of a reaction time study. Electroenceph. Clin. Neurophysiol. 31, 115-127.

Evarts, E.V., 1966. Pyramidal tract activity associated with a conditioned hand movement in the monkey. J. Neurophysiol. 29, 1011-1027.

Evarts, E.V., 1967. Representation of movements and muscles by pyramidal tract neurones of the precentral motor cortex. In Neurophysiological basis of normal and abnormal motor activities. (Eds. Yahr, M.D. and Purpura, D.). Raven Press, Hewlett, N.Y. pp. 215-251.

Evarts, E.V., 1970. Activity of ventralis lateralis neurons prior to movement in the monkey. Physiologist 13, 191.

Evarts, E.V., 1973. As reported in Conference on The Control of Movement and Posture. (Eds. R. Granit and R.E. Burke). Brain Res. 53, 1-28.

Garcia-Austt, E., Bogacz, J., and Vanzulli, A., 1964. Effects of attention and inattention upon visual evoked response. Electroenceph. Clin. Neurophysiol. 17, 136-143.

Gilden, L., Vaughan, H.G. Jr., and Costa, L.D., 1966. Summated human EEG potentials with voluntary movement. Electroenceph. Clin. Neurophysiol. 20, 433-438.

Granit, R., 1972. Constant errors in the execution and appreciation of movement. Brain 95, 649-660.

Granit, R., 1973. Linkage of alpha and gamma motoneurones in voluntary movement. Nature 243, 52-53.

Granit, R., and Kaada, B.F., 1953. Influence of stimulation of central nervous structures on muscle spindles in cat. Acta Physiol. Scand. 27, 130-160.

Hagbarth, K.-E., and Vallbo, Å.B., 1968. Discharge characteristics of human muscular afferents during muscle stretch and contraction. Exp. Neurol. 22, 674-694.

Hagbarth, K.-E., and Vallbo, Å.B., 1969. Single unit recordings from muscle nerves in human subjects. Acta Physiol. Scand. 76, 321-334.

Hammond, P.H., 1954. Involuntary activity in biceps following the sudden application of velocity to the abducted forearm. J. Physiol. 127, 23-25P.

Hammond, P.H., 1956. The influence of prior instruction to the
    subject on an apparently involuntary neuro-muscular response.
    J. Physiol. 132, 17-18P.
Hammond, P.H., Merton, P.A., and Sutton, G.G., 1956. Nervous
    gradation of muscular contraction. Brit. Med. Bull. 12, 214-218.
Harmon, L.D., 1970. Neural subsystems: an interpretative summary.
    In The Neurosciences: Second Study Program. (Ed. F.O. Schmitt).
    Rockefeller Univ. Press, New York. pp. 486-494.
Hufschmidt, H.J., and Hufschmidt, T., 1954. Antagonist inhibition
    as the earliest sign of a sensory-motor reaction. Nature 174, 607.
Humphrey, D.R., Schmidt, E.M., and Thompson, W.D., 1970. Predicting
    measures of motor performance from multiple cortical spike trains.
    Science 170, 758-762.
Karlin, L., Martz, M.J., Brauth, S.E., and Mordkoff, A.M., 1971.
    Auditory evoked potentials, motor potentials and reaction time.
    Electroenceph. Clin. Neurophysiol. 31, 129-136.
Kernell, D., and Wu, C.-P., 1967a. Responses of the pyramidal
    tract to stimulation of the baboon's motor cortex. J. Physiol.
    191, 653-672.
Kernell, D., and Wu, C.-P., 1967b. Post-synaptic effects of cortical
    stimulation on forelimb motoneurones in the baboon. J. Physiol.
    191, 673-690.
Kornhuber, H.H., and Deecke, L., 1964. Hirnpotentialänderungen beim
    Menschen vor und nach Willkürbewegungen, dargestellt mit
    Magnetbandspeicherung und Rückwärtsanalyse. Pflügers Arch. Ges.
    Physiol. 281, 52.
Landgren, S., Phillips, C.G., and Porter, R., 1962. Cortical fields
    of origin of the monosynaptic pyramidal pathways to some alpha
    motoneurones of the baboon's hand and forearm. J. Physiol. 161,
    112-125.
Longuet-Higgins, H.C., 1972. The algorithmic description of
    natural language. Proc. Roy. Soc. B. 182, 255-276.
Luschei, E., Saslow, C., and Glickstein, M., 1967. Muscle potentials
    in reaction time. Exp. Neurol. 18, 429-442.
Marsden, C.D., Merton, P.A., and Morton, H.B., 1972. Servo action
    in human voluntary movement. Nature 238, 140-143.
Marsden, C.D., Merton, P.A., and Morton, H.B., 1973. Latency
    measurements compatible with a cortical pathway for the stretch
    reflex in man. J. Physiol. 230, 58P.
Miller, J.M., and Glickstein, M., 1967. Neural circuits involved
    in visuo-motor reaction time in monkeys. J. Neurophysiol. 30,
    399-414.
Morell, L.K., and Morell, F., 1966. Evoked potentials and reaction
    times: a study of intra-individual variability. Electroenceph.
    Clin. Neurophysiol. 20, 567-575.
Phillips, C.G., Powell, T.P.S., and Wiesendanger, M., 1971.
    Projection from low-threshold muscle afferents of hand and
    forearm to area 3a of the baboon's cortex. J. Physiol. 217,
    419-446.

Phillips, C.G., and Porter, R., 1964. The pyramidal projection
    to motoneurones of some muscle groups of the baboon's fore-
    limb. Progr. Brain Res. 12, 222-242.

Porter, R., and Muir, R.B., 1971. The meaning for motoneurones
    of the temporal pattern of natural activity in pyramidal
    tract neurones of conscious monkeys. Brain Res. 34, 127-142.

Requin, J., 1969. Some data on neurophysiological processes
    involved in the preparatory motor activity to reaction time
    performance. Acta Psychol. 30, 358-367.

Requin, J., and Paillard, J., 1969. Depression of spinal mono-
    synaptic reflexes as a specific aspect of preparatory motor
    set in visual reaction time. Proc. Int. Symp. Bulg. Acad. Sci.,
    pp. 391-396.

Thach, W.T., 1970a. Discharge of cerebellar neurons related to
    two maintained postures and two prompt movements. I. Nuclear
    cell output. J. Neurophysiol. 33, 527-536.

Thach, W.T., 1970b. Discharge of cerebellar neurons related to
    two maintained postures and two prompt movements. II.
    Purkinje cell output and input. J. Neurophysiol. 33, 537-547.

Vallbo, Å.B., 1970. Discharge patterns in human muscle spindle
    afferents during isometric voluntary contractions. Acta
    Physiol. Scand. 80, 552-556.

Vallbo, Å.B., 1971. Muscle spindle response at the onset of
    isometric voluntary contractions in man. Time difference
    between fusimotor and skeletomotor effects. J. Physiol.,
    218, 405-431.

Vaughan, H.G., Jr., and Costa L.D , 1968. Analysis of electro-
    encephalographic correlates of human sensori-motor process.
    Electroenceph. Clin. Neurophysiol. 24, 281-294.

Vaughan, H.G., Jr., Gross, E.G., and Bossom, J., 1970. Cortical
    motor potential in monkeys before and after upper limb
    deafferentation. Exp. Neurol. 26, 253-262.

Wiesendanger, M., 1973. Input from muscle and cutaneous nerves
    of the hand and forearm to neurones of the precentral gyrus
    of baboons and monkeys. J. Physiol., 228, 203-219.

MOTONEURONE PROPERTIES AND MOTOR CONTROL

D. Kernell*

Nobel Institute for Neurophysiology, Karolinska
Institutet, Stockholm, Sweden, and Department of
Neurophysiology, University of Amsterdam, Holland

Firing rate modulation of motor unit contraction is discussed
in relation to recent experiments concerning the properties
and activation patterns of motor units in the first deep lumbrical muscle of the cat's foot (Ducati, Kernell and Sjöholm;
Kernell and Sjöholm; in preparation). Results from these
studies showed that firing rate modulation of motor unit tension was of great importance for gradation of the strength of
contractions elicited in the lumbrical muscle by cortical
stimulation or by pinching the foot pad. It is pointed out that
the extent of firing rate modulation that is produced in a
motoneurone by maintained synaptic activity will partly depend
on the sensitivity of the firing motoneurone to changes in synaptic current intensity. Studies of neurone models suggest
that this sensitivity (i.e. the slope for the relation between
impulse frequency and the intensity of activating current)
would depend markedly on: (i) the size, time course, and
'summing ability' of the permeability changes underlying the
after-hyperpolarization of the neurone, and (ii) the difference
between the threshold potential for spike initiation and the
equilibrium potential for potassium (Kernell, 1968, 1971;
Kernell and Sjöholm, 1973).

*   Present Address: Department of Neurophysiology,
University of Amsterdam, Eerste Constantijn Huygensstraat
20, Amsterdam, Holland.

19

As is well known, the strength of contraction of a mammalian skeletal muscle may be varied by a change in the number of active motoneurones (recruitment control), by a change in the firing rate of already active motoneurones (firing rate modulation), or by a combination of both these mechanisms (Adrian and Bronk, 1929). In the present contribution I would like to discuss questions concerning the modulation of motor unit tension by a control of motoneuronal firing rate. First, I will deal with some recent observations of motor unit discharges. Then I will briefly discuss the results of some theoretical studies concerning the membrane properties which may influence the degree of firing rate modulation in motoneurones.

Previous authors have differed considerably with respect to their general opinions about the relative importance of recruitment and firing rate modulation for the control of muscle contraction (e.g. Adrian and Bronk, 1929; Bigland and Lippold, 1954; Bracchi et al., 1966; Milner-Brown et al., 1973). We have recently made some studies of motor units in a small muscle of the cat's foot. These investigations concerned the contractile properties of the motor units (Ducati, Kernell and Sjöholm, in preparation) as well as the response of their motoneurones to synaptic activation (Kernell and Sjöholm, in preparation). The experiments have given some unusually direct evidence for a powerful firing rate modulation of motor unit tension in contractions evoked via the central nervous system.

Our studies were made on the first deep lumbrical muscle. The total number of motor units in this muscle varied in different animals from as little as 2 to 8 or more (cf. Bessou et al., 1963; Adal and Barker, 1965). It has earlier been shown by Bessou et al. (1963) that the motor units of this muscle vary considerably in strength and contraction speed, and that strong motor units tend to have a briefer twitch contraction time and a more rapidly conducting axon than weaker motor units. In our own studies, we have also found that the strongest and fastest lumbrical motor units tend to be more sensitive to post-tetanic potentiation and fatigue than weaker and slower motor units. It should be noted that even the slowest motor units of the first deep lumbrical muscle generally have twitch contraction times that are briefer than those for motor units of cat soleus (cf. McPhedran et al., 1965).

In our experiments, the cats were anaesthetized with pento-

barbitone (Nembutal, Abbott). With the exception of the first deep
lumbrical muscle, all muscles of the foot and leg were denervated.
Sensory innervation to part of the foot was kept intact. The foot
and the lower leg were immersed in warm liquid paraffin (temperature about 36-38°C). Isometric tension was recorded with the
lumbrical muscle at its optimal length for a twitch. An electromyogram was recorded between two gross electrodes, one
resting on the muscle belly and one on the tendon proximal to the
origin of the muscle. In separate experiments, the amplitude of
single motor unit spikes recorded in this manner was found to be
roughly directly proportional to the maximum tetanic tension of
the corresponding motor unit (cf. Appelberg and Emonet-Dénand,
1967). Every motor unit producing measurable muscle contractions also produced recordable electromyographic activity,
and vice versa (we could measure contractions down to about 10-
20 mg). Thus, with the possible exception of some extremely
small and relatively insignificant units (e.g. motor units innervated by skeleto-fusimotor neurones, and consisting of one or a
few extrafusal fibres, cf. Adal and Barker, 1965), we could
simultaneously record the impulse activity of all the individual
motor units of this muscle. Some of our results concerning
firing rate modulation are demonstrated in Fig. 1.

In each record of Fig. 1, the upper trace shows the electromyogram and the lower trace the isometric tension of the whole
muscle. The muscle contractions were from three different
animals. In Fig. 1A-B the contractions were elicited by prolonged
electrical stimulation of the contralateral motor cortex (stimulus
rate about 200/sec). In Fig. 1A, only one single motor unit was
activated by our stimulus. In this record, the mean tension of
the muscle is about seven times larger when the motor unit fires
at its fastest rate of about 50 impulses/sec than when it is discharging at its slowest rate of about 20 impulses/sec soon after
recruitment (Fig. 1A). The contraction of Fig. 1B is from a
muscle containing only two motor units. After both units have
been recruited there is an increase of firing rate in both motor
units accompanied by a further increase of mean muscle tension
by a factor of about three (Fig. 1B). The contraction of Fig. 1C
was reflexly evoked by pinching the foot pad (cf. Engberg, 1964).
This muscle contained three motor units. Between the recruitment of the second and the third motor unit, the firing rate of the
two active motor units increases and the mean muscle tension is
more than doubled (Fig. 1C). In none of the three contractions of
Fig. 1A-C could the enhancement of tension to any important

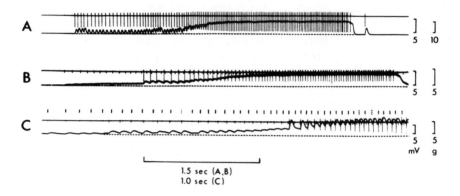

Fig. 1. Contractions elicited in first deep lumbrical
muscles by prolonged electrical stimulation of the contralateral motor cortex (A-B), and by pinching the plantar
cushion of the foot containing the muscle (C). A-C from
three different cats. In each record, upper trace shows
electromyogram, and lower trace isometric tension.
Baseline for myograms (zero active tension) indicated by
interrupted lines (A-C). In A only one motor unit is activated (the other motor units of this muscle were temporarily
blocked or inexcitable while the contraction of A was evoked).
In B, two motor units are activated; the second, larger,
motor unit is recruited at about 1. 35 sec after the beginning
of the record. The smaller motor unit in B continued to fire
throughout the contraction (checked in simultaneous record
at high gain). In C, the stimulation as well as the resulting
impulse activity of a small motor unit had started already
before the beginning of the illustrated record. Occurrence
of impulses in this small motor unit (checked in simultaneous
record at high gain) indicated by vertical bars above record
(dotted bars: probable coincidence of spikes from smallest
and larger motor unit). In C, a second motor unit is recruited at 0. 6 sec, and a third one at 2. 16 sec after the
beginning of the record. Spikes in A-C retouched. The
gradual increase in spike size which accompanies enhancement of tension in A and C might have been due to a change
in the recording situation, caused by the movement of the
muscle. (From unpublished work by Kernell and Sjöholm)

extent to be attributed to potentiation of the contractile machinery.
The post-tetanic potentiation of twitch contraction seen in Fig. 1A
(amplitude of last twitch is about 1.5 times that of the first one)
is relatively small compared with the large total increase of
mean tension during repetitive firing. The motor units of Fig.
1B and C had about the same twitch amplitude just before as just
after the illustrated maintained contractions. Clearly, in all the
three contractions of Fig. 1A-C firing rate modulation of motor
unit contraction was of major importance for the gradation of
muscle tension.

For a quantitative estimate of the relative role of recruitment
and firing rate modulation respectively, one would like to know
what fraction of the maximum tension of a motor unit could be
produced by its recruitment alone. Thus, what tension would be
produced in a lumbrical motor unit if the corresponding motoneurone were firing at its minimum steady rate? A precise
answer to such a question is difficult to give, because the tension
produced in unfused tetani would be expected to depend markedly
on muscle length (cf. Rack and Westbury, 1969), as well as on
the potentiation and fatigue produced in the motor unit by preceding activity. Furthermore, the mean tension produced by a
single lumbrical motor unit firing at a slow rate might perhaps
be somewhat smaller if it were firing alone than if it were taking
part in a slow asynchronous discharge of several motor units
(cf. observations on soleus muscle by Rack and Westbury, 1969).

For motoneurones of the lumbrical muscle, the minimum rate
of steady firing, produced by maintained synaptic activation, was
generally about equal to or slower than the firing rate at which
single twitches of the corresponding motor unit started to sum
(cf. Fig. 1; see also Kernell, 1966b). Thus, as a first approximation, the mean tension produced by recruitment alone might be
assumed to be no larger than roughly half the twitch amplitude.
Among the 18 lumbrical motor units, the twitch-tetanus ratio was
0.20 + 0.08 (mean + S.D.) when the units were relatively unaffected by
potentiation and fatigue, and 0.38 + 0.11 (range 0.24-0.56) when the
units had been potentiated by prolonged and intense preceding activation.
Thus, even in the presence of post-tetanic potentiation, a mean
tension of not more than about 15-25% of the maximum tetanic
tension of a motor unit might be expected to be made available by
recruitment alone (cf. Milner-Brown et al., 1973, for similar
conclusions concerning a human finger muscle). In some of our
animals, 90% or more of the maximum tetanic tension of the

whole muscle could actually be produced in response to cortical
stimulation or pinching of the foot pad.

With regard to the first deep lumbrical muscle, firing rate
modulation of motor unit tension is apparently a powerful and
readily available mechanism for motor control (Fig. 1). In this
respect the lumbrical muscle seems to resemble, for instance,
the human finger muscle recently studied by Milner-Brown et al.
(1973; for other examples of contractions associated with marked
changes in motor unit firing rate see Adrian and Bronk, 1929).
In the lumbrical muscle, firing rate modulation was of importance
also over a range of tensions below that at which all motor units
had been recruited (Fig. 1B-C). In this respect, the lumbrical
muscle appears to differ markedly from cat soleus activated by
the stretch reflex (cf. Denny-Brown, 1929; Granit, 1958;
Grillner and Udo, 1971a, b). Why, then, would muscles differ
from this point of view?

For the interpretation of differences in firing rate modulation
between muscles it is, of course, of major importance to consider the synaptic organization within the respective motoneurone
pools. One should also take into account, however, the cell properties that determine how the respective motoneurones would
respond to a given change in synaptic current. In spinal motoneurones, the relation between firing rate and the intensity of a
stimulating current (the 'f-I relation') has been experimentally
determined with the aid of currents injected into the cell via a
microelectrode (e.g. Granit et al., 1963a; Kernell, 1966b). The
slope of such a f-I relation gives a measure of the 'ease' with
which the firing rate of the neurone in question is altered by
changes in activating current.

We have recently performed a number of investigations concerning the rhythmic properties of various neurone models
(Kernell, 1968, 1971; Kernell and Sjöholm, 1973). These studies
were made in an attempt to understand which membrane properties
would be expected to be of particular importance for the slope of
the f-I relation of motoneurones. The discussion below will
mainly concern firing within the 'primary range' (Kernell, 1965b).

In spinal motoneurones a single soma-dendrite spike is
followed by a prominent after-hyperpolarization, which is mainly
due to a prolonged enhancement of potassium permeability after
the spike (Coombs et al., 1955). It has been suggested that the

after-hyperpolarization is of great importance for the rhythmic properties of motoneurones (e.g. Eccles, 1953, p. 174 ff). This view is supported by theoretical studies, which have shown that many of the rhythmic properties of motoneurones may be imitated by various mathematical models in which spikes are followed by prolonged after-potentials due to enhanced potassium permeability (Kernell, 1968, 1971; Baldissera and Gustafsson, 1971; Baldissera et al., 1973; Kernell and Sjöholm, 1973). Our most recent theoretical studies of this kind were done on various versions of a model based on the equations (Frankenhaeuser and Huxley, 1964) for Frankenhaeuser's voltage clamp data from the amphibian myelinated nerve. We modified the original Frankenhaeuser-Huxley model (1964; 'F-H model') in certain ways in order to make some of its membrane properties (e.g. its after-potentials) more like the known properties of spinal motoneurones (Kernell and Sjöholm, 1972). The models were used for studies concerning steady repetitive firing as well as adaptation. A knowledge of adaptation is actually essential for understanding the factors responsible for the f-I relation of steady discharges in motoneurones.

In spinal motoneurones, there is a brief initial decline of firing rate just after the step-wise onset of a constant stimulating current. This initial adaptation is associated with a marked decline in the slope of the f-I relation (Granit et al., 1963a; Kernell, 1965a, b). After the initial adaptation, which is often largely over following a few initial impulse intervals, the slope of the f-I relation remains constant for prolonged periods of maintained rhythmic firing (Granit et al., 1963b; Kernell, 1965a). A similar initial adaptation, associated with a decline in the slope of the f-I relation, was found also in our modified 'motoneurone-like' versions of the F-H model. In these model versions (Kernell and Sjöholm, 1973), and probably to a great extent in spinal motoneurones as well (e.g. Granit et al., 1963a; Baldissera and Gustafsson, 1971; Calvin and Schwindt, 1972; Kernell, 1972; Baldissera et al., 1973), the initial adaptation is due to a kind of 'summation' of the permeability changes underlying the after-potentials of consecutive spikes (cf. Ito and Oshima, 1962). In our motoneurone-like versions of the F-H model this 'summation' was, however, not a simple algebraic summation of permeability changes. The extent of 'summation', and the degree of initial decline in the slope of the f-I relation, could be altered considerably by simple changes in constants of the equations for potassium permeability (Kernell and Sjöholm,

1973).

A large initial adaptation would be associated with a large initial decline in the slope of the f-I relation. Hence, an increased initial adaptation would lead to a decreased slope of the f-I relation for steady firing. Thus, in our models, the slope of the f-I relation for steady repetitive firing could be markedly decreased by an increased 'summing ability' of the permeability changes underlying the after-hyperpolarization (Kernell and Sjöholm, 1973). Furthermore, in the models the slope of the f-I relation could be markedly decreased by an increased size or slower decline of the permeability changes underlying the after-hyperpolarization, or by an increased difference between the threshold potential for spike initiation and the equilibrium potential for potassium (Kernell, 1968; Kernell and Sjöholm, 1973). Only experiments can, of course, decide to what an extent one or several of these factors actually are of importance for differences in rhythmic properties (f-I relation) between motoneurones.

The resting input resistance is a neuronal property of particular interest for questions concerning the recruitment control of muscle contraction (e.g. Henneman et al., 1965; Kernell, 1966a; Burke, 1968). However, the resting input resistance does not apparently reflect membrane properties of general importance for the firing rate modulation of already recruited motoneurones. Neither in spinal motoneurones (Kernell, 1969), nor in our various neurone models (Kernell, 1968, 1971; Kernell and Sjöholm, 1973) was the slope of the f-I relation markedly affected by simple changes in resting input resistance.

Acknowledgements: This work was supported by the Swedish Medical Research Council (Project No. 14X-2312) and Karolinska Institutets Forskningfonder.

REFERENCES

Adal, M.N. and Barker, D., 1965. Intramuscular branching of fusimotor fibres. J. Physiol. 177, 288-299.
Adrian, E.D. and Bronk, D.W., 1929. The discharge of impulses in motor nerve fibres. Part II. The frequency of discharge in reflex and voluntary contractions. J. Physiol. 67, 119-151.

Appelberg, B. and Emonet-Dénand, F., 1967. Motor units of the
    first superficial lumbrical muscle of the cat. J. Neurophysiol.
    30, 154-160.
Baldissera, F. and Gustafsson, B., 1971. Regulation of repetitive
    firing in motoneurones by the afterhyperpolarization conduc-
    tance. Brain Res. 30, 431-434.
Baldissera, F., Gustafsson, B. and Parmiggiani, F., 1973. Adapta-
    tion in a simple neurone model compared to that of spinal moto-
    neurones. Brain Res. 52, 382-384.
Bessou, P., Emonet-Dénand, F. and Laporte, Y., 1963. Relation
    entre la vitesse de conduction des fibres nerveuses motrices
    et le temps de contraction de leurs unités motrices. Compt.
    Rend. Acad. Sci. (Paris) 256, 5625-5627.
Bigland, B. and Lippold, O.C.J., 1954. Motor unit activity in the
    voluntary contraction of human muscle. J. Physiol. 125,
    322-335.
Bracchi, F., Decandia, M. and Gualtierotti, T., 1966. Frequency
    stabilization in the motor centers of spinal cord and caudal
    brain stem. Amer. J. Physiol. 210, 1170-1177.
Burke, R.E., 1968. Firing patterns of gastrocnemius motor units
    in the decerebrate cat. J. Physiol. 196, 631-654.
Calvin, W.H. and Schwindt, P.C., 1972. Steps in production of
    motoneuron spikes during rhythmic firing. J. Neurophysiol. 35,
    297-310.
Coombs, J.S., Eccles, J.C. and Fatt, P., 1955. The electrical
    properties of the motoneurone membrane. J. Physiol.
    130, 291-325.
Denny-Brown, D., 1929. On the nature of postural reflexes. Proc.
    Roy. Soc. B. 104, 252-301.
Engberg, I., 1964. Reflexes to foot muscles in the cat. Acta
    Physiol. Scand. 62, Suppl. 235, 1-64.
Eccles, J.C., 1953. The neurophysiological basis of mind.
    The Principles of Neurophysiology. Clarendon Press, Oxford.
Frankenhaeuser, B. and Huxley, A.F., 1964. The action potential
    in the myelinated nerve fibre of Xenopus laevis as computed on
    the basis of voltage clamp data. J. Physiol. 171,
    302-315.
Granit, R., 1958. Neuromuscular interaction in postural tone of
    the cat's isometric soleus muscle. J. Physiol. 143,
    387-402.
Granit, R., Kernell, D. and Shortess, G.K., 1963a. Quantitative
    aspects of repetitive firing of mammalian motoneurones, caused
    by injected currents. J. Physiol. 168, 911-931.
Granit, R., Kernell, D. and Shortess, G.K., 1963b. The behavior
    of mammalian motoneurones during long-lasting orthodromic,
    antidromic and trans-membrane stimulation. J. Physiol.
    169, 743-754.
Grillner, S. and Udo, M., 1971a. Motor unit activity and stiff-
    ness of the contracting muscle fibres in the tonic stretch
    reflex. Acta Physiol. Scand. 81, 422-424.

Grillner, S. and Udo, M., 1971b. Recruitment in the tonic stretch reflex. Acta Physiol. Scand. 81, 571-573.

Henneman, E., Somjen, G. and Carpenter, D.O., 1965. Functional significance of cell size in spinal motoneurons. J. Neurophysiol. 28, 560-580.

Ito, M. and Oshima, T., 1962. Temporal summation of after-hyperpolarization following a motoneurone spike. Nature 195, 910-911.

Kernell, D., 1965a. The adaptation and the relation between discharge frequency and current strength of cat lumbosacral motoneurones stimulated by long-lasting injected currents. Acta Physiol. Scand. 65, 65-73.

Kernell, D., 1965b. High-frequency repetitive firing of cat lumbosacral motoneurones stimulated by long-lasting injected currents. Acta Physiol. Scand. 65, 74-86.

Kernell, D., 1966a. Input resistance, electrical excitability, and size of ventral horn cells in cat spinal cord. Science 152, 1637-1640.

Kernell, D., 1966b. The repetitive discharge of motoneurones. In Muscular Afferents and Motor Control. Nobel Symposium I. (Ed. Granit, R.). Almqvist and Wiksell, Stockholm, pp. 351-362.

Kernell, D., 1968. The repetitive discharge of a simple neurone model compared to that of spinal motoneurones. Brain Res. 11, 685-687.

Kernell, D., 1969. Synaptic conductance changes and the repetitive impulse discharge of spinal motoneurones. Brain Res. 15, 291-294.

Kernell, D., 1971. Effects of synapses of dendrites and soma on the repetitive impulse firing of a compartmental neurone model. Brain Res. 35, 551-555.

Kernell, D., 1972. The early phase of adaptation in repetitive impulse discharges of cat spinal motoneurones. Brain Res. 41, 184-186.

Kernell, D. and Sjöholm, H., 1972. Motoneurone models based on 'voltage clamp equations' for peripheral nerve. Acta Physiol. Scand. 86, 546-562.

Kernell, D. and Sjöholm, H., 1973. Repetitive impulse firing: comparisons between neurone models based on 'voltage clamp equations' and spinal motoneurones. Acta Physiol. Scand. 87, 40-56.

McPhedran, A.M., Wuerker, R.B. and Henneman, E., 1965. Properties of motor units in a homogenous red muscle (soleus) of the cat. J. Neurophysiol. 28, 71-84.

Milner-Brown, H.S., Stein, R.B. and Yemm, R., 1973. Changes in firing rate of human motor units during linearly changing voluntary contractions. J. Physiol. 230, 371-390.

Rack, P.M.H. and Westbury, D.R., 1969. The effects of length and stimulus rate on tension in the isometric cat soleus muscle. J. Physiol. 204, 443-460.

FUNCTIONAL SPECIALIZATION IN THE MOTOR UNIT POPULATION OF CAT MEDIAL GASTROCNEMIUS MUSCLE

R. E. Burke, W. Z. Rymer and J. V. Walsh, Jr.

Laboratory of Neural Control, National Institute of
Neurological Diseases and Stroke, National Institutes
of Health, Bethesda, Maryland

The population of motor units making up the medial gastrocnemius (MG) muscle in the cat has been studied as a representative example of a very heterogeneous motor pool. The wide
range in physiological and histochemical characteristics of MG
muscle units, and the details of their interrelation, suggest
that the different motor unit types in the population are
specialized for particular functions and particular patterns
of activity. However, it is clear that the functional activity
of a given muscle unit is controlled by the properties of its
innervating motoneurone, and by the organization of synaptic
input to that cell. In order to provide a clear picture of the
motor unit pool in a heterogeneous muscle, it is thus necessary
to study in detail the interrelations between motoneurone and
muscle unit. The evidence presently available from such
studies indicates that the properties intrinsic to MG motoneurones, and the spatial and functional organization of synaptic input to them, are quite consistent with the patterns of
functional usage for which the different types of muscle units
seem best suited. For example, type S muscle units are
slowly-contracting and extremely resistant to fatigue, the
latter associated with their high oxidative enzyme capacity.
Motoneurones of type S units tend to fire slowly under synaptic
drive, partly due to long durations of the post-spike hyper-
polarizations, and they show little accommodation to steady
input. S units are powerfully excited by monosynaptic con-

nections from group Ia afferents, and are also powerfully
inhibited through segmental interneurones by antagonist Ia
afferents and from cutaneous afferents. All of these observations seem consistent with the conclusion that type S units
participate importantly in movements and postures organized
by many segmental reflexes. Type FR muscle units are also
resistant to fatigue and exhibit high oxidative enzyme capacity,
but these units contract more rapidly than type S and also
produce more tension. The motoneurones of FR units receive
group Ia excitation and inhibition which is almost as powerful
as that seen in type S units, but the polysynaptic inhibition
produced in FR cells by cutaneous afferents is considerably
less potent than in S motoneurones. Rather, in many FR
motoneurones, excitatory effects from skin afferents dominate the postsynaptic response, suggesting that these cells
may receive input from some segmental excitatory interneurones which do not project to cells of S units. Such observations support the idea that FR units may participate in
movements which involve spindle afferent support, like the S
units, but may in addition be activated preferentially by other
input systems. To complete the picture, the fatigue-sensitive
FF muscle units, which are dependent on anaerobic glycolysis,
are innervated by motoneurones with relatively small input
from group Ia afferents but which are also excited by the polysynaptic pathway from low threshold skin afferents, making it
likely that FF units do not participate as readily in movements
supported by gamma drive, but may require other excitatory
systems perhaps called into play in less stereotyped movements.

In both the anatomical and functional senses, motor units are
the quantal elements in movement production (Eccles and
Sherrington, 1930). Each motor unit contains a neural element,
the alpha motoneurone, and a set of muscle fibres innervated
by that motoneurone, referred to here as the "muscle unit". It
has been evident for some time that the populations of motor
units making up many limb and trunk muscles in mammals can
be quite heterogeneous, including units with widely varying contraction speeds and tension outputs (see Burke, 1967, 1973 for
references). Indeed, the physiological properties of the muscle
unit provide the clearest criteria for classification of motor units
into recognizable groups, a necessary first step in any assessment
of possible functional specializations (Burke, 1967; Burke et al.,
1971a, 1973). However, consideration of the issue of functional

specialization within the set of motor units making up a particular heterogeneous muscle also requires attention to the characteristics of the innervating motoneurones, and to the organization of synaptic input to them. In this paper we will attempt to review briefly some of the available evidence suggesting functional specialization within the population of units in the cat medial gastrocnemius (MG), including recent results dealing mainly with the organization of synaptic input to these units.

MUSCLE UNITS

We will begin by summarizing, and to some extent over-simplifying, recent evidence regarding the physiological and histochemical characteristics of MG muscle units (for details, see Burke et al., 1971a, 1973; Burke and Tsairis, 1973a, b). The MG unit population contains two basic types of muscle units, a "fast twitch" group and a "slow twitch" group. The slow twitch group consists of a single type of unit, type S, which is characterized by long twitch contraction times (58-110 msec), small tetanic tension outputs (1.2-12.5 g) and extreme resistance to fatigue during repetitive activation. The muscle fibres belonging to MG type S units are generally small in diameter and have histochemical profiles suggesting high oxidative enzyme capacity and high mitochondrial density, low capacity for anaerobic glycolysis, and low myofibrillar ATPase activity, all of which fit well with their observed physiological properties (cf. Burke and Tsairis, 1973b). In contrast, the fast twitch group contains two major subcategories of muscle units, called types FF and FR, plus a small percentage of intermediate, or "unclassified", units. Type FF units have the shortest twitch contraction times (20-47 msec), the largest tetanic tensions (30-130 g), and are very susceptible to fatigue with only a few hundred impulses. Their muscle fibres are generally large in diameter and have low apparent oxidative enzyme capacity and low mitochondrial density, but exhibit high capacity for anaerobic glycolysis and high myofibrillar ATPase activity. Type FR units also have relatively short contraction times (30-55 msec), produce moderate tension in fused tetani (4.5-55 g) and are much more resistant to fatigue than FF units, but less so than type S units. The muscle fibres of FR units resemble those of FF units except that they are relatively small in diameter and have considerably greater apparent oxidative enzyme capacity and mitochondrial density. "Unclassified" (or "U") units are, in several respects, intermediate between FF and FR units, so that the fast twitch group as a whole (referred to collectively as the "F" group) consists of a spectrum of muscle units with a bimodal distribution of physiological and histochemical characteristics.

The above observations, based on direct matching of physiological and histochemical data in muscle units representative of the entire MG unit population, confirm a number of long-standing suppositions about physiological-histochemical interrelations in mammalian muscle which have been made on the basis of less direct evidence (cf. Close, 1972). The results also fit with some previous suggestions as to possible functional roles played by different motor unit types (cf. e.g. Granit, 1970). Type S units seem best suited for sustained but relatively low-grade tension production such as may be required in maintenance of stable posture, presumably by "tonic" activation at low frequencies. In addition, gastrocnemius type S units can exhibit a "catch" property which is dependent on the interval pattern of motoneurone firing and which may enhance their efficiency in producing tension during sustained activation at relatively low frequencies (Burke et al., 1971b). At the other extreme of the MG unit population, the FF units can produce very high tensions (cumulatively about 80% of the total tetanic tension of the whole muscle) and quick contraction, but they fatigue so rapidly (presumably because of their dependence on anaerobic glycolysis and intrafibre glycogen stores) that they seem specialized only for brief and intermittent (i.e. "phasic") activity. The FR units appear to provide a conceptually rather novel group, combining the advantages of quick contraction and reasonably high tension output plus resistance to fatigue, all of which suit them for activity in sustained repetitive movements such as walking and running at various speeds. Units of the F group do not exhibit a sustained "catch" property. Rather, the non-linear tension enhancement dependent on interpulse interval patterns lasts only a short time in F units, suggesting that they may be best suited to fire in relatively short bursts.

MOTONEURONES

Whether or not the various motor unit types indeed operate along the lines suggested above remains to be demonstrated. However, it should be noted that the pattern of activity of any given motor unit is controlled at the motoneurone by properties intrinsic to the cell itself and by the spatial and functional organization of the synaptic input to the cell. If the different motor unit types subserve functionally distinct roles, there should be recognizable differences between their motoneurones in intrinsic properties and synaptic input.

Direct correlation of motoneurone and synaptic input characteristics with the properties of the innervated muscle unit is possible using the technique of intracellular recording and stimulation in the motoneurone, whereby electrophysiological data can be obtained with conventional methods and then the cell can be stimulated through the penetrating micropipette to cause isolated contractions of its muscle unit (Devanandan et al., 1965; Burke, 1967). In this way, it has been demonstrated that motoneurones of type S units in cat MG exhibit much less tendency for accommodation of firing to transmembrane currents than seen in many F group motoneurones (Burke and Nelson, 1971), a point consistent with the supposed sustained firing role of S units. The duration of post-spike hyperpolarization is in general longer in motoneurones of S units than in F cells (Burke, 1967), consonant with the relatively lower firing frequencies observed in S units under synaptic drive (Burke, 1968b) and with the fact that slowly contracting muscle units function most efficiently with low activation frequencies (Burke, Rudomin and Zajac, unpublished results). Using axonal conduction velocities and motoneurone input resistance values as indices of anatomical cell size (cf. Barrett and Crill, 1971; Burke, 1973), the motoneurones innervating type S muscle units are generally smaller than those of FF or FR units (Burke, 1967; Burke et al., 1973), but the MG motoneurone pool is probably best represented as a spectrum with respect to cell size. Electrophysiological data suggest that the combined electrotonic length of the dendrites in large and smaller alpha motoneurones is about the same, irrespective of motor unit type (Burke and ten Bruggencate, 1971). The latter two points are of importance in the interpretation of synaptic potential data (cf. Burke, 1973).

SYNAPTIC ORGANIZATION

The results of analyzing synaptic input organization to MG motor units, identified only as belonging to F and S unit groups (Burke, 1968a, b; Burke et al., 1970), have been discussed in a recent review in relation to other evidence regarding central

nervous system control of different motor unit types (Burke,
1973). We have recently renewed this type of investigation in
order to define possible differences in synaptic organization in
FF, U and FR subdivisions of the F unit group. The recent
results are completely compatible with earlier data and represent an extension of, rather than a revision of, the earlier work
since we have been able to show that the motor units called "type
S" in the earlier work were essentially identical to units identified
now as type S on the basis of somewhat different criteria (cf.
Burke et al., 1973).

Three categories of afferent systems have been studied, using
methods described in detail elsewhere (Burke, 1968a; Burke et
al., 1970): (a) group Ia muscle spindle afferents; (b) presumed
vestibulospinal tract fibres; and (c) cutaneous afferents in the
ipsilateral sural nerve. There is a clear correlation between
unit type and the peak amplitude of the composite monosynaptic
EPSP produced by stimulation of group Ia afferents in the muscle
nerve to which the recorded unit belongs (the homonymous nerve).
As shown in the histograms in Fig. 1, the homonymous Ia EPSP
is largest on the average in type S units, somewhat smaller in
FR units, still smaller in U units, and finally considerably
smaller in type FF units. These new results permit an important conclusion to be drawn from a previous study of firing
patterns of F and S motor units in the decerebrate cat (Burke,
1968b), in which it was shown that some F units could be activated by MG stretch (thus participating in the classical stretch
reflex). Such stretch responsive F units exhibited relatively
large homonymous Ia EPSPs and were probably largely, if not
exclusively type FR motor units. It had been clear previously
that the type S units were intensely active in decerebrate rigidity.
Thus the fatigue resistant FR and S units both appear to participate in stretch reflexes in the decerebrate cat, while the fatigue
sensitive FF units with their less powerful Ia excitatory input
probably do not participate to any extent in such reflexes. Whether
or not the FF units can be activated by other synaptic systems in
the decerebrate state remains to be demonstrated.

A similar basic pattern of input organization is apparent in the
relation between unit type and the maximum amplitude of disynaptic inhibition produced in MG motoneurones by group I volleys
in the antagonist tibialis anterior and extensor digitorum longus
nerves (abbreviated here "TA"). Quantitative study of this synaptic system is complicated by the fact that the Ia inhibitory inter-

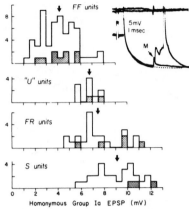

Fig. 1. Peak amplitude of homonymous Ia EPSPs in identified
MG motoneurones. Inset record: Typical record showing
blockade of antidromic invasion of the recorded motoneurones
by hyperpolarizing current pulse passed through the recording
micropipette. Intracellular trace (lower) shows M spike
(arrow) preceding the Ia EPSP. EPSP amplitude measured
from the first peak after subtraction of small distortion caused
by the M spike (cf. Burke, 1968a). Upper trace is cord dorsum
potential at the L7 dorsal root entry. Histograms: Distributions
of amplitude of composite homonymous Ia EPSPs in 119 MG
motoneurones, identified as to the type of muscle unit innervated by each cell. Arrows indicate the mean value of each
distribution. Hatched bars indicate sample of units in a
single animal, showing that pooling data from different animals
did not distort the relation.

neurones mediating the effect are for the most part "gated off"
in anaesthetized, low spinal animals such as used for these
experiments (cf. Burke et al., 1970). However, transmission
through the pathway can be facilitated by conditioning volleys to
descending (probably largely rubrospinal) axons coursing in the
ipsilateral dorsolateral funiculus in the lower thoracic spinal
cord (Fig. 2, inset records; see Hongo et al., 1969). Assuming
that the DQ conditioning produces equal facilitation of the antagonist Ia pathway to motor units of different types, an assumption
with some previous support (Burke et al., 1970), there is a clear
correlation evident in the graph in Fig. 2 between the disynaptic
IPSP amplitude (abscissa) and (a) the unit type (denoted by the
different symbols); and (b) the amplitude of Ia monosynaptic
EPSPs recorded in the same cells (ordinate). Thus, both mono-

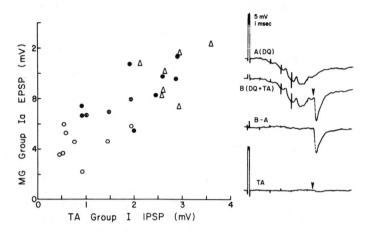

Fig. 2. Inset records: Computer averages (20 trials in each) of intracellular potential in a type S MG motoneurone, showing the effect of five shocks to the surgically isolated ipsilateral dorsolateral quadrant (DQ) of the cord at Th13 on the disynaptic IPSP evoked by a single volley in the tibialis-extensor digitorum longus nerve (TA). Membrane potential - 60 mV. TA stimulus alone (lowest record; TA) produced a barely detectable disynaptic IPSP (arrow: stimulus strength just maximal for group I). Conditioning train to the dorsolateral quadrant (DQ) facilitated production of a large disynaptic IPSP (DQ+TA: arrow). Digital substraction of DQ alone (A) from DQ plus TA (B) yielded record of the disynaptic IPSP alone (B-A). Graph: plot of the maximum amplitude of the TA disynaptic Ia IPSP after DQ conditioning (abscissa) against the amplitude of the homonymous Ia EPSP recorded in the same cell (ordinate). Membrane potential in each case was between -60 and -75 mV. Each point on the graph denotes a different motoneurone, with motor unit type indicated by the symbols: FF - 0; "U" - ⊗; FR - ●; S - △.

synaptic excitation and disynaptic inhibition produced in MG motoneurones by activation of group Ia afferents is more powerful (in terms of composite PSP amplitudes) in the S and FR motoneurones innervating muscle units with high fatigue resistance and high oxidative enzyme capacity.

There is a significant positive correlation between motoneurone input resistance values and the amplitude of Ia EPSPs in gastrocnemius motoneurones (Burke, 1968a, b), but, as has been dis-

cussed elsewhere in detail (cf. Burke, 1973), the larger Ia
EPSPs in small alpha motoneurones is not due to their high input
resistance per se. Rather, the controlling factors appear to be:
(a) the density of synaptic terminations belonging to the active
system; (b) the absolute postsynaptic conductance change produced
by each active synapse; (c) the spatial distribution of the active
synapses over the receptive membrane of the motoneurone; and
(d) the electrotonic scaling factors present in the set of neurones
under consideration. These points have been developed further
in a rather rigorous model formulation by Zucker (1973).
Parsimony of hypothesis has led us to choose the factor of
synaptic density as probably controlling the observations on composite PSP amplitudes (Figs. 1 and 2; see also Burke, 1968a,
1973).

In light of the above discussion, recent observations on the
amplitude of monosynaptic EPSPs evoked in MG motoneurones
by stimulation of the ipsilateral ventral spinal quadrant are of
interest. In these experiments, the surgically isolated ventral
quadrant (VQ) was stimulated with single shocks in the low
thoracic cord (cf. Grillner and Lund, 1968), producing in most
MG cells a small monosynaptic EPSP (Fig. 3, inset records).
The peak amplitude of VQ EPSPs (abscissa in the graph in Fig. 3)
is rather poorly correlated with unit type and with Ia EPSP amplitude (ordinate), in contrast to results such as shown in Fig. 2.
The mean values for VQ EPSP amplitude in FF and FR units in
this sample is the same (about 0.77 mV; note arrow on abscissa)
while that in the type S units is about 1.1 mV. The difference
between mean VQ EPSPs between FF and S unit groups is thus
considerably smaller in percentage than that between the same
unit groups with regard to Ia EPSP amplitude (arrows on the
ordinate). Most, if not all, of such VQ EPSPs are probably produced by activation of lateral vestibulospinal tract fibres descending in the ventral funiculus (Grillner et al., 1970). While it
is difficult to formulate a functional interpretation of these results,
especially in view of the small amplitude of the VQ EPSPs in all
MG units, the lack of a strong correlation between unit type and
VQ EPSP amplitude does illustrate the fact that the input resistance of the postsynaptic motoneurones is not the only critical
factor in determining the amplitude of composite PSPs recorded
at the cell soma.

We have recently re-examined a previously described (Burke
et al., 1970) relation between the predominant synaptic effect

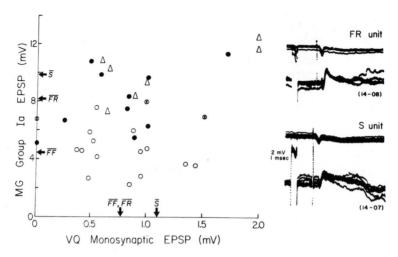

Fig. 3. Inset records: Photographically superimposed traces
of monosynaptic EPSPs produced in two identified MG motoneurones by single shock stimulation of surgically isolated
ipsilateral ventral cord quadrant (VQ) at Th13 level. Units
obtained serially in the same animal. Upper traces show cord
dorsum potential, with arrival of volley in the most rapidly
conducting fibres at L7 segment. Graph: plot of the amplitude
of maximum VQ monosynaptic EPSP (abscissa) against amplitude of homonymous Ia EPSP (ordinate) in the same identified
MG motoneurones. Unit type denoted by symbols as in Fig. 2.
Membrane potential of cells included was between -55 and
-75 mV. Arrows along the abscissa and ordinate indicate the
mean values of the respective EPSPs in identified unit groups.
Mean VQ EPSP was the same in FF and FR unit groups.

(i. e. excitation versus inhibition) produced in identified MG
motoneurones by volleys in the ipsilateral sural nerve. Analysis
of such effects is complicated because the pathways involved are
polysynaptic (trisynaptic at minimum, see Lundberg, 1969a) and
because the polysynaptic sural PSPs contain both excitatory and
inhibitory components. Excitatory components occur with the
shorter latency and inhibitory PSPs arrive beginning a few
milliseconds later. Despite the analytic problems, there is a
clear statistical difference between the predominant synaptic
effect produced by relatively low threshold sural afferents in F
and S unit groups. The inset records in Fig. 4 show sural PSPs
in three identified MG motoneurones, obtained sequentially in the

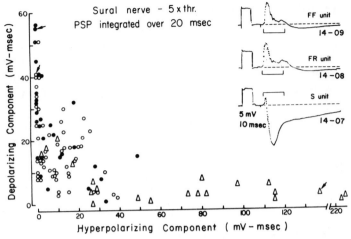

Fig. 4. Inset records: Computer averages (20 responses each) of polysynaptic PSPs evoked in three identified MG motoneurones by stimulation of the ipsilateral sural nerve at five times threshold for the most excitable fibres in the nerve. Units obtained sequentially in the same animal, with membrane potential between -60 and -70 mV in each cell. The brackets in each record show 20 msec epoch after PSP onset which was integrated digitally to produce data such as shown in the graph. Graph: Plot of the area of depolarizing component of the polysynaptic sural PSP (ordinate) and the hyperpolarizing component (abscissa), integrated over the initial 20 msec of the PSP (as in insets) from PSPs in 105 identified MG motoneurones. Each point denotes a different unit and symbol key same as in Figs. 2 and 3. Membrane potential in each unit included was between -60 and -75 mV at the time of recording the sural responses. Points corresponding to the specimen records in the inset are denoted by arrows on the graph.

same animal and recorded under essentially identical conditions. The records illustrate the striking difference in predominant effect which can be observed. The graph in Fig. 4 presents an attempt to display results obtained from a large sample of identified MG units, illustrating the integrated area (in mV-msec) under the PSP voltage-time curve for the depolarizing component (ordinate) versus the hyperpolarizing component (abscissa) from sural PSPs produced by a single shock at five times threshold for the most excitable fibres in the nerve. In about 70% of the F

group (FF, FR and "U"), the area of the early depolarizing
component exceeds that of the later hyperpolarization while the
reverse is true for 86% of the S units. While the interpretation
of such results cannot be taken very far since the measurable PSP
represents a summation of mixed effects, the predominance of
inhibitory components in S units is striking and in many S units
the early excitation is either small or virtually absent. It
appears reasonable to conclude that motoneurones belonging to
the MG nucleus do not necessarily all receive qualitatively identical inputs, at least with regard to the sets of last-order interneurones conveying excitatory effects from sural afferents. It
seems probable that some of the excitatory interneurones which
project to motoneurones of the F group do not reach some of the
S cells.

In a previous study, it was suggested that the excitatory components in the sural PSPs are produced by special pathways separate from those generating the inhibitory components (Burke et
al., 1970). We have now obtained some evidence supporting this
notion. Preceding the sural volley with a short conditioning train
of stimuli to the surgically isolated dorsolateral quadrant (DQ) of
the thoracic cord (after total removal of the dorsal columns) produces suppression of the inhibitory component in sural PSPs without apparent changes in the excitatory component. Suppression
of the inhibitory components can be quite profound and long-lasting,
as shown in Fig. 5. The DQ stimulation used in this experiment
is, of course, quite non-specific, but it can be suggested that the
long-lasting inhibitory depression is probably due largely to the
dorsolateral reticulospinal inhibitory system which inhibits interneuronal transmission from the flexor reflex afferents (FRA) to
both flexor and extensor alpha motoneurones (Engberg et al.,
1968). The effect of DQ conditioning is qualitatively the same
(i.e. suppression of inhibitory components in the complex sural
PSPs) in all of the MG unit types, although it is less dramatic in
many F cells because of the smaller amplitude of the inhibitory
components.

The available evidence suggests that the interneurones transmitting excitatory effects from low threshold sural afferents to
MG motoneurones form a specialized pathway separate from the
FRA segmental system. Recent work in Lundberg's laboratory
has suggested that some of these interneurones may also convey
effects from the rubrospinal tract to motoneurones (Hongo et al.,
1972). The relatively powerful effects produced by this system of

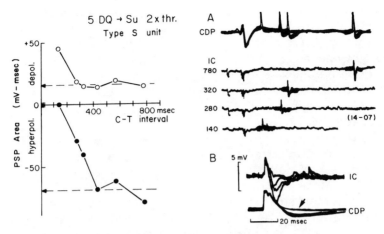

Fig. 5. Effect of five conditioning shocks to surgically isolated
dorsolateral quadrant (DQ) on the polysynaptic response evoked
by sural stimulation at two times threshold. Same S unit illustrated in Fig. 4; membrane potential -60 mV. A - CDP-cord
dorsum potential at L7 dorsal root entry showing intervals
between DQ train (first response) and subsequent sural volleys.
Photographically superimposed records at four different con-
ditioning-testing (CT) intervals). IC - Intracellular records
corresponding to A, showing suppression of inhibitory component of sural PSP with decreasing CT intervals. CT intervals
in msec given with each trace. Calibration pulse = 5 mV, 10
msec. B - Superimposed records of sural PSPs corresponding
to records in A, but shown on expanded amplification and time
scales. Note suppression of CDP P wave (arrow) corresponding
to the 140 msec CT interval, in which there was apparent complete suppression of the sural inhibitory component. Note also
that the excitatory component of the sural PSP is apparently
unaffected by DQ conditioning. Graph - Average areas of depolarizing and hyperpolarizing components of sural PSPs
measured for several responses at each of the indicated CT
intervals following DQ conditioning. Suppression of inhibitory
component begins with an interval of about 350 msec and is
apparently complete at 140 msec. The area of the excitatory
component is unchanged except for responses at 140 msec CT
interval, when suppression of the inhibitory component revealed
underlying depolarizing component. Areas of control responses
indicated by arrows and dashed lines.

segmental interneurones in motoneurones of F units, including
both FF and FR units (cf. Fig. 4), may indicate the existence of
a pathway for selective activation of units in the F group. Such a
pathway might operate in the production of movements organized
in patterns other than those available through the more stereotyped segmental reflex pathways. The FRA inhibitory pathway,
on the other hand, appears to be very much a part of the segmental
reflex apparatus and, viewed in this light, it may be appropriate
that its effects are most powerful among the S units which are also
very effectively tied into the reflex pathways from muscle proprioceptive afferents. Of course, it must be recognized that these
suggestions are quite tentative since they are based on the results
of non-selective electrical stimulation in anaesthetized preparations. The effects of polysynaptic pathways in motoneurones are
also very dependent on the experimental conditions under which
they are measured (Eccles and Lundberg, 1959).

While the above suggestions must remain tentative, there can
be little doubt that the organization of group Ia input to MG motor
units, both via direct monosynaptic excitatory connections and
through the disynaptic inhibitory pathway from antagonists, fits
well with the conclusion that S and FR motor units are the "prime
movers" in muscular activity organized through segmental reflex
mechanisms. Many such movements, of which stepping is an
important example, appear to involve alpha-gamma coactivation
(Granit, 1970), and the input from muscle spindles probably forms
a large part of the excitatory drive supporting and controlling the
total pattern of muscle activation (Lundberg, 1969b). The available evidence suggests that the organization of the entire motor
unit system in the cat MG, including the critical factor of synaptic
input, is consistent with the functional roles which appear to be
best suited to the mechanical and biochemical characteristics of
the involved muscle units. Of particular interest is the set of
observations relating to the FR units, which is consistent with
their probable role in both reflexly organized movements as well
as in less stereotyped (i.e. "phasic") movements.

REFERENCES

Barrett, J.N., and Crill, W.E., 1971. Specific membrane resistivity of dye-injected cat motoneurons. Brain Res. 28, 556-561.

Burke, R.E., 1967. Motor unit types of cat triceps surae muscle. J. Physiol. 193, 141-160.

Burke, R.E., 1968a. Group Ia synaptic input to fast and slow twitch motor units of cat triceps surae. J. Physiol. 196, 605-630.

Burke, R.E., 1968b. Firing patterns of gastrocnemius motor units in the decerebrate cat. J. Physiol. 196, 631-654.

Burke, R.E., 1973. On the central nervous system control of fast and slow twitch motor units. In New Developments in Electromyography and Clinical Neurophysiology. Vol. 3, Karger, Basel, pp.69-94.

Burke, R.E., Jankowska, E., and ten Bruggencate, G., 1970. A comparison of peripheral and rubrospinal synaptic input to slow and fast twitch motor units of triceps surae. J. Physiol. 207, 709-732.

Burke, R.E., Levine, D.N., Tsairis, P., and Zajac, F.E., 1973. Physiological types and histochemical profiles in motor units of the cat gastrocnemius. J. Physiol. In press.

Burke, R.E., Levine, D.N., Zajac, F.E., Tsairis, P., and Engel, W.K., 1971a. Mammalian motor units: Physiological-histochemical correlation in three types in cat gastrocnemius. Science 174, 709-712.

Burke, R.E., and Nelson, P.G., 1971. Accommodation to current ramps in motoneurons of fast and slow twitch motor units. Internat. J. Neurosci. 1, 347-356.

Burke, R.E., Rudomin, P., and Zajac, F.E., 1971b. Catch property in single mammalian motor units. Science 168, 122-124.

Burke, R.E., and ten Bruggencate, G., 1971. Electrotonic characteristics of alpha motoneurones of varying size. J. Physiol. 212, 1-20.

Burke, R.E., and Tsairis, P., 1973a. Anatomy and innervation ratios in motor units of cat gastrocnemius. J. Physiol. In press.

Burke, R.E., and Tsairis, P., 1973b. The correlation of physiological properties with histochemical characteristics in single muscle units. Ann. N.Y. Acad. Sci. In press.

Close, R., 1972. Dynamic properties of mammalian skeletal muscles. Physiol. Rev. 52, 129-197.

Devanandan, M.S., Eccles, R.M., and Westerman, R.A., 1965. Single motor units of mammalian muscle. J. Physiol. 178, 359-367.

Eccles, J.C., and Sherrington, C.S., 1930. Numbers and contraction-values of individual motor-units examined in some muscles of the limb. Proc. Roy. Soc., B. 106, 326-357.

Eccles, R.M., and Lundberg, A., 1959. Supraspinal control of interneurones mediating spinal reflexes. J. Physiol. 147, 565–584.

Engberg, I., Lundberg, A., and Ryall, R.W., 1968. Reticulospinal inhibition of transmission in reflex pathways. J. Physiol. 194, 201–223.

Granit, R., 1970. The Basis of Motor Control. Academic Press, N.Y.

Grillner, S., Hongo, T., and Lund, S., 1970. The vestibulospinal tract. Effects on alpha motoneurones in the lumbosacral spinal cord in the cat. Exp. Brain Res. 10, 94–120.

Grillner, S., and Lund, S., 1968. The origin of a descending pathway with monosynaptic action on flexor motorneurones. Acta Physiol. Scand. 74, 274–284.

Hongo, T., Jankowska, E., and Lundberg, A., 1969. The rubrospinal tract. II. Facilitation of interneuronal transmission in reflex paths to motoneurones. Exp. Brain Res. 7, 365–391.

Hongo, T., Jankowska, E., and Lundberg, A., 1972. The rubrospinal tract. IV. Effects on interneurones. Exp. Brain Res. 15, 54–78.

Lundberg, A., 1969a. Convergence of excitatory and inhibitory action on interneurones in the spinal cord. In The Interneuron. Univ. Calif. Press, Los Angeles. pp. 231–265.

Lundberg, A., 1969b. Reflex Control of Stepping. Proc. Norwegian Acad. Sci. Lett., Universitetsforlaget, Oslo.

Zucker, R.S., 1973. Theoretical implications of the size principle of motoneurone recruitment. J. Theor. Biol. 38, 587–596.

SOMATOTOPIC CONNECTIVITY OR SPECIES RECOGNITION CONNECTIVITY?

R. J. Wyman

Yale University, New Haven, Connecticut

The vertebrate genome does not have enough DNA to specify independently all the connections in the nervous system. Large numbers of nerve cells must be hooked up by a single genetic specification. One task of neurophysiology is to find out what these genetic commands are. An approach is to look for regularities in the connections of large groups of cells. One of these regularities is somatotopic projection - neighbouring presynaptic cells connect with neighbouring postsynaptic cells. A different assumption, often held by spinal cord researchers, is that large numbers of nerve cells are grouped into different "species" (e.g. the motoneurones innervating a single muscle), and that all members of a species have similar connections.

This paper distinguishes "classes" of nerve cells (possible "classes" are alpha motoneurones, Renshaw cells, ventral spinal cerebellar tract cells, slow motoneurones, flexor motoneurones, etc.) and species (species refers to cells whose connections are specific for the muscle in whose control pathway they find themselves, e.g. medial gastrocnemius motoneurones, pyramidal cells controlling plantaris motoneurones). The paper suggests that connectivity in the spinal cord can be accounted for by a somatotopic organization by "class" without further specification of connections by species.

In this theory motoneurones which have anatomically neighbouring somato-dendritic arborizations have more similar synaptic connections (even though they innervate different muscles) than motoneurones that are anatomically distant in the cord (even though they innervate the same muscle).

Eccles' data on 1A connections is reconsidered in view of this theory and a reformulation of size principle is offered based on this theory. Experimental tests of the theory are proposed.

The vertebrate genome does not have enough DNA to specify, independently, all the connections in the nervous system. There are more than a million neural connections for each base pair in the whole human genome. If the whole genome is used only to specify neural connections, then the average (1000 base pairs) gene would specify about a billion connections. If single genes are specifying millions or billions of connections at once, then researchers must find regularities of connectivity of this order of magnitude.

The vertebrate literature suggests two different ways in which these "rules of specification" may be written by the genome. Researchers on sensory systems generally find that their nerve cells are connected by somatotopic projections. This has led to gradient theories of neural specification - large numbers of nerve cells find their proper connections by sorting themselves out along a gradient.

On the other hand, researchers on motor systems tend to assume that neurones are grouped into different "species". The large number of members of a 'species' all follow the same rules of connectivity. A typical species would be all the motoneurones innervating a single muscle (the Sherringtonian motoneurone pool). Connections are appropriate for each 'species' and one of the tasks of neurophysiology is to find out which species connects to which other species and with what average size synaptic potential. A classic example of this is Eccles et al. study of the monosynaptic (1957) and disynaptic (1961) connections of different 'species' of motoneurones.

The species assumption has led motor systems researchers to a different view of neural specification. Since motoneurones to different muscles are intermixed in the motor columns of the cord (Romanes, 1964), ingrowing fibres must have a way of recognizing which species of motoneurone they are about to synapse, or not synapse, with. This leads to theories of cellular recognition by surface properties. As Eccles (1964) puts it, "the highly specific motoneuronal connections" require that pre- and postsynaptic fibres "have a complementary specificity whereby synaptic connections are attracted and maintained". In this theory there is some molecule, or a density of molecules, or a mosaic array of molecules, on the surface of one species of neurones which is different from that on the surface of any other species.

Now the gradient theory of connectivity and the surface recognition theory of connectivity are quite different. They may both be correct, but we should at least consider, for parsimony's sake, whether only one is correct. I would like to suggest that the connectivity in the spinal cord can be accounted for by a somatotopic organization without further specification of connections by species. Somatotopic is not precisely the right word to use here, since most neural connections are not involved in mapping the body surface. Perhaps a more general term would be "topological" connectivity, meaning that contiguous cells of the presynaptic class connect with contiguous cells of the postsynaptic class. The genetic, or ontogenetic, instructions then specify a region in which to synapse, but not the particular cells on which to synapse.

In cases where two motoneuronal groups are anatomically separated in the cord, predictions from the two theories are not easy to distinguish. However, in the cat spinal cord "the cells innervating a single muscle are intermingled with cells supplying the other muscles" (Romanes, 1964). Thus, Romanes (1964) shows medial and lateral gastrocnemius, soleus, tibialis posterior and popliteus intermixed in a single column; and extensor digitorum brevis, peroneus 2 and 3, extensor digitorum longus, tibialis anterior and peroneus longus intermixed in another column. The critical question is - can presynaptic fibres distinguish among the different species of motoneurones when the motoneurones are intermingled; or are the connections made indiscriminantly with all motoneurones sitting in a given locus.[1]

1   Unfortunately neuronal migration is one further complicating factor. Neuronal groups that form their connections when anatomically distinct may, during ontogeny, migrate to inter-mixed positions.

    The experimental data (Eccles et al., 1957) from which
Eccles (1964) argues for specificity of connection is not really
adequate to prove the specificity. Eccles et al. (1957) report
the average size of EPSPs generated in different species of
motoneurone by a given input. Differences in the average EPSP
may only be a result of the fact that the average location of the
different species of motoneurones is different. Thus Romanes
(1951) shows that although medial gastrocnemius (MG) and
lateral gastrocnemius (LG) intermix in part of their range, they
are separate in part and the average location for the two types
of motoneurone is different. Mendell and Henneman (1971)
found that MG 1As synapse on a smaller percentage of LG cells
than on MG cells, but the LG cells which sit in the same region
as the MG cells are equally likely to receive MG 1A synapses.
The lower average LG EPSP to a MG 1A volley would then be
due to the smaller percentage of LG cells contacted and the
possibility that synapses with distant LG cells would tend to
be out on the dendrites, and thus have smaller EPSPs.

    Of course, the 1As, like other fibres, may ramify into
more than one region of the cord (Scheibel and Scheibel, 1969),
and thus are not restricted to synapsing only with neighbours
of homonymous motoneurones.

    The evidence of Asanuma and Sakata (1967) on descending
cortical control is also not definitive on the question of
specificity of connections. We do not know whether the forelimb motor nuclei in cats are intermixed or separate for the
muscles that can be individually activated from the cortex. If
the greater separateness of motor nuclei in primates is related
to the greater manipulative use of the limb, then we should
expect cat forelimbs to have more separate motor nuclei than
their hindlimbs.

    A recent paper on the size principle (Wyman et al., 1974)
has shown how experimental data that is usually interpreted in
a connectivity by species framework may possibly be better
interpreted in a connectivity by place theory. The size principle
asserts that a group of motoneurones is recruited in order of
increasing size. Henneman et al. (1965a, b) suggest that size
principle holds for all the motor neurones to a given muscle.
However, their experiments may be interpreted quite differently.
They recorded units in L7 and S1 ventral root filaments without
identification of the muscle of termination of the axon. They

evoked stretch reflexes, flexor reflexes and crossed reflexes, they stimulated electrically in the motor cortex, basal ganglia, cerebellum and brain stem (Somjen et al., 1965). These stimuli must certainly have recruited fibres to many muscles in the leg. (Romanes, 1951, shows axons to 22 muscles, ranging from gluteus to plantaris, exiting in these roots). Yet in every case, Henneman and co-workers found that size principle held for these very mixed groups of fibres.

On the surface, then, size principle seems to hold for all the fibres which exit in a single rootlet, independently of the muscle of termination of the fibres. Wyman et al. (1974) checked to see if a unique order of recruitment held for the fibres to a given muscle by recording single units myographically in the muscle. Bursts were elicited in a number of different muscles by using a range of mechanical stimuli. In many cases units were recruited in a fixed order, but in many cases they were not. In 70% of pairs of gastrocnemius units, either unit could start or end a burst. In 48% of pairs either unit could have runs of firing of at least 10 spikes while the other was totally inactive.

Although these experiments of Wyman et al. (1974) were only exploratory in nature, they suggest that size principle may hold less well for the collection of units in a single muscle, than for the collection of units in a single ventral root filament. What is common to the units in a single ventral root filament is that their somas probably sit very closely together, while the various motoneurones to a given muscle are spread out in a column that may be 5 to 10 mm long. It is possible then that size principle holds for those motoneurones whose somas lie together, but not for those whose axons terminate together.

Now size principle can be explained by assuming that pre-synaptic fibres send on the average an equal number of synapses to all the members of a postsynaptic group. In that case, the smallest ones, with the highest input resistance, will fire first. Thus, if size principle holds for the group of motoneurones that sit together, then that group has all the same input connections.

Strong evidence for a place theory of connectivity comes from the above mentioned results of Mendell and Henneman (1971). They found that each MG 1A synapsed on virtually all the MG motoneurones. LG motoneurones sitting outside the MG region received fewer synapses. However, for LG motoneurones sitting in the same rostro-caudal extent as the MG motoneurones, they could find no statistically significant difference in the percentage of motoneurones synapsed with, nor in amplitude of EPSP.

It is known from many studies that there is at least a rough somatotopic organization of the cord. The motoneurone columns are arranged in a somatotopic way, descending cortical control is somatotopic, sensory inflow arrives somatotopically. The question is whether there is, in addition to, or within, this somatotopic organization also an organization by neurone "species". I am suggesting that there is not. If within the somatotopic organization there were divergence at each synaptic station, then in local regions we should expect to find the kind of local uniformity of input which I am suggesting explains the size principle phenomena.

For instance, 1A fibres enter the cord with a somatotopic organization, at least by dermatone. They each turn and run longitudinally, dropping branches into the motoneurone region every 100 to 200 μ for several millimeters (Scheibel and Scheibel, 1969). Thus each 1A may send an axo-somatic synapse to all motoneurones (independent of species) in a longitudinal path over a length of several millimeters. It will make further synapses on the dendrites of motor neurones with somas outside this region. Thus a single 1A fibre may have uniformly large synaptic actions on motoneurones in the central part of its range, and decreasing synaptic actions on motoneurones lying further away.

When the effects of all the 1As are summed we would see an overall somatotopic gradation, but for motoneurones sitting within a millimeter or so of each other in a longitudinal direction, the input might be quite uniform. Other input arrives via interneurones that ramify in different planes. This input might be received quite uniformly by different species of motoneurones lying in the proper plane. Thus a size principle organization based on place may be a corrolary of a somatotopic organization when the synaptic fields of individual elements are large and overlapping.

It is possible to speculate even further. Henneman et al. (1965) find size principle to hold very generally. It holds for

ipsilateral, contralateral and descending pathways, for flexor
muscles and for extensor muscles. One way to maintain size
principle for the polysynaptic pathways is for size principle
and local uniformity of input to hold for each synaptic step in
the pathways. That is, not only would sensory and motor cells
be topologically connected, but the various kinds of interneurones also.

I don't mean to go overboard in questioning "species"
recognizability. By 'species', in this paper, I mean any cells
whose connections are supposed to be specific for the <u>muscle</u>
in whose control pathway they find themselves. I do not mean
that larger 'classes' are not distinguishable, i.e. alpha motoneurones, gamma motoneurones, Renshaw cells and some ventral
spinal cerebellar tract cells are all spatially intermixed, but
they apparently receive quite different connections. It may be
that flexor and extensor motoneurones, even though usually
lying in distinct locations may have distinct connections in
border zones where they intermix. Also, the evidence of
Eccles et al. (1957) that quadriceps 1As send a larger projection
to soleus motoneurones than to the gastrocnemius motoneurones
intermixed with them, may indicate that "slow" motor neurones
may be distinguishable from "fast" (see also Burke et al.,
1970).

I would like to point out that several areas of neurophysiology,
which usually invoke a species recognition theory, are more
simply explained by a topologic type of connectivity without
additional species recognition. (1) During ontogeny motoneurones differentiate and sprout axons in a particular spatiotemporal order. The first axons to sprout will reach the most
proximal muscles first and exclude later developing neurones.
As the wave of differentiation passes dorsally in the cord the
successive sprouting axons will innervate more and more distal
muscles (Romanes, 1941). Thus neuromuscular innervation
does not require nerve-muscle species recognition. (2) In
nerve regeneration, in mammals, there is no specificity in the
establishment of connections between motor nerves and muscles
(see Jacobson, 1970, p. 273 ff. for a summary of the evidence).
(3) A shifting focus of motor cortex activation would correspond
to a shifting focus of spinal activation. At each new focus a
different mix of motoneurone "species" would be recruited and
hence the direction of motion of the limb would shift. (4) Reflex
sign can be simply accounted for as in (3) by the somatotopic

matching of sensory and motor pathways; individual muscles
do not have to be specifically controlled.

In summary, somatotopic (or topologic) connectivity,
without species recognition, is a very appealing hypothesis
to apply to motor systems as well as sensory systems. It is
also an easy hypothesis to test. One test is through size
principle, as suggested by Wyman et al. (1974). A more direct
test would be to see how similar the input is for pairs of
heteronymous motoneurones that are neighbours in the cord,
and compare that with the input similarity for pairs of
homonymous motoneurones that are quite separate in the cord.

REFERENCES

Asanuma, H., and Sakata, H., 1967. Functional organization of a
    cortical efferent system examined with focal depth stimulation
    in cats. J. Neurophysiol. 30, 35-54.
Burke, R.E., Jankowska, E., and Ten Bruggencate, G., 1970. A
    comparison of peripheral and rubrospinal synaptic input to
    slow and fast twitch motor units of triceps surae. J. Physiol.
    207, 709-732.
Eccles, J.C., 1964. The Physiology of Synapses. Springer-Verlag,
    Berlin.
Eccles, J.C., Eccles, R.M., Iggo, A., and Ito, M., 1961. Distri-
    bution of recurrent inhibition among motoneurones. J. Physiol.
    159, 479-499.
Eccles, J.C., Eccles, R.M., and Lundberg, A., 1957. The convergence
    of monosynaptic excitatory afferents on to many different species
    of alpha motoneurones. J. Physiol. 137, 22-50.
Henneman, E., Somjen, G., and Carpenter, D.O., 1965a. Functional
    significance of cell size in spinal motoneurones. J. Neuro-
    physiol. 28, 560-580.
Henneman, E., Somjen, G., and Carpenter, D.O., 1965b. Excitability
    and inhibitability of motoneurons of different sizes. J.
    Neurophysiol. 28, 599-620.
Jacobson, M., 1970. Developmental Neurobiology. Holt, Rinehart and
    Winston, N.Y.
Mendell, L.M., and Henneman, E., 1971. Terminals of single IA
    fibers: location, density, and distribution within a pool of 300
    homonymous motoneurons. J. Neurophysiol. 34, 171-187.
Romanes, G.J., 1941. The development and significance of the cell
    columns in the ventral horn of the cervical and upper thoracic
    spinal cord of the rabbit. J. Anat. 76, 112-130.
Romanes, G.J., 1951. The motor cell columns of the lumbro-sacral
    spinal cord of the cat. J. Comp. Neurol. 94, 313-363.

Romanes, G.J., 1964. The motor pools of the spinal cord. In Organization of the spinal cord. (Ed. Eccles, J.C., and Schade, J.P.). Prog. Brain Res. 11, 93–119. Elsevier, Amsterdam.

Scheibel, M.E., and Scheibel, A.B., 1969. Terminal patterns in cat spinal cord III. Primary afferent collaterals. Brain Res. 13, 417–443.

Somjen, G., Carpenter, D.O., and Henneman, E., 1965. Responses of motoneurons of different sizes to graded stimulation of supra-spinal centers of the brain. J. Neurophysiol. 28, 958–965.

Wyman, R.J., Waldron, I., and Wachtel, G., 1974. Lack of fixed order of recruitment in motoneuron pools. In Press.

PHYSIOLOGICAL ESTIMATES OF THE NUMBERS AND SIZES OF MOTOR UNITS IN MAN

A. J. McComas, R. E. P. Sica, A. R. M. Upton,
D. Longmire and M. R. Caccia

Department of Medicine (Neurology) and the Medical
Research Council Group in Developmental Neuro-
biology, McMaster University Medical Centre,
Hamilton, Ontario

The results and uncertainties of histological methods of
determining the numbers of motor units in various human
muscles are reviewed. An electrophysiological technique
employing graded nerve stimulation is also described and
the underlying assumptions are pointed out; the technique
depends on comparing the sizes of individual motor unit
potentials with that of the maximal muscle response. The
electrophysiologically-derived values for the extensor
digitorum brevis (EDB), thenar, hypothenar and soleus
muscles are reported for healthy subjects below the age
of 60. Beyond the age of 60, there is a progressive loss
of functioning motor units which has been attributed to
motoneurone failure. The sizes of the motor units have
been assessed in terms of the evoked potential amplitudes
and twitch tension of individual motor units; both methods
indicate that there is a considerable variation in this
parameter. Attention is drawn to the marked spurt in
contractile force which affects motor units in males at
puberty. Finally, an attempt has been made to determine
the proportions of motor units with 'fast' and 'slow'
twitches within various human muscles and possible

correlations with results of histochemical staining have
been sought.

NUMBER OF MOTOR UNITS

Histological Methods

The determination of the numbers of human motor units,
although ostensibly a mundane preoccupation, is one which has
recently shed new light on the probable nature of several neuromuscular diseases (see, for example, McComas et al., 1971 a).
In this presentation, however, the results of studies on patients
will be ignored and instead we shall concentrate entirely on the
findings in healthy subjects. Two experimental approaches will
be considered - one histological and the other physiological. Of
the two, the histological is the older and has involved the
counting of axons in the muscular branches of various peripheral
nerves. The most important of the very few studies undertaken
in man is undoubtedly that of Feinstein et al. (1955) who investigated several muscles and obtained, amongst others, the values
set out in Table 1. Interesting and useful though such values are,
it is important to recognize that they are based on several major
assumptions. The first of these concerns the normality of the
subjects from whom the specimens were taken, prior to death.
The mere absence of overt neuromuscular disease is certainly
an insufficient criterion since the peripheral nervous system is
affected in most metabolic disorders as well as by any illness
sufficiently prolonged and severe to produce cachexia. For this
reason the most suitable post-mortem specimens of peripheral
nerve are those taken from supposedly healthy young adults
suffering sudden accidental death. A second difficulty encountered in anatomical studies is that, although it is known from
animals and human studies that the alpha motor fibres are among
the largest in a peripheral nerve, the diameters of the smallest
alpha fibres are uncertain. In the case of a nerve for which the
histogram of axon diameters is bimodal, it is assumed that all
the alpha fibres are contained within the population of large
diameter axons. This is not necessarily so, however, and
furthermore, many muscular nerve branches do not yield
bimodal distributions of axon diameters. Even for the same
nerve a distribution may be bimodal in one subject and unimodal

SPECIES	MUSCLE	NUMBER OF MOTOR UNITS	MUSCLE FIBRES/UNIT	AUTHOR
Man	Ext. rectus	2,970	9	Feinstein et al. (1955)
"	Platysma	1,096	25	"
"	1st Lumbrical	96*	108	"
"	1st Dorsal Interosseus	119	340	"
"	Brachioradialis	333*	> 410	"
"	Tibialis ant.	445	562	"
"	Med. gastrocnemius	579	1,934	"
Baboon	Abductor pollicis brevis	43	220	Wray (1969)
"	Med. gastrocnemius	292	790	"

Table 1. Numbers and sizes of motor units in man and baboon, as determined from histological studies (* = averaged values).

in another. Nor is it possible for the electrophysiologist to
help the anatomist for, although the impulse conduction velocities of the slowest alpha motor axons can be measured
accurately in man by a collision technique (Hopf, 1962), the
appropriate conversion factor relating axon diameter to conduction velocity is uncertain (Boyd and Davey, 1968). Again,
even if the sizes of the alpha fibres were known, it would still
be necessary to assume a certain value for the proportions of
fibres within this range which were alpha motor as opposed to
sensory in function. This proportion is difficult to determine
as the detailed investigations of Boyd and Davey (1968) in
the cat have shown. These authors found that the alpha motor
fibres comprised as much as 73% of the large fibres in the
peroneus longus, while for the popliteus muscle the corresponding value was only 44% (calculated from Table 7 of Boyd
and Davey, 1968). In their calculations, Feinstein et al.
(1955) had assumed that 60% of the large fibres were alpha
motor on the basis of a post-mortem study of a single muscle
in a patient with severe poliomyelitis. However, from the
careful study of Wray (1969) in the abductor pollicis brevis
and medial gastrocnemius muscles of the baboon, it would
appear that 50% is a better value to use for the proportion of
alpha motor axons within the large fibre population of a primate muscle nerve. Further uncertainty in anatomical
studies results from the fact that up to half of the axons may
divide before the nerve enters the muscle belly (Eccles and
Sherrington, 1930; Wray, 1969). Unless this branching is
allowed for the number of motor axons will be over-estimated.
Finally, it is important to bear in mind that most of the values
of Feinstein et al. (1955) are derived from observations on
one muscle only and it is certainly possible that there may be
considerable variation in innervation among individuals
corresponding to that found in the baboon by Wray (1969). In
the only other extensive examination of human motor units
of which we are aware, material was obtained from stillborn
infants by Christensen (1959). For reasons which are not
apparent, some of her derived values are improbably large
in relation to those of other studies in man (Feinstein et al.,
1955; see also below) and lower mammals. For example,
approximately six thousand motor units were estimated for
the opponens pollicis alone; the values for larger muscles
are more reasonable, however.

If a conclusion is to be drawn from anatomical studies of

post-mortem material it is that, far from providing accurate
estimates of motor unit populations, they are themselves susceptible to appreciable errors and may not be very much more
reliable than the electrophysiological estimates to be described
below.

Electrophysiological Methods

Electrophysiological methods may, or may not, be more
accurate for estimating numbers of motor units than the anatomical ones, but they undoubtedly have three major advantages.
They are fast, they are repeatable, and above all, they yield
data on living subjects. The method to be described is one
which has been in continuous use for five years in the author's
laboratory. Its principle is extremely simple and involves comparing the amplitudes of individual motor unit potentials with
that of the maximum muscle response (M wave) evoked by nerve
stimulation. Since the motor unit potentials vary considerably
in size, it is necessary to obtain an average value from a sample
of potentials. Such a sample could be obtained during a weak
voluntary contraction, but it is known that under these circumstances the motor units recruited would be relatively small
and therefore not representative of the total population (Milner-
Brown et al., 1973). For this reason, and also for technical
convenience, we have preferred to employ graded electrical
stimulation of peripheral nerve as a method for investigating
the electrical activity of single motor units. The muscle first
chosen for this type of experiment was the extensor digitorum
brevis (EDB) since it possessed certain favourable features
(Fig. 1). Firstly, because of the isolated position of this muscle
on the dorsum of the foot, its electrical evoked responses could
be recorded with little contamination from the only other muscles
supplied by distal part of the deep peroneal nerve, i.e. the dorsal interossei. Secondly, the end-plates within the muscle were
grouped in a band which ran transversely across the proximal
third of the muscle belly. This arrangement made it possible
to record simultaneously from all the end-plate zones of the
fibres using one large electrode attached to the overlying skin.
The advantage of this recording system was that it ensured all
the evoked motor unit potentials would summate algebraically
with each other; thus, each newly recruited motor unit would
be expected to enlarge the evoked muscle action potential.

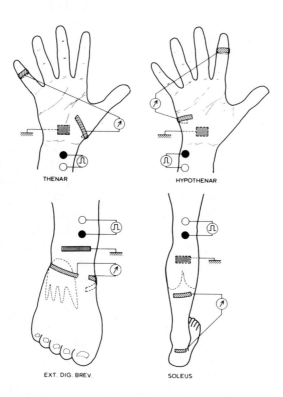

Fig. 1. Experimental arrangements used for estimating numbers of motor units in various muscles or muscle groups. A filled circle denotes the cathode of each pair of stimulating electrodes. The stigmatic and reference electrodes used for recording are indicated by hatched lines. Interrupted lines show outlines of EDB and gastrocnemius muscles, as well as electrodes, or parts of electrodes, attached to the opposite aspects of the various limbs.

Finally, the EDB muscle had a relatively thin and flattened belly so that the component motor units should have been reasonably equidistant from an overlying recording electrode. This being so, any differences in motor unit potential amplitude would mainly reflect inequalities in the numbers of muscle fibres within those units rather than the varied positions of respective unit territories within the muscle belly.

Fig. 1 shows the stimulating and recording arrangement used for estimating the numbers of motor units in EDB. Unlike the original study (McComas et al., 1971), we now prefer to have the reference electrode on the inner aspect of the foot and level with the stigmatic electrode. This modification results in a smaller stimulus artefact, and is convenient if the number of motor units in the medial plantar muscles are to be estimated subsequently, for the reference electrode can then be used as a stigmatic one.

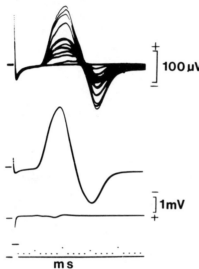

Fig. 2. Recordings used to estimate the number of motor units in the EDB muscle of a 25 year old healthy female control subject. At top, there are eleven discernible increments in the responses evoked by weak graded stimulation of the peroneal nerve; the average increment size is $34 \mu V$. The maximum evoked response is 7.1 mV (middle trace) and hence the estimated number of motor units is 208.

Fig. 2 shows how the evoked muscle response enlarges in an incremental manner as the stimulus intensity, initially sub-threshold, is gradually increased. Each of these increments is thought to represent the excitation of an additional motor unit. After about ten such increments have been detected, their mean size is calculated and is assumed to be the mean amplitude of the motor unit potentials sampled. The number of motor units is then found by dividing this mean value into the maximal response recorded from the muscle following a strong stimulus to the

nerve. The answer obtained is, of course, a very gross approximation of the true motor unit population since it depends on two
important assumptions - the adequacy of the sample of units and
the identification of each response increment with the activation
of an additional motor unit.

First, is the sample of units representative? By using a
collision technique, and also by comparing the responses of the
most and least excitable units in each sample, it was shown that
the electrical stimuli did not preferentially activate the axons
innervating the largest motor units in the muscle - as might have
been anticipated on theoretical grounds. Furthermore, it is
possible to compensate for inaccuracy in the determination of
mean motor unit potentials in individual subjects by pooling the
estimated numbers of units for all the normal subjects examined.
Secondly, does each response increment correspond to the excitation of an additional motor unit? Here the problem is more
difficult for axons with similar thresholds may be expected to
fire in different combinations when stimuli of similar intensities
are repeated ('alternation' phenomenon, see McComas et al.,
1971b). Notwithstanding these analytical difficulties, the results
in any one subject are reasonably reproducible, for in the subject who was examined on eleven different occasions the values
ranged from 167 to 243 units (mean 203, S.D. ± 28 units).

Recently we have extended the motor unit counting technique
to other muscles and muscle groups; these are (i) the thenar
muscles innervated by the median nerve, (ii) the hypothenar
muscles, and (iii) the soleus. The arrangements of the stimulating and recording electrodes for each experimental situation
are shown in Fig. 1. (see also Sica et al., 1973).

Table 2 shows the mean number of motor units estimated in
each of these muscles of muscle groups in healthy volunteer
subjects below the age of 60. It is of interest that the median-
innervated thenar muscles have also been studied independently
by Brown (1972), who obtained a mean value of 253 ± 34 units.
This result is significantly smaller than our own value but is
possibly accounted for by Brown's use of smaller recording
electrodes since these could have biased the results in favour
of the muscle lying immediately underneath them (abductor
pollicis brevis).

How well do these results correlate to anatomical studies?

ESTIMATED MOTOR UNIT POPULATIONS
Mean ± S. D. (n)

Extensor digitorum brevis	208 ± 66 (111)
Thenar group	340 ± 87 (67)
Hypothenar group	380 ± 79 (77)
Soleus	801 ± 167 (18)

Table 2. Numbers of motor units estimated electro-
physiologically in control subjects below the age of 60.

In the case of EDB two values are available from specimens of
the lateral terminal branch of the deep peroneal nerve obtained
post-mortem from victims of road accidents. If 50% of the
fibres larger than 8μ are considered to be alpha-motor, then the
corresponding values are 365 and 280. Although both values are
within the normal range of physiological values for EDB, they
are well above the mean value (208 units); however, the anatomical estimates would have included those fibres running through
EDB to supply some of the dorsal interossei. In the case of
soleus there are no anatomically-determined values available
and probably the most relevant observation is the estimate of
579 units obtained for the medial gastrocnemius muscle by
Feinstein et al. (1955). Unfortunately, the situation for the
thenar and hypothenar muscles is equally unsatisfactory since
Christensen's (1959) estimate of six thousand units for the
opponens pollicis, a thenar muscle, is far too large. Again,
the only data of relevance are those of Feinstein et al. (1955)
who calculated that there are roughly 100 motor units in each of
two other intrinsic muscles of the hand, the first dorsal interosseus and the first lumbrical. Among the thenar muscles there
are usually two (the short abductor and opponens) supplied
entirely by the median nerve and one (the short flexor) in which
the innervation is shared with the ulnar nerve. If Feinstein et
al.'s (1955) value of about 100 units per intrinsic muscle is
applicable, then both the electrophysiological estimates of 253
(Brown, 1972) and 340 (Sica et al., 1973) appear reasonable.
Similarly, for the four hypothenar muscles (abductor, opponens,
short flexor and palmar) an estimate of 380 units is certainly of
the correct order, especially if the rather small sizes of these

muscles are taken into account.

Effects of Age

One of the interesting problems which can be studied in healthy subjects is the nature of the neuromuscular changes during ageing. It is a common observation that in the elderly there is a reduction in muscle strength and that this is associated with some degree of generalised muscle atrophy. The most careful studies to date, those of Gutmann and his colleagues in the rat, have suggested that there is a random loss of muscle fibres and that, although transmitter release from the nerve terminal is also affected in the case of other fibres (Gutmann et al., 1971), the numbers of motor units is actually unchanged. The evidence for the latter conclusion was the previous finding of a normal number of motor axons in the nerve to the rat soleus muscle (Gutmann and Hanzlíková, 1966). Such a conclusion may have been premature, however, for the mere presence of an axon need not necessarily imply normal function. In fact, recent electrophysiological studies of motor units in aged rats have shown that in most animals a selective loss of functioning motor units does occur (Caccia, unpublished observations).

In healthy subjects of various ages the loss of motor unit function with age is especially striking. This is well seen in Fig. 3, which shows the numbers of motor units in 167 EDB muscles of 157 subjects, all of whom were considered to be in good health for their ages. Before the age of 60 little, if any, denervation appears to have taken place. Beyond 60, however, there was a progressive loss of functioning motor units which was complete, or almost so, in some of the eldest subjects. Since our original description of this neural ageing phenomenon in EDB (Campbell and McComas, 1970; see also Campbell et al., 1973) we have observed its occurrence in the thenar and hypothenar muscles. Interestingly, the thenar and EDB muscles are more severely affected than the hypothenar group. Why there should be this difference in the case of the hand muscles is unknown - it clearly cannot be related to the lengths of the nerve axons since these are similar, nor is it likely that any "non-specific" factor such as ischaemia of the spinal cord or peripheral nerves is at play. Our own suggestion, for which we have no direct evidence, is that the longevity of the motoneurones is specified genetically and may differ from one motoneurone pool

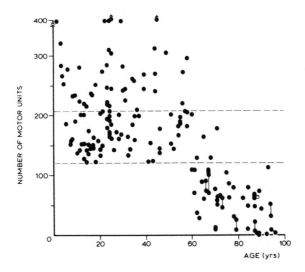

Fig. 3. Estimated numbers of motor units in 157 healthy control subjects of various ages. Bilateral results in same subjects indicated by paired values. Upper interrupted line indicates mean number of motor units in controls below the age of 60 (111 units). Lower line represents lower limit of control range (120 units).

to another within the same spinal cord, as well as from species to species.

Before leaving the subject of age, it is of some interest to consider the numbers of motor units in very young muscles. In the cat it now appears that, at birth, a substantial proportion of muscle fibres are supplied by more than one motoneurone but that, within a few weeks, the secondary innervation is lost (Bagust et al., 1973). From studies on the rat (Reier and Hughes, 1972), it is probable that these changes are associated with a degeneration of motoneurones in the ventral horn, such as occurs in the developing tadpole (Hughes, 1961). If this early motoneurone loss is shown to be common to man as well, then it will be of interest to determine its time course in neonates. The electrophysiological motor unit counting technique would provide one possible approach though the inaccuracies inherent in the method would require the sampling of a large population of infants.

SIZES OF HUMAN MOTOR UNITS

One prediction from the results of motor unit studies in animals is that the sizes of the units in human muscles will vary considerably. There are two ways in which this variation can be detected, of which one is to measure the twitch tensions of individual motor units. The other is to record the potentials of single motor units using large electrodes suitable for summing the activities of all the component muscle fibres. In Fig. 4,

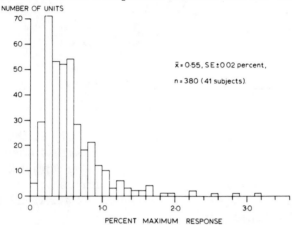

Fig. 4. Amplitudes of 280 motor unit potentials recorded from EDB muscles of 41 control subjects below the age of 60. Results have been expressed in terms of the maximum evoked response, rather than as absolute values (from McComas et al., 1971b; courtesy of the Editor of the Journal of Neurology, Neurosurgery and Psychiatry).

which shows the results obtained by the last method for EDB, it can be seen that the amplitudes of evoked motor unit potentials vary considerably (ranging from .07 to 3.15% of maximal M wave). Since the amplitudes should be directly proportional to the numbers of muscle fibres in the respective motor units, it is probable that the motor unit sizes vary by a similar amount.

So far as measurements of motor unit twitch tensions are concerned, there are now two sets of data available - one by Sica and McComas (1971) for EDB and the other by Milner-Brown et al. (1973) for the first dorsal interosseus muscle. It is interesting that quite different methods were used in these studies for while Sica and McComas used weak, indirect stimulation to

excite the motor axons with lowest thresholds, Milner –Brown et
al. were able to recognize the twitches of individual motor units
during a voluntary contraction. In theory, neither method is
ideal for the stimulation method might be expected to favour the
largest axons, although in practice this does not seem too true
(see McComas et al., 1971b). Conversely, the volitional
method would not be able to detect these units which only fire
during maximal contractions and limit their discharges to a few
impulses. Such units, usually yielding large spikes during recordings with concentric needle electrodes, are well known to
clinical electromyographers. Nevertheless, with both methods

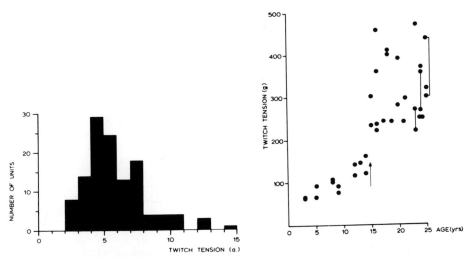

Fig. 5. Left: Twitch tensions of 122 motor units in EDB
muscles of 31 control subjects below the age of 60 (from
Sica and McComas, 1971). Right: Maximal EDB twitch
tensions in healthy boys of different ages (from McComas
et al., 1973; both illustrations reproduced by courtesy of
the Editor of the Journal of Neurology, Neurosurgery and
Psychiatry).

it has been possible to demonstrate substantial variations in
motor unit twitch tension. In the case of EDB the tensions were
found to range from 2 to 14 g (Fig. 5) while for the interosseus
muscle the corresponding values were 0.1 to 10 g. Large differences have also been reported for other mammalian muscles; for
example, in the cat gastrocnemius, Burke (1967) found that the
motor unit twitch tensions varied from 0.2 to 97 g, a 500-fold
range.

Motor Unit Twitch Speeds

For a detailed analysis of motor units within a human muscle, it is necessary to determine the numbers and sizes of units not only within the whole population, but also within the various sub- groups which can be recognized on the basis of differences in histochemical staining properties or in isometric twitch speed. Thus, it has long been known from animal studies that the twitch speeds of individual motor units may differ considerably, even in the same muscle, and there is now good evidence to indicate that the same is also true of man. Fig. 6 shows the contraction

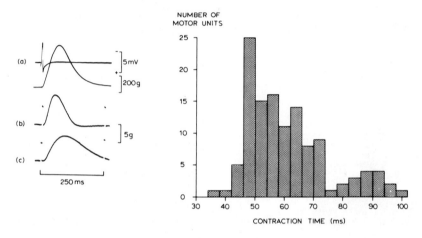

Fig. 6. Left: a - Maximal evoked M wave and isometric twitch of EDB muscle; b and c - averaged twitch responses from a 'fast' and a 'slow' motor unit respectively. Right: Contraction times of 122 motor units in control subjects (from data of Sica and McComas, 1971).

times of 122 single motor units in the EDB muscles of 31 healthy control subjects below the age of 60; it can be seen that the values range from 35 to 98 ms (Sica and McComas, 1971). In the first dorsal interosseus muscle, Milner-Brown et al. (1973) have ob- tained very similar values (30 to 100 ms). In the EDB muscle there was a suggestion that the values fell into two groups, with a separation at about 75 ms, but in Milner-Brown et al.'s (1973) results there is no clear evidence of a multimodal distribution. Sica and McComas further found that the 'fast' units were more plentiful than the 'slow' ones in EDB. Although these authors did not find a correlation between twitch tension and twitch speed, Milner-Brown et al. (1973) were able to demonstrate one in two of their three subjects. In other mammalian muscles it is now established that the motor units generating the largest tensions have fast twitches while relatively weak units may be fast or slow (Burke, 1967).

What of other human muscles? Previously McComas and Thomas (1968) had used a surface recording technique to examine both EDB and the first dorsal interosseus muscle and had obtained contraction times for the whole muscles of 67.1, S.E. ± 3.3 and 64.9 ± 3.3 ms respectively. However, when the same technique was employed for the gastrocnemius and facial muscles the results differed considerably, being 117.6 ± 6.5 ms for the former and 42.6 ± 4.3 ms for the latter. From this study it might have been predicted that the facial muscles would be found to contain muscle fibres, which with myosin ATP-ase staining, were predominantly of type II. From a recent histochemical investigation by Johnson et al. (1973) of 'fresh' post-mortem material, it would appear that this is indeed the case for the orbicularis oculi, but not for frontalis. McComas and Thomas (1968) could not be certain which of the eyebrow muscles they were recording from, though the orientation of their transducer system suggested that the frontalis was mainly involved. However, since the most obvious muscle response following stimulation of the facial nerve at the zygoma is eyelid closure, it may well have been the orbicularis oculi, rather than the frontalis, which had contributed most to the evoked twitches. In the case of the mechanical recordings from the lateral gastrocnemius belly it is unlikely that any other muscle was significantly involved; therefore, in this muscle the slow twitch appears to be generated by evenly mixed populations of type I and type II fibres. In contrast, the soleus muscle, which has an equally slow twitch (Buller et al., 1959) is composed mainly of type I fibres (Johnson et al., 1973) and this association would have been anticipated from animal experiments.

It is of interest to enquire at what age, in man, the differentiation of muscle fibres in terms of their twitch speeds is complete. In the kitten it appears from the work of Buller et al. (1960) that at birth all muscles have slow twitches and that several weeks are required for the 'fast' muscles to acquire their characteristic twitch velocities. In man it has not been

possible to carry out a similar study because of the technical
problems involved in studying the twitches of infants. On the
basis of contraction time measurements in young children,
however, it would appear that this parameter has assumed its
adult values by the age of three, though twitch relaxation is still
rather slow (Sica and McComas, 1971). Twitch studies in
children are interesting for another reason since they demonstrate the remarkable increase in muscle strength which occurs
at puberty, presumably under the influence of circulating tes-
tosterone (McComas et al., 1973). Whether this increase
reflects changes throughout the whole spectrum of motor units,
or whether certain types of unit are preferentially enhanced is
not clear. If the diameters of the muscle fibres are any guide,
the similarity of the sizes of type I and type II fibres in the
adult suggests that both types are involved at puberty (Brooke
and Engel, 1969). Nevertheless, it is certainly possible that
relatively subtle changes, affecting the packing density or the
fine structure of the myofibrils, are involved.

In conclusion, physiological studies of human muscle, although inevitably subjected to various technical limitations,
have nevertheless progressed remarkably during the past decade. It is to be hoped that future studies will not be used simply
as further extensions of animal investigations, but will instead
be tailored to the particular advantages of the human preparation. In this context, we are especially mindful of the recent,
and most elegant, studies of motor unit recruitment during voluntary contraction by Milner-Brown et al. (1973). It also
seems quite likely that man may become the preparation of
choice for examining the effects of use and disuse on the neuromuscular system. In any event, the usefulness of human
studies, far from having been exhausted, would seem to be
capable of considering expansion in the foreseeable future.

Acknowledgments: We are grateful to Irene Csatari for secretarial
services and to Bernice Crompton, Judy Leon (supported by the
Muscular Dystrophy Association of Canada) and Trevor Blogg for
technical assistance.

REFERENCES

Bagust, J., Lewis, D.M. and Westerman, R.A., 1973. Polyneuronal innervation of kitten skeletal muscle. J. Physiol. 229, 241-255.

Boyd, I.A. and Davey, Mary R., 1968. Composition of Peripheral Nerves. Edinburgh: Livingstone.

Brooke, M.H. and Engel, W.K., 1969. The histographic analysis of human muscle biopsies with regard to fibre types. I. Adult male and female. Neurology (Minneap.) 19, 221-233.

Brown, W.F., 1972. A method for estimating the number of motor units in thenar muscles and the changes in motor unit count with ageing. J. Neurol. Neurosurg. Psychiat. 35, 845-852.

Buller, A.J., Eccles, J.C. and Eccles, R.M., 1960. Differentiation of fast and slow muscles in the cat hind limb. J. Physiol. 150, 399-416.

Buller, A.J., Dornhorst, A.C., Edwards, R., Kerr, D. and Whelan, R.F., 1959. Fast and slow muscles in mammals. Nature (Lond.) 183, 1516-1517.

Burke, R.E., 1967. Motor unit types of cat triceps surae muscle. J. Physiol. 193, 141-160.

Campbell, M.J. and McComas, A.J., 1970. The effects of ageing on muscle function. Fifth Symposium on Current Research in Muscular Dystrophy and Related Disorders (Abstracts). Muscular Dystrophy Group of Great Britain: London.

Campbell, M.J., McComas, A.J. and Petito, F., 1973. Physiological changes in ageing muscles. J. Neurol. Neurosurg. Psychiat. 36, 174-182.

Christensen, E., 1959. Topography of terminal motor innervation in striated muscles from stillborn infants. Amer. J. Phys. Med. 38, 65-78.

Eccles, J.C. and Sherrington, C.S., 1930. Numbers and contraction-values of individual motor units examined in some muscles of the limb. Proc. Roy. Soc. B. 106, 326-356.

Feinstein, B., Lindegaard, B., Nyman, E. and Wohlfart, G., 1955. Morphologic studies of motor units in normal human muscles. Acta Anat. 23, 127-142.

Gutmann, E. and Hanzlíková, V., 1966. Motor unit in old age. Nature 209, 921-922.

Gutmann, E., Hanzlíková, V. and Vyskočil, F., 1971. Age changes in cross striated muscle of the rat. J. Physiol. 216, 331-343.

Hopt, H.C., 1962. Untersuchungen uber die Unterschiede in der Leitgeschwindigkeit motorischer Nervenfasern beim Menschen. Dtsch. Z. Nervenheilk. 183, 579-588.

Huges, A., 1961. Cell degeneration in the larval ventral horn of xenopus laevis (Daudin). J. Embryol. Exp. Morphol. 9, 269-284.

Johnson, M.A., Polgar, J., Weightman, D. and Appleton, D., 1973. Data on the distribution of fibre types in thirty-six human muscles. An autopsy study. J. Neurol. Sci. 18, 111-129.

McComas, A.J. and Thomas, H.C., 1968. Fast and slow twitch muscles in man. J. Neurol. Sci. 7, 301-307.

McComas, A.J., Sica, R.E.P. and Campbell, M.J., 1971a. 'Sick' motoneurones. A unifying concept of muscle disease. Lancet 1, 321-325.

McComas, A.J., Sica, R.E.P. and Petito, F., 1973. Muscle strength in boys of different ages. J. Neurol. Neurosurg. Psychiat. 36, 171-173.

McComas, A.J., Fawcett, P.R.W., Campbell, M.J. and Sica, R.E.P., 1971b. Electrophysiological estimation of the number of motor units within a human muscle. J. Neurol. Neurosurg. Psychiat. 34, 121-131.

Milner-Brown, H.S., Stein, R.B. and Yemm, R., 1973. The orderly recruitment of human motor units during voluntary isometric contractions. J. Physiol. 230, 359-370.

Reier, P.J. and Hughes, A., 1972. Evidence for spontaneous axon degeneration during peripheral nerve maturation. Amer. J. Anat. 135, 47-152.

Sica, R.E.P. and McComas, A.J., 1971. Fast and slow twitch units in a human muscle. J. Neurol. Neurosurg. Psychiat. 34, 113-120.

Sica, R.E.P., McComas, A.J., Upton, A.R.M. and Longmire, D., 1973. Motor unit estimations in small muscles of the hand. J. Neurol. Neurosurg. Psychiat. In press.

Wray, Shirly, H., 1969. Innervation ratios for large and small limb muscles in the baboon. J. Comp. Neurol. 137, 227-250.

CONTRACTILE AND ELECTRICAL PROPERTIES OF NORMAL AND MODIFIED HUMAN MOTOR UNITS

R. B. Stein and H. S. Milner-Brown

Department of Physiology, University of Alberta, Edmonton, Canada

By signal averaging the twitch tensions and the early time course of a twitch from single human motor units can be measured during voluntary, isometric contractions. Under normal conditions motor units with increasingly large twitch tensions are recruited during increasing voluntary contractions. This orderly pattern of recruitment is irretrievably lost following accidental severance of a nerve, even though the regenerated motor units eventually return to approximately normal size.

In the partial denervation that results from pressure or en-entrapment neuropathies, motor axons are thought to sprout collaterals which innervate other muscle fibres. This leads to an increase in EMG amplitudes although the twitch tensions measured under these conditions are actually reduced. Similarly, in motor neurone disease greatly increased EMG amplitudes are associated with near normal twitch tensions. Enlarged motor units may be much more susceptible to fatigue, and therefore less efficient units for generating maintained forces.

Regular use of a muscle to exert large, brief forces leads to a nearly synchronous activation of motor units even during maintained contractions. Disuse of a muscle leads to a loss of this synchronization.

Over the past two years we have used signal averaging to measure the contractile as well as the electrical properties of human motor units during voluntary, isometric contractions. This technique has permitted us to gain some insight into the normal organization of the human neuromuscular system and the ways in which this organization can be altered by various disease processes. It has also permitted a comparison between voluntary control in man and reflex studies in animals. Many of the basic results on the normal organization of the human neuromuscular system have now appeared in print (Milner-Brown et al., 1973a, b, c). These will be reviewed briefly here before discussing how this organization can be modified.

SIGNAL AVERAGING

The method is basically quite simple and was developed independently by Buchthal and Schmalbruch (1970) and by our group (Stein et al., 1972). We have now used it to study nearly a thousand motor units under a variety of conditions without encountering major difficulties. The use of signal averaging permits signals which are locked in time to one another to be extracted from those which are uncorrelated. The signals used in this application are the impulses from single motor units, the force exerted by a muscle, and the surface electromyogram (EMG). Needle electrodes were inserted into a muscle and positioned so as to reliably record the impulses from a single motor unit when it was voluntarily activated. Conventional needle electrodes used in electromyography have been modified somewhat to improve their selectivity for single units (Milner-Brown et al., 1973a), and subjects were provided with auditory and visual feedback to help them in controlling single motor units. The impulses from a single unit were used to trigger a signal averager or a general purpose laboratory computer and the force correlated in time with these impulses was determined. Assuming that the motor units in a muscle discharge independently of one another (this assumption will be considered in the section on Synchronization), the force correlated to the impulses gives a measure of the magnitude and time course of the contractions generated by a single motor unit. Even when a subject is instructed to exert just enough force to produce a maintained activity of a motor unit (threshold force), impulses occur at a rate of 7-8/sec. This is sufficient to produce the appearance of a somewhat fused contraction (see Fig. 1).

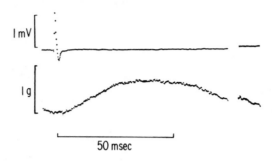

Fig. 1. Average voltage recorded by a needle electrode from a single motor unit during voluntary contraction (upper trace) and the average force generated by the motor unit (lower trace). A predetection facility in the tape recorder permitted the sweeps of a signal averager to be started some time before the impulses from the motor unit. From these traces a measure of the twitch tension, contraction time (time from the EMG signal to the peak of the contraction) and half-relaxation time could be obtained.

Nonetheless, measurements from such records give a measure of the twitch tension, contraction time and often the half-relaxation time for single motor units. This technique has been used mainly in a relatively small muscle, the first dorsal interosseus muscle of the hand, and the subsequent results apply specifically to this muscle. However, the same technique may be applied to as large a muscle as soleus (unpublished observations). Somewhat more averaging is required to obtain as clean a trace from larger muscles. It is also helpful to filter out unwanted components at both high and low frequencies (Milner-Brown et al., 1973a).

ORDER OF RECRUITMENT

When different motor units were examined in normal human subjects, an orderly pattern of recruitment was observed. Motor units which became active at increasingly large voluntary force levels, generated increasingly large twitch tensions (Fig. 2A). A double logarithmic plot has been used in Fig. 2 because of the wide range of twitch tensions and threshold forces observed. The slope of the best-fitting straight line on this plot is close to unity. A value close to unity has generally been observed (Milner-Brown et al., 1973b), and implies that there is a nearly linear relation

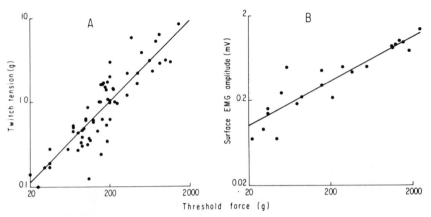

Fig. 2. Twitch tensions (A) and peak-to-peak surface EMG amplitudes (B) produced by single motor units in one subject as a function of the force at which the motor units were recruited (threshold force). The computed best-fitting straight lines shown on these log-log plots had slopes of (A) 0.945 $\pm$ 0.065 and (B) 0.518 $\pm$ 0.051 (slope $\pm$ S. E.). The difference in slope on these plots indicates that the surface EMG amplitudes increased less than linearly with the twitch tension of a motor unit.

between the twitch tension a unit generates and the voluntary force level at which it becomes active.

The voltage recorded by surface electrodes was measured simultaneously in most experiments, and was also averaged to determine the contribution of each unit to the surface EMG. The peak-to-peak amplitudes contributed by different motor units are shown in Fig. 2B and an orderly pattern of recruitment is also evident for the surface EMG. There was often more scatter in the EMG data, presumably because the contribution of a unit to the surface EMG depends more on the position of the unit in the muscle than does the measured twitch tension. The best-fitting slope is significantly smaller in Fig. 2B than in Fig. 2A (the data in both parts of this Fig. are from the same subject). This result has been consistently observed, and implies that the contribution of a unit to the surface EMG increases less than linearly with its twitch tension. Possible explanations for this result will be considered elsewhere (Stein and Milner-Brown, in preparation).

The orderly recruitment of increasingly large motor units is often observed in animal experiments with increasing reflex stimulation (Henneman, 1968) and has been referred to as the 'size principle'. It was encouraging to demonstrate that this principle applies also to voluntary contractions in man. The generality of the size principle is a controversial topic (see articles by Wyman et al. and Burke et al. in this volume). We have found one condition where it does not hold. If a nerve is completely severed and surgically repaired, the nerve will regenerate and within a few months begin to reinnervate the muscles involved. In examining a number of patients in whom regeneration had taken place, we found that the twitch tensions generated by motor units eventually returned to approximately their original size. (Since the injuries were unilateral, the other hand served as a control.) However, the orderly pattern of recruitment never returned. This is illustrated in Fig. 3 for four patients at different stages of

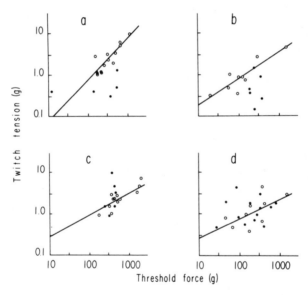

Fig. 3. Twitch tensions produced by single motor units from 4 patients with previous complete severance of their ulnar nerves as a function of the threshold force at which the motor units were recruited. Above - early stage of regeneration (about 6 months); below - advanced stage of regeneration (about 2 years). The computed best-fitting straight lines shown on these log-log plots are for the normal hands only. Normal (O), abnormal (●).

regeneration. The normal hands (open circles) showed an orderly pattern of recruitment (straight lines), but in no case was the slope of computed best-fitting straight lines for the abnormal hands (filled circles) significantly different from zero, even when about 2 years had been allowed for regeneration (lower parts of Fig. 3). Thus, the orderly pattern of recruitment is established during normal development, but cannot be re-established if the physical pathway from the nerve to the muscle is disrupted in an adult.

To explain this result, one might assume that larger motoneurones begin to grow axons at an earlier stage of development, and hence are able to innervate more muscle fibres. An analogous situation would be the earlier myelination of large fibres in developing nerves.

Different types of fibres are known to reach and innervate end organs at different times during development. For example, Diamond and Miledi (1962) found miniature end-plate potentials in rat muscles 5 days before birth, indicating the establishment of innervation by alpha motoneurones at this time. Primary muscle spindle afferents also have begun to cause the differentiation of intrafusal muscle fibres 3 days before birth in the rat (Zelená, 1964).

Innervation by smaller motor and sensory fibres only occurs after birth. Afferents which supply Golgi tendon organs (and which are somewhat smaller than primary muscle spindle afferents) are seen 3 days after birth. The gamma motoneurones can be distinguished 5-10 days after birth, and the smaller secondary muscle spindle afferents also appear about this time (Zelena, 1964). Thus, there appears to be a correlation between the size of different fibre types and their order of innervation. Whether this correlation holds within a given fibre type, the population of alpha motoneurones, remains to be tested. As indicated above, this hypothesis could explain the relation between the size of a motoneurone and the number of muscle fibres it innervates. It would then account for the 'size principle' in normal muscles, since larger motoneurones will have lower input impedances and require stronger synaptic currents to activate them (Kernell, 1965; Burke, 1968).

Given an even start following nerve section in later life, nerve fibres of different size grow at similar rates (Gutmann et al., 1942; Lubinska, 1964), and the number of muscle fibres innervated would then be random.

RELATION BETWEEN SURFACE EMG AND FORCE

It has been known for over 20 years (Bayer and Flechtenmayer, 1950; Lippold, 1952; Inman et al., 1952) that if the surface EMG is rectified and filtered there is a linear relation between surface EMG and force. We have confirmed this relation in the first dorsal interosseus muscle under our experimental conditions (see also Stephens and Taylor, 1972), though the basis for the relation remains uncertain. Indeed, our finding of a non-linear relation between the twitch tension of single units and their contributions to the surface EMG (Fig. 2) further obscures the basis of this linear relation. The slope of the linear relation between rectified surface EMG and force is increased during fatigue (Edwards and Lippold, 1956; Lippold et al., 1960) and in various disease states (Lenman, 1969), so that more EMG activity is required to produce the same force.

The basis for this increase has been investigated at the unit level in a number of patients with a unilateral neuropathy involving pressure or entrapment of the ulnar nerve as it passes the elbow joint. Approximately 10 motor units were analyzed from the affected and from the control hands in each patient. Under these conditions the orderly pattern of recruitment is retained, presumably because the physical pathway along the nerve to the muscle is not disrupted. It is well known to neurologists that EMG potentials recorded by a needle electrode under these conditions are enlarged. This finding, together with histological evidence (Coërs and Woolf, 1959), suggests that surviving motor axons can sprout new collaterals to innervate muscle fibres which become denervated following blockage of their motor axons.

We have found that the average surface EMG contributed by units in these patients is also increased. Most of our patients were unilaterally affected, and the other hand again served as a control. This is illustrated in Fig. 4, in which the ratios of the mean surface EMG amplitude on the affected side to that on the control side have been plotted (interrupted lines) for a number of patients. Most of these ratios are substantially greater than 1, indicating that the EMG amplitudes were larger on the affected side. The ratios of the mean twitch tension for motor units on the affected side relative to that on the normal side are also plotted in Fig. 4

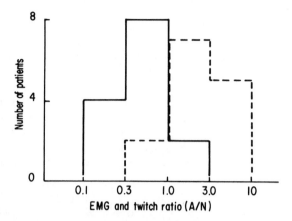

Fig. 4. Ratios of mean twitch tensions (solid lines) and mean EMG amplitudes (interrupted lines) for motor units in abnormal (A) and normal (N) hands of 14 patients with unilateral ulnar neuropathies. The EMG amplitudes in the affected hands are larger on average while the twitch tensions are smaller.

on the same scale. Note that most of the ratios are less than 1, indicating that the twitch tensions are smaller on the affected side, even though the EMG amplitudes are increased.

Similarly, in patients with motor neurone disease, we have found greatly increased EMG amplitudes associated with approximately normal twitch tensions. There is also an increase in the contraction times and half-relaxation times for units in these disease states. These changes in the twitch tension and time course in the abnormal motor units might be explained if the motor units in these muscles are much more easily fatigued than normal units. Although there were few overt signs of fatigue in these patients, our procedure does involve the maintenance of a steady force for a couple of minutes while signal averaging was carried out for each unit.

McComas et al. (1971) found that the twitch tensions of motor units were increased in patients with motor neurone disease using stimulation techniques. These techniques require only a minimal number of action potentials to be elicited from a given unit in a muscle at rest, and presumably would not fatigue the motor units. The simplest conclusion from these experiments is that motor units enlarged by collateral sprouting may give larger twitches transiently, but that they fatigue readily and are less efficient contractile units for providing maintained forces. McComas et al. (1973) have recently shown that enlarged motor units in chronic hemiplegic patients show marked fatigue within 1 sec after beginning stimulation at 30/sec. Similar tests could be carried out for patients with ulnar neuropathies and motor neurone disease to test whether fatigue is also prominent in these patients.

SYNCHRONIZATION

For our averaging techniques to measure the twitch tension of single motor units accurately, the impulses from different motor units must be generated independently. Any tendency for 2 or more motor units to discharge synchronously would increase the tension measured by averaging above the true twitch tension of the single unit and might alter the measured time course. Therefore, we tested for synchronization in several ways (Milner-Brown et al., 1973a) and found that there were marked differences between individuals. Most individuals showed no evidence of synchronization, and data from these subjects were suitable for studying the contractile properties of motor units. Other normal individuals showed a tendency for synchronization in nearly all their motor units. Using different methods, Buchthal and Madsen (1950) estimated that 15-20% of normal subjects showed synchronization, and our data are consistent with this estimate.

The method which we use routinely to test for synchronization utilizes recordings from needle and surface electrodes, as illustrated schematically in Fig. 5. Impulses from single motor units recorded by a needle electrode are again used to trigger a signal averager, and the surface recordings are averaged with and without rectification. If there is no synchronization (each motor unit fires independently), then by averaging the surface EMG without rectification, the contribution of a single unit to the surface recordings (Fig. 5B) can be measured, as discussed previously. There will be no net contribution from other units since AC recording is employed. However, if averaging is carried out after full-wave rectification (Fig. 5C), negative deflections will be reversed in sign, and there will be a net contribution from other units. This contribution will be about 0.8 times the root mean square voltage (σ) of the surface EMG (Milner-Brown et al., 1973a), and is shown by a horizontal line in Fig. 5C. In addition,

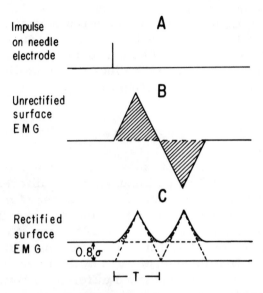

Fig. 5. Schematic representation of a test for synchronization of motor units using the surface EMG. If a signal averager is triggered by impulses from a single unit (A) recorded by a needle electrode, a waveform (B) is obtained by directly averaging the surface EMG. When impulses in different motor units are generated independently (no synchronization), this average will simply represent the voltage generated by the single unit which is recorded by the surface electrodes - the area is indicated by diagonal lines in (B). If averaging is done after rectification (C), there will be a net contribution to the average of (1) the waveform in (B) after rectification, (2) the ongoing activity of other units (0.8σ, see explanation of notation in text) and (3) a partial summation of these two (dotted area). However, if the discharge of several units tends to be grouped (synchronization) over a period greater than T, a broader and larger increase in the rectified surface EMG will be observed than can be accounted for by (1) to (3) above.

there will be a small degree of summation between the contribution of the single unit and that due to activity in other motor units (the degree of summation can be calculated and is indicated by the dotted area in Fig. 5C). If the discharge of several units tends to be grouped over a period of time (synchronization), there will be a

broader and larger increase in the rectified signal than can be
accounted for by this small degree of summation. The dotted area
in Fig. 5C is only 0.08 times as large as the shaded area in Fig.
5B. Values of the ratio between these two areas, which we call
"synchronization ratios", have been measured for a large number
of motor units in both normal subjects and patients with pressure
and entrapment neuropathies. Values above 0.2 have been assumed
to indicate a significant degree of synchronization. Typical results
from a patient who showed evidence of synchronization on his control side are shown in the upper part of Fig. 6. When averaging

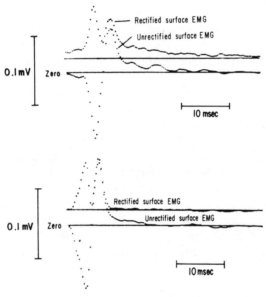

Fig. 6. Experimental trace of an averaged rectified surface
EMG superimposed on an unrectified surface EMG, for eval-
uating synchronization ratios in a patient with a unilateral ulnar
neuropathy: (above - normal hand; below - affected hand). The
horizontal lines indicate voltages of zero and the mean values
of the rectified surface EMG.

was done after rectification, an increased response was observed
for a period of several msec before and after the occurrence of
impulses in a single motor unit and the synchronization ratio (0.8)
was much larger than could be accounted for by the small degree
of summation expected. Interestingly, synchronization was much
less prominent or absent on the affected side (lower part of Fig. 6).
This pattern was observed consistently in the 5 patients tested who

showed evidence of synchronization in the motor units on the control side.

This finding of a reduced synchronization of motor units in ulnar neuropathies raises a more fundamental question. Why do some individuals show synchronization while others do not? We noted that most of the patients who showed synchronization were involved in manual jobs which required large, brief forces to be exerted. One normal subject who showed a high degree of synchronization regularly lifted weights. Perhaps the regular use of these muscles to exert large, brief forces leads, not only to hypertrophy of the muscles involved, but also to changes in the central nervous system. These changes result in motor units being activated nearly synchronously, even during the generation of steady forces where this synchronization is not required.

To test this hypothesis, 5 other weightlifters were examined. All showed clear evidence of synchronization. If 20% of the population show synchronization, as Buchthal and Madsen (1950) suggest, then the chance of finding synchronization in each of 6 individuals chosen at random would be less than 0.0001. Since all 6 subjects who lifted weights showed synchronization in most of their motor units, this provides strong evidence for the hypothesis. The mechanisms are unknown whereby near maximal, brief use of a muscle could lead to changes in the patterning of motor output (synchronization) even during maintenance of steady forces, and whereby disuse could abolish these changes.

CONCLUSION

These studies on the contractile and electrical properties of normal and modified motor units in man have led to three intriguing sets of hypotheses which can be tested further in human and animal experiments:

(1) Early outgrowth of axons from large motoneurones during development leads to the normal, orderly recruitment of motor units according to size. Simultaneous outgrowth of motor fibres after nerve section leads to a random recruitment of motor units following regeneration.

(2) Although in partially denervated muscles motor fibres can sprout new collaterals, the enlarged motor units that result are

more easily fatigued than those in normal muscles. Thus, they can only provide functional compensation for brief periods of time.

(3) Regular use of muscles to exert large, brief forces leads to a grouping or a synchronization of motor units which persists even when the muscle is exerting a maintained level of force. Discontinuation of this regular use leads to a reduction in synchronization.

Acknowledgement: Many of the experiments on normal motor units were done in collaboration with Dr. R. Yemm. The studies on patients with neuropathies and motor neuron disease were done in collaboration with Dr. R. Lee. This research was supported by grants from the Medical Research Council of Canada and the Muscular Dystrophy Association of Canada. Fig. 1 has been reproduced from Brain Research while Fig. 5 has been reproduced from the Journal of Physiology.

REFERENCES

Bayer, H., and Flechtenmayer, C., 1950. Ermüdung und Aktionspannung bei der isometrischen Muskelcontraktion des Menschen. Arbeitsphysiol. 14, 261-270.

Buchthal, F., and Madsen, A., 1950. Synchronous activity in normal and atrophic muscle. Electroencephalogr. Clin. Neurophysiol. 2, 425-444.

Buchthal, F., and Schmalbruch, H., 1970. Contraction times and fibre types in intact human muscles. Acta Physiol. Scand. 79, 435-452.

Burke, R.E., 1968. Group Ia synaptic input to fast and slow twitch motor units of cat triceps surae. J. Physiol. 196, 605-630.

Coërs, C., and Woolf, A.L., 1959. The Innervation of Muscle. Blackwell, Oxford.

Diamond, J., and Miledi, R., 1962. A study of foetal and new-born rat muscle fibres. J. Physiol. 162, 393-408.

Edwards, R.G.,and Lippold, O.C.J., 1956. The relationship between force and integrated electrical activity in fatigued muscle. J. Physiol. 132, 677-681.

Gutmann, E., Gutmann, L., Medawar, P.B., and Young, J.Z., 1942. The rate of regeneration of nerve. J. Exp. Biol. 19, 14-44.

Henneman, E., 1968. Peripheral mechanisms involved in the control of muscle. In Medical Physiology, 12 edn., C.V. Mosby Co., St Louis. pp. 1697-1716.

Inman, V.T., Ralston, H.J., Saunders, J.B. de C.M., Feinstein, B., and Wright, E.W. Jr., 1952. Relation of human electromyogram to muscular tension. Electroencephalogr. Clin. Neurophysiol. 4, 187-194.

Kernell, D., 1966. Input resistance, electrical excitability and size of ventral horn cells in cat spinal cord. Science 152, 1637-1640.

Lenman, J.A.R., 1969. Integration and analysis of the electro-
   myogram and related techniques. In Disorders of Voluntary
   Muscle. 2nd edn. Churchill, Lond. pp. 843–876.
Lippold, O.C.J., 1952. The relation between the integrated
   action potentials in a human muscle and its isometric tension.
   J. Physiol. 117, 492–499.
Lippold, O.C.J., Redfearn, J.W.T., and Vučo, J., 1960. The
   electromyography of fatigue. Ergonomics 3, 120–131.
Lubińska, L., 1964. Axoplasmic streaming in regenerating and in
   normal nerve fibers. Prog. Brain Res. 13, 1–66.
McComas, A.J., Sica, R.E.P., Campbell, M.J. and Upton, A.R.M.,
   1971. Functional compensation in partially denervated muscles.
   J. Neurol. Neurosurg. Psychiat. 34, 453–460.
McComas, A.J., Sica, R.E.P., Upton, A.R.M., and Aguilera, N.,
   1973. Functional changes in motoneurones of hemiparetic patients.
   J. Neurol. Neurosurg. Psychiat. 36, 183–193.
Milner-Brown, H.S., Stein, R.B., and Yemm, R., 1973a. The contractile properties of human motor units during voluntary, isometric
   contractions. J. Physiol. 228, 285–306.
Milner-Brown, H.S., Stein, R.B., and Yemm, R., 1973b. The orderly
   recruitment of human motor units during voluntary isometric
   contractions. J. Physiol. 230, 359–370.
Milner-Brown, H.S., Stein, R.B., and Yemm, R., 1973c. Changes in
   firing rate of human motor units during linearly changing
   voluntary contractions. J. Physiol. 230, 371–390.
Stein, R.B., French, A.S., Mannard, A., and Yemm, R., 1972. New
   methods for analysing motor function in man and animals. Brain
   Res. 40, 187–192.
Stephens, J.A., and Taylor, A., 1972. Fatigue of maintained vol-
   untary muscle contraction in man. J. Physiol. 220, 1–18.
Zelená, J., 1964. Development, degeneration and regeneration of
   receptor organs. In Mechanisms of Neural Regeneration. (Eds.
   Singer, M. and Schade, J.P.). Elsevier Publishing Co., Amsterdam.
   Prog. Brain Res. 13, 175–211.

CRUSTACEAN MOTOR UNITS

H. L. Atwood

Department of Zoology, University of Toronto
Toronto, Ontario

The principles of motor control seen in crustaceans differ
in several important respects from those found in mammals
and other higher vertebrates. In crustaceans, the number of
motor units in a muscle is small, and in muscles with more
than one motor unit, the innervation fields of the different
motor axons overlap. Thus, recruitment of different motor
units is less important as a mechanism of tension control
than in vertebrates. Crustacean muscle fibres and neuromuscular synapses show a wide range of performance, and it
is therefore possible for a motor axon to recruit different
parts of a motor unit by appropriate sequences of nerve impulses. In addition, it is common for crustacean muscle
fibres to produce continuously variable tension rather than
values between twitch and tetanus levels. Peripheral inhibitory
input can serve to eliminate certain parts of a motor unit from
contraction, to grade tension, or to alter the speed of contraction of a motor unit. Some features of crustacean motor
control are similar to those found in vertebrates. Examples
include the occurrence of phasic and tonic motor axons, the
"size principle" of motor axon recruitment, and recruitment
of slower parts of a muscle during low level activity. The
differences between the crustacean and vertebrate motor systems may reflect the large difference in the number of cells
available in their nervous systems. Higher vertebrates, by
virtue of the larger number of neurones they possess, do not
have to depend on some of the mechanisms for grading tension
found in crustacean muscles.

Even casual observations of the activities of crustaceans and other arthropods is sufficient to show that these animals can command a range of movement equal to, or even surpassing that found in mammals and other vertebrates. Among crustaceans, there are muscles specialized for speed which are equal in frequency of response to the fastest mammalian muscles (Mendelson, 1969). Other muscles are intrinsically far slower and on a cross-sectional area basis, stronger than mammalian muscles (Jahromi and Atwood, 1969). The delicate and complicated manoeuvres performed by some crustaceans and other arthropods further attest to their powers of motor control. Thus, it is worth-while to enquire into the mechanisms of motor control in these animals, and to establish which mechanisms they share with mammals and other vertebrates, and which are different.

Two outstanding differences between crustaceans and higher vertebrates have become apparent from work on their respective neuromuscular systems. First, crustaceans employ far fewer motor neurones to control their muscles than do the vertebrates; and of those they employ, some have a direct inhibiting effect on the muscle, rather than an excitatory effect. This economical use of motor neurones limits severely the number of motor units available for recruitment during muscular contraction. Second, by way of compensation, crustaceans and some other arthropods have developed a greater range of response and a wider diversity of components at the level of the muscle fibre and the neuro-muscular junction, than have the higher vertebrates. They are therefore able to produce a wide range of movement and force within a single motor unit, and to develop different types of motor unit for different purposes.

In what follows, I will elaborate on these points by reviewing the organization and properties of crustacean motor units, and by making comparisons with motor units of higher vertebrates. The crustaceans discussed here are mostly decapods, but from what little is known of other groups, it seems likely that most of the underlying principles of organization found in decapods will apply to the other groups as well.

PROPERTIES OF MUSCLE FIBRES

Crustacean muscle fibres are very diverse in their structure and in their electrical and contractile properties (Atwood et al.,

1965; Atwood, 1972, 1973). The primary structural differentiation appears to be the length of the sarcomere, which varies from about 2 μm to about 14 μm in different muscle fibres. In general, the short sarcomere fibres are often electrically excitable and fast contracting, while the long sarcomere fibres are often not completely electrically excitable and develop slow but powerful contractions (Jahromi and Atwood, 1969, 1971). Biochemical differences also exist between the different fibre types (Morin and McLaughlin, 1973). Examples of crustacean muscle fibre performance are given in Figs. 1 and 2.

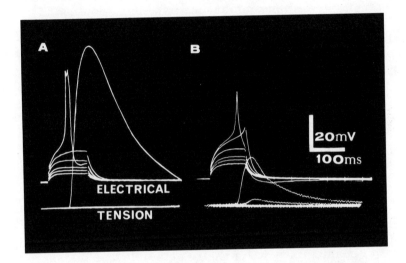

Fig. 1. Electrical and mechanical responses of single muscle fibres in a crustacean leg muscle (from Atwood et al., 1965). The fibres were stimulated directly with square pulses of current supplied through a microelectrode. The first fibre (A) developed an all-or-nothing spike and a twitch contraction at a critical level of membrane potential; the second fibre (B) showed graded electrical responses and graded contractions.

Depending upon its location and function, a particular muscle may be composed of a uniform population of muscle fibres, or a mixture of many types.

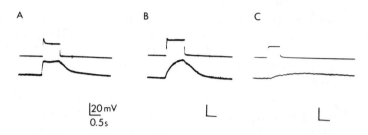

Fig. 2. Electrical and mechanical responses of three muscle fibres in crustacean leg muscles. None of these fibres generated an electrically excited membrane response. Tension in (A) developed more rapidly than in (B) and (C), for a similar type of stimulation. Resting sarcomere length of the first fibre (A) was shorter than for the second and third fibres (B and C). (From Jahromi and Atwood, 1971).

PROPERTIES OF AXONS AND SYNAPSES

Efferent axons supplying crustacean muscles fall primarily into two categories: excitatory and inhibitory. All muscles receive at least one excitatory axon, and most also receive inhibitory innervation.

Some of the excitatory axons can be classed as phasic or tonic, depending upon their firing patterns and their reaction to prolonged stimulation. The phasic axons are usually rather large, and often generate large postsynaptic potentials which fatigue rapidly with repeated stimulation. They normally fire brief bursts of impulses which produce rapid movements. The tonic axons are usually smaller, fire in more prolonged bursts or tonically, fatigue less rapidly, and generate smaller excitatory postsynaptic potentials on the average than do phasic axons.

The "size principle" of motor axon recruitment, well known in vertebrate motor systems (Henneman, 1968; Henneman et al., 1965) seems to occur also in crustaceans. Thus the tonic motor axons are more continuously active than phasic motor axons, which normally require strong stimuli to the animal before they become active. Within a group of motor axons supplying a crustacean muscle, the largest are generally the ones tending to fire in bursts, while the smaller ones are more tonically active. These features are apparent in the five motor axons (and one inhibitor) supplying the slow flexor muscles of the crayfish abdomen (Kennedy and Takeda, 1965b).

Some tonic axons provide a wide range of neuromuscular synapses to different muscle fibres. Some of these synapses release a substantial amount of transmitter for each impulse while others release very little unless facilitated by high frequencies of stimulation (Atwood, 1967; Bittner, 1968; Atwood and Bittner, 1971). Differences in transmitter output are also seen, though less strikingly, in phasic axons (e.g. Atwood and Hoyle, 1965).

The different types of synapse appear to be morphologically as well as physiologically distinct. Thus, many synapses of phasic axons have few synaptic vesicles, a feature which may correlate with rapid fatigue (Atwood and Johnston, 1968). Among tonic axons, synapses releasing little transmitter at low frequencies of stimulation appear to be smaller than those releasing a lot (Sherman and Atwood, 1972).

ORGANIZATION OF MOTOR UNITS

Many muscles consist of only a single motor unit. In the stomach of crabs and lobsters and in the walking legs also, there are motor units consisting of two or more discrete muscles (Fig. 3). The two muscles supplied by the opener-stretcher motor axon in the walking legs can be operated independently by virtue of separate inhibitory innervation; but in the stomach, there is no inhibitory supply, and the different muscles of a motor unit always contract together if stimulation is intense enough.

The stomach motor unit of Fig. 3 and the fibres of the leg muscle diagrammed in Fig. 4 both illustrate two principles which seem to occur commonly in the organization of crustacean motor units. First, different parts of the motor unit can be recruited by different frequencies of impulses in the motor axon, by virtue of the physiological properties of the synapses. Those releasing a lot of transmitter at low frequencies of stimulation cause their muscle fibres to contract at relatively low frequencies, whereas those which liberate substantial transmitter only after facilitation by a high frequency train of impulses produce contraction in their muscle fibres only when impulse frequency is high. (Often, such fibres contract only when electrically excited membrane responses are generated, as in the example of Fig. 4.)

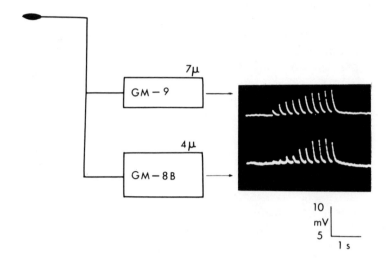

Fig. 3. A "motor unit" in the stomach of the blue crab
Callinectes. Muscles GM-9 and GM-8B are supplied by one
axon. The synaptic potentials of GM-9 show less facilitation
than do those of GM-8B. Correlated with this, the fibres of
GM-9 have a longer sarcomere length and slower contraction
than do those of GM-8B. These results were obtained in
collaboration with Dr. C. K. Govind.

A second principle is the matching of synapses with muscle
fibres, such that the long sarcomere, slow contracting parts of
the motor unit are recruited first (Atwood, 1965; Sherman and
Atwood, 1972). There is an interesting parallel here with
mammalian muscles in some of which the slower contracting
motor units are recruited earliest during a voluntary contraction
(Milner-Brown et al., 1973).

Muscles receiving more than one motor axon, such as the
closer and bender muscles of the leg, usually show overlap of the
motor units governed by each axon (Fig. 5). The same organizational feature is found in muscles of the crayfish abdomen and
uropod (Kennedy and Takeda, 1965a, b; Parnas and Atwood, 1966;
Larimer and Kennedy, 1969), and in lobster swimmeret muscles
(Davis, 1968). Sometimes, as in crayfish abdominal muscles,
the axons supplying a muscle are all phasic or all tonic, and the
contractions evoked by the different axons are all similar. In
abdominal muscles, the phasic axons supply short sarcomere,

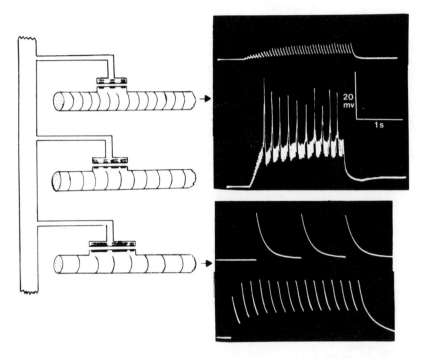

Fig. 4. Matching of synapse and muscle fibre in a singly
motor innervated crab leg muscle, the stretcher of Grapsus
(from Atwood and Bittner, 1971). The more rapidly contracting muscle fibres (with shorter sarcomeres) show small
postsynaptic potentials with a high degree of facilitation. In
the top two electrical records, responses of such a fibre to
stimulation of the motor axon at 20 Hz and at 60 Hz are shown;
small facilitating postsynaptic potentials are seen, which generate large secondary graded responses, and contractions in
the muscle fibre, at the higher frequency. The more slowly
contracting fibres (with the longer sarcomeres) show large,
poorly facilitating postsynaptic potentials, usually without
secondary graded responses. The lower two electrical records
show responses to stimulation of the motor axon at 1 Hz and at
5 Hz; contraction of the muscle fibre occurred at the latter
frequency. Thus, many of the slower fibres are recruited for
contraction at low frequencies of impulse discharge in the
motor axon, whereas the more rapidly contracting fibres are
recruited only at higher frequencies.

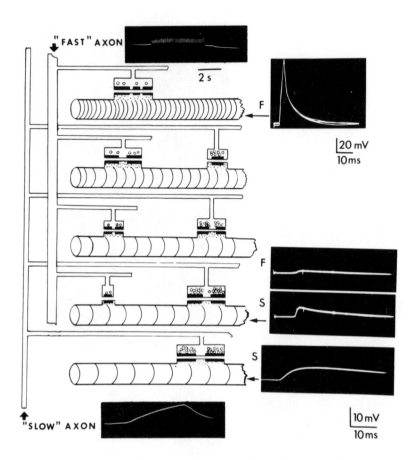

Fig. 5. Arrangement of synapses and muscle fibres in a crab
leg muscle (closer of Carcinus; Atwood, 1963) supplied by two
motor axons, a phasic or "fast" axon and a tonic or "slow"
axon. The tension responses evoked by the two axons differ
greatly at low frequencies of stimulation, as shown in the
topmost and lowest recordings. This is brought about by recruitment of the more rapidly contracting fibres by the phasic
axon, and of slowly contracting fibres by the tonic axon. The
innervation fields of the two axons overlap, so that many
fibres share both, as shown in the electrical records.

rapidly contracting muscle fibres, and the tonic axons supply long
sarcomere slower fibres. The fibres are grouped into separate
phasic and tonic muscles (Kennedy and Takeda, 1965a; Parnas and

Atwood, 1966). In the doubly innervated muscles of walking legs, there is sometimes a mixture of fibres, and the more phasic axon ("fast axon" of Wiersma's terminology; see Wiersma, 1961) innervates most heavily the short sarcomere fibres of the muscle, while the more tonic axon ("slow axon") innervates most heavily the longer sarcomere, slower fibres (Atwood, 1963; 1965). Thus, in spite of the extensive overlap of innervation, the two axons produce different types of contraction at low frequencies of impulse activity (Fig. 5). As the frequency of impulses along either axon increases, the evoked contractions of the muscle become more similar to each other as more of the "intermediate" doubly innervated fibres are recruited.

In the swimmeret muscles of the lobster (Davis, 1968, 1969), a number of synergistic motor units, acting in parallel, can be recruited during activity. Both the number of motor units, and their firing rates, can be varied to provide different levels of tension. In this case, the organization is more like the vertebrate situation than in most other appendages.

From the above examples, it can be seen that the performance of a "motor unit" is crucially dependent upon the frequency of impulses arriving along a motor axon. The impulse pattern serves both to recruit different parts of the motor unit and to govern tension in parts already recruited. Furthermore, within a motor unit there may be fibres with a twitch-tetanus type of contractile response, and others in which there is no twitch, but a continuously graded tension output which is a function of the average membrane depolarization set up by the postsynaptic potentials.

PATTERN SENSITIVITY

Sensitivity of crustacean muscles to particular patterns of nerve impulses has been demonstrated in several instances. One of the axons to the crayfish slow abdominal flexor muscles normally fires in a short burst pattern, and the muscle develops tension more effectively with this pattern of input than with a more regular pattern. The neuromuscular synapse may be the source of the pattern sensitivity (Gillary and Kennedy, 1969).

A "catch" mechanism (a maintained increase in tension) is apparent in many crustacean muscles when an extra impulse is

interjected into a steady train. The catch mechanism seems to
reside in the muscle rather than in the neuromuscular synapse
(Wilson and Larimer, 1968). The reasons for the versatility of
crustacean motor units are partly evident from these factors
alone, without even considering the action of the inhibitory system.

PLASTICITY

A further factor contributing to the overall performance of
crustacean motor units is the effect of previous bouts of stimulation. Most crustacean excitatory synapses show some degree
of short term facilitation and post-tetanic potentiation. In some
phasic units, long lasting depression is seen after even a single
impulse (Bruner and Kennedy, 1970) or a few closely spaced
ones (Hoyle and Wiersma, 1958). Prolonged activity of a phasic
motor axon soon leads to a drastic reduction of its post-synaptic
potentials (Fig. 6); however, the fatigue is less rapid when the
stimuli are delivered in bursts, as occur naturally, instead of
equally spaced (unpublished observation). This phenomenon
represents a further example of pattern sensitivity.

The low output synapses of tonic axons show long-term facilitation rather than fatigue when stimulated for a prolonged period
of time (Fig. 6). After prolonged stimulation, transmitter output
for succeeding bursts of impulses is considerably greater than
before the stimulation. This condition can persist for over an
hour at some synapses. The elevated transmitter output appears
to be linked to sodium accumulation by the nerve terminals
(Sherman and Atwood, 1971). It is interesting to note that high
output terminals of the same axon often show long term facilitation first, then fatigue as stimulation continues (Fig. 6).
Evidently, the supply of transmitter is not enough to meet the
demands of prolonged secretion at such terminals.

It is not yet known whether the crustaceans make use of long
term facilitation in operating their motor units. Casual observations indicate that muscles taken for study from animals which
were active just before a limb was removed, show larger excitatory postsynaptic potentials than muscles taken from quiescent
animals. Thus, long term facilitation may play a part in the
animal's normal activity.

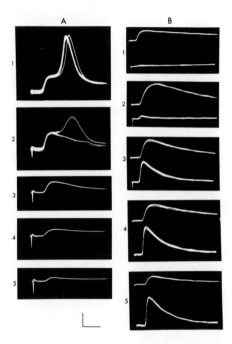

Fig. 6. Plasticity of phasic (A) and tonic (B) postsynaptic potentials during maintained stimulation. The phasic axon (to the extensor muscle of the leg of Pachygrapsus) was stimulated at 1 Hz and the tonic axon at 10 Hz. Initially, the phasic axon generated a large postsynaptic potential with a large secondary response, but with continued stimulation, the response became greatly reduced. The tonic axon (to the stretcher muscle of Pachygrapsus) generated both large, poorly facilitating (top records in each picture) and small, highly facilitating (bottom records) postsynaptic potentials. With continued stimulation, the former first increased substantially, then declined, while the latter showed a large continued increase. In (A) pictures were taken at 1 min (1), 5 min (2), 10 min (3), 15 min (4) and 20 min (5) after the start of stimulation, while in (B), the pictures were taken at 1 min (1), 10 min (2), 20 min (3), 30 min (4), and 40 min (5). Calibrations: voltage = 20 mV (A), 10 mV (B); time, 10 msec.

INHIBITION

The inhibitory axons, if present, make neuromuscular synapses with the fibres of the muscle they supply. Inhibitory input is not always equal to all fibres of a muscle. In leg muscles, the more rapidly-contracting fibres tend to respond less well than the slower fibres to stimulation of inhibitory axons (Atwood et al., 1967). In singly-motor-innervated opener and stretcher muscles of crab and crayfish legs, the properties of the "specific" inhibitory nerve terminals seem to be "matched" to those of the excitatory nerve terminals; muscle fibres with small, facilitating excitatory postsynaptic potentials also show small, facilitating inhibitory postsynaptic potentials, while muscle fibres with large excitatory postsynaptic potentials also show large inhibitory postsynaptic potentials (Atwood and Bittner, 1971). These features of organization provide for more effective inhibitory regulation of slow contractions than of fast ones, in muscles consisting of a single motor unit.

A corollary of the organization described above is that the speed of contraction of a motor unit supplied by a single tonic axon should increase with inhibition, since the slower contracting muscle fibres would be suppressed. A high frequency of inhibition would be required to suppress the more rapidly contracting fibres recruited by high-frequency bursts of impulses in the excitatory axon. Direct evidence for an increase in speed of response during inhibition has been provided by studies of Bush (1962), who found that changes in tension of a crab opener muscle could occur more rapidly during inhibition.

In leg muscles supplied by phasic as well as tonic axons, the contractions elicited by the phasic axons are often incompletely inhibited (Wiersma, 1961; Atwood et al., 1967). The inhibitory axons have little electrical effect on fibres heavily innervated by the phasic axons, and probably do not supply them with much innervation. In phasic muscles of the crayfish abdomen, the inhibitory axons can regulate the size of a "twitch" by decreasing the electrical responses set up by the phasic axons (Atwood et al., 1967); however, the contractions cannot be completely suppressed. These observations further support the idea that inhibition is more effective in regulating tonic contractions, where small adjustments in muscle tension are required.

In some muscles, but not in all (Kennedy and Evoy, 1966), the inhibitory axons make axo-axonal synapses with the terminals of the excitatory axon, thereby allowing for presynaptic inhibition (Dudel and Kuffler, 1961; Atwood and Jones, 1967). The inhibitory impulses must be timed to arrive just before the excitatory impulses in order to depress the output of excitatory transmitter substance and thereby reduce muscle tension. It has recently been shown that phase-coupling of inhibitory to excitatory impulses does, in fact, occur in at least one crab, Uca (Spirito, 1970). Here, the specific inhibitor to the stretcher muscle is stronger presynaptically than the specific inhibitor to the opener muscle. Inhibitory impulses to the stretcher muscle normally precede the excitatory impulses, thereby activating axo-axonal inhibitory synapses and reducing electrical excitation and tension in the muscle fibres. By contrast, inhibitory impulses to the opener muscle normally follow excitatory impulses, thereby producing effective postsynaptic inhibition via inhibitory neuromuscular synapses.

In the crayfish claw opener muscle and the claw opener muscle of Carcinus, which also shows presynaptic inhibition, there does not appear to be any phase-locking of excitatory and inhibitory impulses. Rather, the contractions of the muscle are regulated by the overall level of inhibitory bombardment, which is, in turn, subject to control from stretch receptors (Bush, 1962; Wilson and Davis, 1965).

In muscles with two inhibitory axons, such as the stretcher and opener muscles of crab legs, one of the axons may be specialized for postsynaptic inhibition and the other for presynaptic inhibition. The pattern of specialization may vary from one species to another, as shown in Fig. 7. The consequences of these differences in organization for muscle performance have not yet been worked out. However, it may turn out that the "common inhibitor" which rarely fires when the animal is constrained in an experimental set up (Bush, 1962), normally serves to increase the speed of response in the leg by eliminating the slower contracting fibres from participation during vigorous activity. The "common inhibitor" has more effect on the slower contracting fibres of both stretcher and closer muscles, and little or no effect on the faster fibres, in the crabs Grapsus, Pachygrapsus and Gecarcinus (Atwood et al., 1967; Atwood and Bittner, 1971; and unpublished).

Among the various other roles which inhibitory axons can play, uncoupling of excitatory facilitation and muscle tension is probably functionally important. In Fig. 8 A, an example is given of the effects of stimulating the inhibitory axon during a train of impulses in an excitatory axon. The excitatory postsynaptic potentials decrease progressively in size as the inhibitory system facilitates.

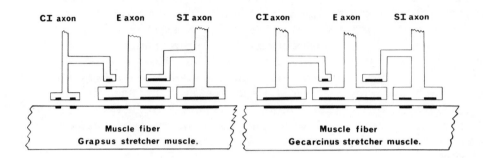

<u>Fig. 7.</u> Specialization of two inhibitory axons of crab leg (stretcher) muscles. Representative slowly contracting muscle fibres of two crabs are shown, with synaptic connections elucidated by electrical recording. In Grapsus, the common inhibitory (CI axon) has a weak postsynaptic effect and very little presynaptic effect, while the specific inhibitor (SI axon) has a powerful effect both pre- and postsynaptically. In Gecarcinus, the common inhibitor has a stronger postsynaptic effect than the specific inhibitor, but a weaker presynaptic effect. In this case, the two axons are specialized for the two types of inhibition.

However, excitatory facilitation proceeds in spite of the inhibition, for when inhibition is released, the excitatory potentials immediately become larger than before the inhibition. This effect is analogous to the action of the clutch in an automobile, and permits more rapid generation of tension at a given instant in time. Examples of this effect in muscle potentials of a freely moving animal are presented in Fig. 8B (see also Atwood and Walcott, 1965).

The above discussion serves to show that inhibitory axons can alter the performance of crustacean motor units by regulating tension, by affecting the recruitment of different parts of a motor unit, and by altering overall speed of contraction in various ways. The functional properties of crustacean motor units are thereby greatly extended. It is significant that inhibitory mechanisms are most prominent in muscles used for a wide range of varied movements, such as those in the walking legs. Inhibition is not present

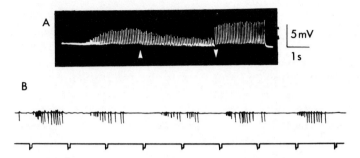

Fig. 8. Possible role of inhibition in uncoupling muscle tension from facilitation. In (A), a train of motor impulses was delivered to the stretcher muscle of Grapsus: Inhibition was delivered between the points marked by the two arrowheads. The excitatory postsynaptic potentials declined during inhibition (indicating inhibitory facilitation), but rebounded to greater than pre-inhibition amplitude as soon as inhibition was terminated, indicating continued excitatory facilitation during the period of inhibition. Muscle potentials recorded from the stretcher muscle of a freely walking crab, Cancer (B) appear to show the same phenomenon: the potentials are small at the beginning of a burst, then suddenly increase in size, probably corresponding with the release of intense inhibition. Time marker, 1 sec.

in some muscles used for routine repetitive movements, such as those of the stomach or scaphognathites.

COMPARISON OF CRUSTACEAN AND
MAMMALIAN MUSCLES

The muscles of crustaceans share some features with mammalian (and other higher vertebrate) muscles, but differ from them in important respects. These points have been made in the above discussion and are summarized below.

The most important shared features include: (1) Development of phasic and tonic motor neurones and the "size principle" of motor neurone recruitment. (2) Development of a range of different muscle fibres. (3) Recruitment of the slower part of a muscle during low-level activity. (4) Use of impulse frequency as a tension-regulating mechanism.

The more important differences between the crustacean motor
systems and those of higher vertebrates seem to be: (1) The relative unimportance of recruitment of different motor units in
crustaceans and consequently, the relatively greater importance
of the motor nerve impulse pattern. (2) The ability of many
crustacean muscle fibres to give continuously graded tension output without a lower limit imposed by the twitch. (3) The greater
variability and wider range of response of most crustacean neuromuscular synapses. (4) The additional flexibility imparted to
crustacean muscles by peripheral inhibitory regulation. (5) The
commonly found overlap of innervation fields in arthropods, and
the general lack of this feature in higher vertebrates.

Obviously, the vertebrate and arthropod schemes represent
two divergent but successful approaches to the problem of motor
control. The arthropod solution, with its emphasis on flexibility
at the muscle fibre and neuromuscular synapse levels, seems to
have been partly dictated by the limited number of cells available
in the nervous system. Each motor and inhibitory neurone carries
a relatively large share of responsibility for a particular muscle.
The higher vertebrates, with their more numerous neurones, can
afford to sacrifice some of the versatility available in the muscle
cell and the neuromuscular synapse. It is noteworthy that some of
the crustacean features (eg. multiply-innervated tonic muscle
fibres) appear in the muscles of lower vertebrates, but these
features become less and less evident as the evolutionary tree of
the vertebrates is ascended, and as the number of neurones
available increases.

REFERENCES

Atwood, H.L., 1963. Differences in muscle fibre properties as a
    factor in "fast" and "slow" contraction in Carcinus. Comp.
    Biochem. Physiol. 10, 17-31.
Atwood, H.L., 1965. Excitation and inhibition in crab muscle
    fibres. Comp. Biochem. Physiol. 16, 409-426.
Atwood, H.L., 1967. Variation in physiological properties of
    crustacean motor synapses. Nature 215, 57-58.
Atwood, H.L., 1972. Crustacean muscle. In The Structure and
    Function of Muscle. Volume 1, Part 1. (Ed. G.H. Bourne)
    Academic Press, N.Y., pp. 421-489.
Atwood, H.L., 1973. An attempt to account for the diversity of
    crustacean muscle. Amer. Zool. 13, 357-378.

Atwood, H.L., and Bittner, G.D., 1971. Matching of excitatory and inhibitory inputs to crustacean muscle fibers. J. Neurophysiol. 34, 157-170.

Atwood, H.L., and Hoyle, G., 1965. A further study of the paradox phenomenon of crustacean muscle. J. Physiol. 181, 225-234.

Atwood, H.L., Hoyle, G., and Smyth, T., 1965. Mechanical and electrical responses of singly innervated crab-muscle fibres. J. Physiol. 180: 449-482.

Atwood, H.L., and Johnston, H.S., 1968. Neuromuscular synapses of a crab motor axon. J. Exp. Zool. 167, 457-470.

Atwood, H.L., and Jones, A., 1967. Presynaptic inhibition in crustacean muscle: axo-axonal synapse. Experientia 23, 1036-1038.

Atwood, H.L., Parnas, I., and Wiersma, C.A.G., 1967. Inhibition in crustacean phasic neuromuscular systems. Comp. Biochem. Physiol. 20, 163-177.

Atwood, H.L., and Walcott, B., 1965. Recording of electrical activity and movement from legs of walking crabs. Can. J. Zool. 43, 657-665.

Bittner, G.D., 1968. Differentiation of nerve terminals in the crayfish opener muscle and its functional significance. J. Gen. Physiol. 51, 731-758.

Bruner, J., and Kennedy, D., 1970. Habituation: Occurrence at a neuromuscular junction. Science 169, 92-94.

Bush, B.M.H., 1962. Peripheral reflex inhibition in the claw of the crab, Carcinus maenas, J. Exp. Biol. 39, 71-88.

Davis, W.J., 1968. The neuromuscular basis of lobster swimmeret beating. J. Exp. Zool. 168, 363-378.

Davis, W.J., 1969. The neural control of swimmeret beating in the lobster. J. Exp. Biol. 50, 99-117.

Dudel, J., and Kuffler, S.W., 1961. Presynaptic inhibition at the crayfish neuromuscular junction. J. Physiol. 155, 543-562.

Gillary, H.L., and Kennedy, D., 1969. Neuromuscular effects of impulse pattern in a crustacean motoneuron. J. Neurophysiol. 32, 607-612.

Henneman, E., 1968. Peripheral mechanisms involved in the control of muscle. In Medical Physiology, 12th edition (Ed. Mountcastle, V.B.) C.V. Mosby Co., St. Louis, pp. 1697-1716.

Henneman, E., Somjen, G., and Carpenter, D.O., 1965. Functional significance of cell size in spinal motoneurons. J. Neurophysiol. 28, 560-580.

Hoyle, G., and Wiersma, C.A.G., 1958. Excitation at neuromuscular junctions in Crustacea. J. Physiol. 143, 403-425.

Jahromi, S.S., and Atwood, H.L., 1969. Correlation of structure, speed of contraction, and total tension in fast and slow abdominal muscle fibers of the lobster (Homarus americanus) J. Exp. Zool. 171, 25-38.

Jahromi, S.S., and Atwood, H.L., 1971. Structural and contractile properties of lobster leg-muscle fibers. J. Exp. Zool. 176, 475-486.

Kennedy, D., and Evoy, W.H., 1966. The distribution of pre- and post-synaptic inhibition at crustacean neuromuscular junctions. J. Gen. Physiol. 49, 457–468.

Kennedy, D., and Takeda, K., 1965a. Reflex control of abdominal flexor muscles in the crayfish. I. The twitch system. J. Exp. Biol. 43, 211–227.

Kennedy, D., and Takeda, K., 1965b. Reflex control of abdominal flexor muscles in the crayfish. II. The tonic system. J. Exp. Biol. 43, 229–246.

Larimer, J.L., and Kennedy, D., 1969. Innervation patterns of fast and slow muscle in the uropods of crayfish. J. Exp. Biol. 51, 119–133.

Mendelson, M., 1969. Electrical and mechanical characteristics of a very fast lobster muscle. J. Cell Biol. 42, 548–563.

Milner-Brown, H.S., Stein, R.B., and Yemm, R., 1973. The orderly recruitment of human motor units during voluntary isometric contractions. J. Physiol. 230, 359–370.

Morin, W.A., and McLaughlin, E., 1973. Glycogen in crustacean fast and slow muscle. Amer. Zool. 13, 435–445.

Parnas, I., and Atwood, H.L., 1966. Phasic and tonic neuromuscular systems in the abdominal extensor muscles of the crayfish and rock lobster. Comp. Biochem. Physiol. 18, 701–723.

Sherman, R.G., and Atwood, H.L., 1971. Synaptic facilitation: Long-term neuromuscular facilitation in crustacean muscles. Science 171, 1284–1250.

Sherman, R.G., and Atwood, H.L., 1972. Correlated electrophysiological and ultrastructural studies of a crustacean motor unit. J. Gen. Physiol. 59, 586–615.

Spirito, C.P., 1970. Relfex control of the opener and stretcher muscles in the cheliped of the fiddler crab, Uca pugnax. Z. Vergl. Physiol. 68, 211–228.

Wiersma, C.A.G., 1961. The neuromuscular system. In The Physiology of Crustacea, Volume 2. (Ed. Waterman, T.H.). Academic Press, N.Y., pp. 191–240.

Wilson, D.M., and Davis, W.J., 1965. Nerve impulse patterns and reflex control in the motor system of the crayfish claw. J. Exp. Biol. 43, 193–210.

Wilson, D.M., and Larimer, J.L., 1968. The catch property of ordinary muscle. Proc. Nat. Acad. Sci. U.S.A. 61, 909–910.

SKELETOMOTOR AND FUSIMOTOR ORGANIZATION IN AMPHIBIANS

R. S. Smith, G. Blinston and W. K. Ovalle*

The Neurophysiology Laboratory, Department of
Surgery, University of Alberta, Edmonton, Canada

This paper discusses recent findings pertinent to the skeletomotor and fusimotor organization in the tailless amphibia.
Recent work in this laboratory has led to the morphological
identification of five types of extrafusal muscle fibres in the
hindlimb muscles of frogs and toads. Three of the types (Types
1, 2 and 3) stain darkly for myosin-ATPase but may be distinguished by their diameters and the pattern of staining for
SDHase. Two of the types (Types 4 and 5) stain lightly for
myosin-ATPase and may be distinguished by their reaction for
SDHase. The five types of fibres show ultrastructural differences in myofibril cross-sectional areas, mitochondrial size
and content, glycogen and lipid droplet content, the structure
of the Z and M band and in the complexity of the sarcotubular
system. We postulate that Types 1, 2 and 3 are variants of the
fast or twitch fibre while Types 4 and 5 are slow fibres. The
contractile properties of single motor units in the iliofibularis
muscle of Xenopus laevis allow the fast motor units to be separated into three types while slow motor units are divisible
into two types. The fast motor units are supplied by large diameter motor axons (> 10μm diameter) while the slow motor
units are supplied by small diameter axons (< 10μm diameter).
Two structural and functional types of intrafusal muscle fibres
have previously been described in the amphibia. The two types
are separately innervated by large and small motor axons.

---

* Present Address: Department of Anatomy, University of
British Columbia, Vancouver, British Columbia.

Schemes for the motor organization of amphibian skeletal
muscle will be proposed based on the available information.

The primary object of this paper is to discuss the organization
of skeletal muscle in the amphibia. This means that we wish to
consider what different kinds of muscle fibres and motor units are
present, what kinds of intrafusal muscle fibres exist, and how the
motor innervation of the motor units is related to that of the intrafusal muscle fibres. The discussion will be restricted to the Anura
since only a very small amount of work has been done on urodele
musculature. However, the Anura are of great intrinsic interest
since these are the most primitive vertebrates to contain muscle
spindles. Thus, one would like to think that an understanding of
the organization of the skeletal muscle of frogs and toads will
contribute towards the understanding of the role the muscle spindle
has to play in the control of movement, not only of amphibians,
but also the more highly evolved vertebrates.

EXTRAFUSAL MUSCLE FIBRES

The division of amphibian skeletal muscle fibres and motor
units into two categories is well accepted (see reviews by Peachey,
1961 and Hess, 1970). Fast muscle fibres are supplied by large
diameter motor axons and, when stimulated, propagate an action
potential and develop a transient increase in tension (a 'twitch').
Slow muscle fibres are multiply innervated by motor axons of
small diameter; these muscle fibres do not normally propagate an
action potential and contract in a graded fashion in response to
trains of stimuli.

Much recent evidence indicates that the organization of Anuran
muscle cannot be fully explained in terms of two fibre types alone.
There is ample evidence for a variety of both fast and slow muscle
fibres. Fast muscle fibres of various types have been described
on both physiological and histochemical grounds (Orkand, 1963;
Nasledov, 1966; Lännergren and Smith, 1966; Engel and Irwin,
1967; Asmussen and Kiessling, 1970). The fast fibres appear to
be organized into at least two kinds of fast motor units (Smith and
Lännergren, 1968). There is some evidence that slow muscle
fibres may not all have the same kinds of electrical properties
(Shamarina, 1962, 1963) and slow motor units in Xenopus laevis
have been divided into two groups on the basis of their contractile
properties (Smith and Lännergren, 1968).

In an attempt to clarify this situation, Smith and Ovalle (1973) have examined the histochemical and ultrastructural varieties of fast and slow muscle fibres in various hindlimb muscles of Xenopus laevis. Muscles from Rana pipiens and Bufo woodhousei were also examined histochemically to confirm that there were no noticeable differences between the various types of Anura. The results are summarized in Table 1. In the muscles iliofibularis and flexor tarsi, five different kinds of muscle fibres could be distinguished. Three types (Types 1, 2 and 3) stained darkly in the histochemical reaction for myosin ATPase. Two types (Types 4 and 5) showed little or no reaction for myosin ATPase. In serial sections each of the five fibre types could be distinguished on the basis of their density of staining for, and the distribution of, succinic dehydrogenase (SDHase). Correlated electron microscopy showed that the five fibre types could also be distinguished by their ultrastructure. Features of significance were: the mean myofibril cross-sectional area, mitochondrial size and content, glycogen and lipid content, the structure of the Z and M bands, and the complexity of the sarcotubular system. In conjunction with the results already reported in the literature, we considered these observations sufficient to justify the proposition that the skeletal muscle of the Anura can be described in terms of five types of muscle fibres, Types 1, 2 and 3 being varieties of fast fibres, while Types 4 and 5 are varieties of slow fibres.

It should be mentioned, however, that not all hindlimb muscles contained all five kinds of muscle fibres. This could be anticipated from the results of earlier histochemical studies (Lännergren and Smith, 1966; Engel and Irwin, 1967; Asmussen and Kiessling, 1970). In our work, there were two major types of muscles. The first type which included the muscles iliofibularis, semitendinosus, tibialis anterior, gastrocnemius, rectus internus, the adductors brevis, longus and magnus, the flexor tarsi, contained all five types of muscle fibres. These muscles showed a characteristic zoned pattern (Fig. 1) in which fibres of Type 1 were concentrated in a peripheral area distant from the entry of the nerve into the muscle. Deeper in these muscles the number of Type 2 fibres increased, while close to the entry of the nerve trunk, fibres of Types 3, 4 and 5 were mixed together. The second major category of muscles contained fibres of Types 1 and 2 only and showed no zoning. Muscles of this type were: sartorius, rectus externus, semimembranosus, triceps, rectus internus major and minor, rectus femoris anticus, extensor cruris brevis and peroneus. Small muscles such as the extensor digiti IV longus and piriformis

MUSCLE FIBRE TYPES	1	2	3	4	5
Myosin ATPase Staining	Dark	Dark	Dark	Pale	Clear
SDHase Staining	Pale	Dark	Very Dark	Pale	Clear
Muscle Fibre Diameter (μm)	169.0 ± 17.8	145.0 ± 17.6	76.7 ± 12.1	60.7 ± 5.4	44.0 ± 7.7
Myofibril Cross-Section (μm^2)	3.3 ± 1.0	1.1 ± 0.3	0.7 ± 0.2	2.8 ± 1.2	5.4 ± 2.5
Mitochondrial Volume (%)	2.5	11.1	17.4	4.1	1.3
Glycogen and Lipid Droplet Content	Low	High	Very High	Low	Very Low
Z Band	Thin; Square Lattice; Straight	Moderately Thick; Straight Lattice; Straight	Moderately Thick; Square Lattice; Straight	Thick; Square Lattice; Jagged	Thick; Irregular Lattice; Jagged
M Band	Straight	Straight	Straight	Irregular When Present	Absent

Table 1. A summary of the histochemical and structural characteristics of five types of muscle fibres in the hindlimb muscles of Xenopus laevis. Numerical values are for the iliofibularis and flexor tarsi muscles. Where appropriate values are given as mean $\pm$ S. D. Fiber diameters estimated from random selections of equal number, n = 20. Myofibril cross-sectional areas, n = 50, for each sample (from Smith and Ovalle, 1973).

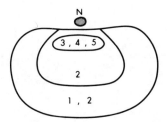

Fig. 1. Typical arrangement of the five muscle fibre types in
a zoned muscle. Types 1 and 2 are found at the outer surface
with Type 1 predominating. Type 2 fibres are clustered at the
centre of the muscle. Types 3, 4 and 5 are mixed together
within the Type 2 zone and are close to the entry of the nerve
trunk, N. Spindles are found among and close to the aggregation of fibres of Types 3, 4 and 5.

contained fibres of Types 2, 3, 4 and 5.

MOTOR UNITS

If the hypothesis is valid that the organization of hindlimb muscles in the Anura may be described in terms of five types of muscle fibres, then five corresponding types of motor units should be
present. If this were not true, then the types of fibres we
have described would be merely structural variants having little
direct significance for the arrangement of muscular systems controlling movement.

Earlier results of the examination of the isometric contraction
of motor units in the iliofibularis muscle of Xenopus laevis in response to the stimulation of single motor axons (Smith and Lännergren,
1968) indicated that four kinds of motor units could be distinguished;
two varieties of fast motor units and two varieties of slow units
(Fig. 2, parts 1, 2, 4 and 5).

Blinston and Smith are now repeating and extending this work.
The presence of the four kinds of motor units previously observed
has been confirmed, and in addition, we have detected a third type
of fast motor unit. The five types of motor units we number 1 to 5,
implying in doing so that each is composed of the similarly numbered
types of muscle fibres of Table 1. This position is at the moment

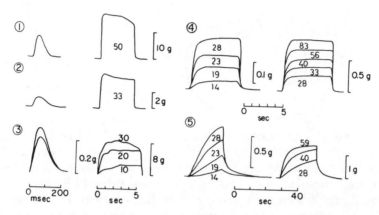

Fig. 2. Mechanical activity of single motor units in the iliofibularis muscle in response to stimulation of single motor
axons. The circled numbers 1-5 refer to the motor unit types
described in the text. Twitch responses to single stimuli for
the fast motor units (Types 1, 2 and 3) are illustrated in the
left-hand column. Two consecutive twitch responses of the
Type 3 motor unit are superimposed. The remaining records
illustrate the response to continuous stimulation. The number
on each trace illustrates the rate of stimulation in stimuli/sec.
Abscissae and ordinates are located respectively below and to
the right of the group of records to which they refer. The traces
for motor unit Types 1, 2, 4, and 5 are adapted from Smith
and Lännergren (1968).

hypothetical, both with respect to the types of muscle fibres included
in the various motor units and with respect to the homogeneity of the
units. A brief description of the properties of the five types of motor
units is given below and is illustrated by Fig. 2. At the present time
the total information is based on observations of 20 single motor
units in male animals and 25 units in female animals. Ranges for
the various values are given since we do not yet have sufficient
observations to justify statistical statements. However, each type
of unit may be recognized by its qualitative characteristics.

Type 1 motor units are located in the periphery of the iliofibularis muscle and are supplied by the largest motor axons (17-23
μm diameter). These are large fast motor units with maximum
tetanic tensions varying from 17-23 g in male animals and 30-55 g

in the larger female animals. Characteristic of these units is a
high twitch-tetanus ratio (0. 3-0. 6) and very rapid fatigue on
maintained stimulation.

Type 2 units are located in the central portion of the muscle,
are supplied by axons with diameters ranging from 9-19 μm (14-
19 μm in female animals), and are fast with maximum tensions
of 1-16 g in males and 15-40 g in females. Characteristic of
these units is a lower twitch-tetanus ratio (0. 1-0. 3) and a lesser
susceptability to fatigue than exhibited by the Type 1 units.

The units which we call Type 3 have unusual properties which
do not seem to have been reported before. This type of unit is
located in the core of the muscle and is supplied by motor axons
of diameters 13-16 μm. Typical isometric contractile responses
are shown in Fig. 2, part 3. Stimulation of a single motor axon
to this type of motor unit   produced a small twitch response whose
amplitude fluctuated with successive stimuli. A small biphasic
longitudinal current record could simultaneously be recorded at
the surface of the muscle. On tetanic stimulation the amplitude
of the longitudinal current record increased and large tetanic
tensions were developed. The twitch-tetanus ratio was thus very
small, varying from 0. 01-0. 07. We believe that this type of motor
unit is made up of muscle fibres with properties similar to those
described by Orkand in 1963. He reported that some muscle
fibres of the tonus bundle (the central portion) of the iliofibularis
muscle of the frog, Rana temporaria, did not respond with a
propagated action potential, and hence did not twitch, following
a single stimulus to the motor nerve.   Orkand obtained evidence
that the quantal contribution to the end-plate potential was smaller
for these fibres than for other fast fibres. It has not been suggested before that these fibres might be gathered together as
motor units; however, our observations would be completely consistent with this point of view.

The two types of slow units, 4 and 5, are supplied by axons of
diameters, respectively, of 6-10 μm and 4-7 μm. Both types of
units produce small tensions (maximum 0. 1-2 g) in a graded
fashion in response to repetitive stimulation (Fig. 2, parts 4 and 5).
The Type 4 units, however, develop tension much more rapidly
than do the Type 5 units. Type 4 units also show an unusual potentiation of tension on maintained stimulation at 20-30 stimuli/sec
(Smith and Lännergren, 1968).

It is of interest to note that the responses of units of Types 1, 2 and 3, if analyzed in a manner similar to that described by Mannard and Stein (1973), may all be quite well described in terms of a linear second-order system with corner frequencies decreasing through units 1-3 from 5.5 Hz to 2.0 Hz. The damping ratios do not appear to be very different and vary from 0.9-1.1. In contrast, units of Types 4 and 5 are very non-linear and cannot be adequately described in such terms.

The supposition that motor units of Types 1-5 are composed of muscle fibres of Types 1-5 is unproven at present. Some support for this idea may be drawn from the cited literature, but these arguments will not be developed here. The point we wish to make is that the available information on the properties of muscle fibres and on the properties of motor units lends crédance to the idea that the extrafusal organization of amphibian hindlimb muscles can be described in terms of five types of motor units.

INTRAFUSAL MUSCLE FIBRES

The spindles of the muscle extensor digiti IV longus contain two types of intrafusal fibres (Smith, 1964a, b; Page, 1966; see also review by Smith and Ovalle, 1972). One type tends to be of larger diameter, propagates an impulse, and contracts rapidly. The other is of small diameter, is also capable of propagating an impulse but contracts more slowly. The large and small intrafusal muscle fibres are separately innervated by large and small diameter motor nerves respectively (Gray, 1957; Smith, 1964a). Page (1966) has described structural differences between the intrafusal muscle fibres: one has a structure resembling that of the fast group of extrafusal fibres while the other ultrastructurally resembles the Type 4 extrafusal fibre described above. Other muscles which contain the slow varieties of extrafusal muscle fibres, e.g. the iliofibularis, probably also contain the two kinds of intrafusal muscle fibres (Brown, 1971). On the other hand, muscles which do not contain slow fibres (e.g. the sartorius) have spindles which lack one of these two types of intrafusal fibres (Brown, 1971), namely those which are supplied by small diameter motor axons. A point which probably has a bearing on the motor organization of zoned muscles of the amphibia is that spindles are found exclusively in the core of the muscles close to the aggregation of fibres of Types 3, 4 and 5.

THE ORGANIZATION OF THE MUSCLES

What may be called the classical scheme for the organization of amphibian skeletal muscle developed from the work of Katz (1949), Gray (1957) and Eyzaguirre (1957, 1958). This scheme is shown diagramatically in Fig. 3. A set of fast motor units is

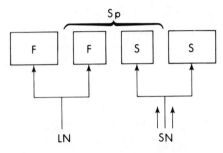

Fig. 3. Schematic diagram of the 'classical' concept of the organization of muscle in frogs and toads. Sp, spindle; F, fast motor units or intrafusal muscle fibres; S, slow motor units or intrafusal muscle fibres; LN, large diameter motor nerves; SN, small diameter motor nerves. Multiple arrows on the right, above SN, indicate polyneuronal innervation to the slow muscle fibre system.

innervated by large diameter motor axons and a set of slow motor units is innervated, probably polyneuronally, by small diameter motor axons. Some of the fast motor units share their innervation with one class of intrafusal muscle fibres (presumably fast fibres) while some of the slow motor units share their innervation with a second class of intrafusal muscle fibres (presumably slow fibres). Other motor units may be composed of extrafusal fibres only, but have similar properties to those which contain intrafusal fibres. Such units are not shown in Fig. 3 and subsequent figures.

The scheme of Fig. 1 has the merit of simplicity but does not agree with all the facts known today. A major difficulty is that no slow muscle fibres of the well-known type (Peachey and Huxley, 1962; Page, 1965; and Type 5, Table 1) have ever been demonstrated in the muscle spindle. Thus, the scheme is supported mainly by the observations that (1) large and small diameter motor axons innervate the spindle, (2) skeleto-fusimotor innervation is the norm in amphibian muscle (Gray, 1957), and (3) large motor axons innervate fast extrafusal muscle fibres while small motor axons innervate slow muscle fibres (Peachey, 1961; Barker, 1968).

In 1968 Barker reviewed the motor organization of vertebrate skeletal muscle and, taking more recent work into account, proposed the organizational scheme shown in Fig. 4. At this time,

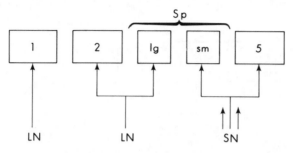

Fig. 4. Concept of the organization of anuran skeletal muscle after Barker (1968). 1, 2 and 5, muscle fibre types as in Table 1. lg. and sm., large and small intrafusal muscle fibres respectively. Other symbols as in Fig. 3.

fast fibres which correspond to types 1 and 2 (Table 1) had been described histochemically. It was also known that two types of intrafusal fibres existed, one of which had unexpected properties; the two types of intrafusal fibres are now referred to as the large and small intrafusal fibres in order to avoid specific implications regarding their structure and function. In Barker's scheme large intrafusal muscle fibres are co-innervated with fast muscle fibres of Type 2 while the small intrafusal muscle fibres are co-innervated with slow muscle fibres (Type 5, Table 1).

The organizational schemes of Figs. 3 and 4 are hypothetical, and certainly the introduction of five kinds of extrafusal muscle fibres and motor units does not simplify the situation. However, a scheme can be drawn up which embodies the most likely arrangement for these five types (Fig. 5). In this scheme muscle fibres and motor units of Type 1 are not co-innervated with the intrafusal fibres. This is a supposition which follows partly from the unfavourable position of spindles in zoned muscles to receive collaterals from the appropriate axons, and partly from the lack of Type 1 fibres in the extensor digiti IV longus in which the spindle does receive innervation from large motor axons. We propose that muscle fibres and motor units of Type 2 do participate in common innervation with the large intrafusal muscle fibres. In

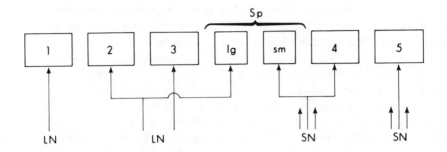

Fig. 5. Hypothetical scheme for the organization of skeletal muscle. 1-5, muscle fibre and motor unit types as in Table 1 and Fig. 2. For Xenopus laevis, LN indicates motor axons with diameters greater than 10 µm; SN motor axons with diameters less than 10 µm. Other symbols as for Figs. 3 and 4.

fact, in muscles containing extrafusal muscle fibre Types 1 and 2 only, such as the sartorius, one presumes that only the large intrafusal fibre is present in the spindle (Brown, 1971) and that this is co-innervated with motor units of Type 2.

The small intrafusal muscle fibre receives its motor innervation from small diameter axons and is structurally similar to the Type 4 extrafusal muscle fibre. We assume, provisionally, that Type 4 muscle fibres and motor units are co-innervated with the small intrafusal muscle fibre. It should be noted, however, that the small intrafusal fibre stains darkly for myosin ATPase (Smith and Ovalle, 1972) while the fibre Types 4 and 5 both stain lightly for this enzyme. This may reflect the influence of the sensory inner-vation on the properties of intrafusal muscle fibres. An additional problem is that the small intrafusal fibre is capable of propagating an impulse. Whether the Type 4 fibres with which we suppose the spindle is co-innervated can normally propagate an impulse is not known, but this seems unlikely judging from the contractile res-ponses of either of the slow motor units described above. Once again, it is quite possible that the intrafusal fibres have some pro-perties which are distinct from those of the extrafusal fibres with which they share motor axons.

One might well ask what is the significance of such hypothetical organizational schemes. The answer, as we see it, has several levels. At the level of the biology of amphibian muscle, we see such

a scheme as a step towards the rationalization of many separate
reports of muscle fibres with various properties (e.g. Burke and
Ginsborg, 1956; Shamarina, 1962, 1963; Orkand, 1963;
1966). At the level of the control of skeletal muscle in the amphibia the prediction is that some types of motor units must be activated at the same time as the muscle spindle while other types of
motor units do not participate in this very primitive form of
"alpha-gamma linkage". This could mean that two forms of motor
acts take place in the frog: those, as in jumping or in maintained
steady posture, which are essentially 'open loop' in nature and
those movements which are more finely controlled and require
modulation or load compensation by sensory feedback. Finally
at the broader level of the organization of skeletal muscle in the
vertebrates we find that the organization is often viewed in over-
simplified terms and is not fully understood in any vertebrate (see
Barker, 1968, and Laporte, this Symposium). The proposal of
Fig. 5 may be no more complicated than the organization of the
extraocular muscles of mammals which themselves contain a
number of fibre types (Mayr, 1971) and could well be homologues
of certain amphibian muscles.

Acknowledgement: This work was supported by the Muscular Dystrophy
Association of Canada.

REFERENCES

Asmussen, G., and Kiessling, A., 1973. Die Muskelfasersorten des
    Frosches: Ihre Identifikation und die gesetzmässigkeiten ihrer
    Anordnung in der Skelettmuskalatur. Acta Biol. Med. (Ger.) 24,
    871-889.
Barker, D., 1968. L'innervation motrice du muscle strie des
    vertebres. Actual. Neurophysiol. 8, 23-71.
Brown, M.C., 1971. A comparison of the spindles in two different
    muscles of the frog. J. Physiol. 216, 553-563.
Burke, W., and Ginsborg, B.L., 1956. The electrical properties of
    the slow muscle fibre membrane. J. Physiol. 132, 586-598.
Engel, W.K., and Irwin, R.L., 1967. A histochemical-physiological
    correlation of frog skeletal muscle fibers. Amer. J. Physiol.
    213, 511-518.
Eyzaguirre, C., 1957. Functional organization of neuromuscular
    spindle in the toad. J. Neurophysiol. 20, 523-542.
Eyzaguirre, C., 1958. Modulation of sensory discharges by efferent
    spindle excitation. J. Neurophysiol. 21, 465-480.
Gray, E.G., 1957. The spindle and extrafusal innervation of a frog
    muscle. Proc. Roy. Soc. Lond. B 146, 416-430.

Hess, A., 1970. Vertebrate slow muscle fibers. Physiol. Rev. 50, 40-62.

Katz, B., 1949. The efferent regulation of the muscle spindle in the frog. J. Exp. Biol. 26, 201-217.

Lännergren, J., and Smith, R.S., 1966. Types of muscle fibres in toad skeletal muscle. Acta Physiol. Scand. 68, 263-274.

Mannard, A., and Stein, R.B., 1973. Determination of the frequency response of isometric soleus muscle in the cat using random nerve stimulation. J. Physiol. 229, 275-296.

Mayr, R., 1971. Structure and distribution of fibre types in the external eye muscles of the rat. Tissue and Cell 3, 433-462.

Nasledov, G.A., 1966. Electrical excitability of different types of frog skeletal muscle fibers. Fed. Proc. Trans., Suppl. 25, T 443.

Orkand, R.K., 1963. A further study of electrical responses in slow and twitch muscle fibers of the frog. J. Physiol. 167, 181-191.

Page, S.G., 1965. A comparison of the fine structures of frog slow and twitch muscle fibres. J. Cell Biol. 26, 477-497.

Page, S.G., 1966. Intrafusal muscle fibres in the frog. J. Microsc. 5, 101-104.

Peachey, L.D., 1961. Structure and function of slow striated muscle. In Biophysics of Physiological and Pharmacological Actions. (Ed. Shanes, A.M.) Amer. Assoc. Adv. Sci., Wash. D.C. pp. 391-411.

Peachey, L.D., and Huxley, A.F., 1962. Structural identification of twitch and slow striated muscle fibers of the frog. J. Cell Biol. 13, 177-180.

Shamarina, N.M., 1962. Electric response of 'tonic' muscle fibers of the frog skeletal musculature. Nature 193, 783-784.

Shamarina, N.B., 1963. Electrical response of tonic skeletal muscle fibres to rhythmical stimulation. In The Effect of Use and Disuse on Neuromuscular Functions. (Eds. Gutmann, E. and Hnik, P.) Elsevier, Amsterdam pp. 499-514.

Smith, R.S., 1964a. Activity of intrafusal muscle fibres in muscle spindles of Xenopus laevis. Acta Physiol. Scand. 60, 223-239.

Smith, R.S., 1964b. Contraction in intrafusal fibres of Xenopus laevis following stimulation of their motor nerves. Acta Physiol. Scand. 62, 195-208.

Smith, R.S., and Lännergren, J., 1968. Types of motor units in the skeletal muscle of Xenopus laevis. Nature 217, 281-283.

Smith, R.S., and Ovalle, W.K., 1972. The structure and function of intrafusal muscle fibers. In Muscle Biology Vol. I (Ed. Cassens, R.G.) Marcel Dekker Inc. N.Y. pp. 147-227.

Smith, R.S., and Ovalle, W.K., 1973. Varieties of fast and slow extrafusal muscle fibers in amphibian hind-limb muscles. J. Anat. In press.

EVIDENCE FOR COMMON INNERVATION OF BAG AND CHAIN MUSCLE FIBRES IN CAT SPINDLES

Y. Laporte and F. Emonet-Dénand

Laboratoire de Neurophysiologie, Collège de France
Paris

Several investigations will be described which show that in cat spindles static axons frequently supply both nuclear bag and nuclear chain intrafusal muscle fibres: (1) histological study of the intrafusal distribution of static axons in teased silver stained spindles in which the motor innervation was reduced to a single axon after degeneration of all the other motor axons; (2) identification of intrafusal muscle fibres by intracellular injection of Procion Yellow or by depletion of their glycogen content; (3) cinematography of the contraction of intrafusal muscle fibres elicited by single static axons.

The simple model of spindle motor innervation proposed by Boyd and Matthews according to which bag and chain fibres are to a large extent separately innervated (bag fibres by dynamic axons and chain fibres by static ones) must be modified. Only that part of the model concerning dynamic axons should be retained, since direct evidence indicates that these axons almost exclusively supply bag fibres.

Recent observations using various techniques show that in many muscle spindles there is a common innervation of nuclear bag and nuclear chain muscle fibres. Evidence from each of these techniques will be reviewed in subsequent sections of this paper.

DEGENERATION EXPERIMENTS

In normal spindles, it is practically impossible to trace the distribution of a single fusimotor axon to the muscle fibres that it innervates because of the intermingling of the several axons which supply these fibres. To overcome this difficulty, spindles were prepared in which all but one of the fusimotor axons had degenerated.

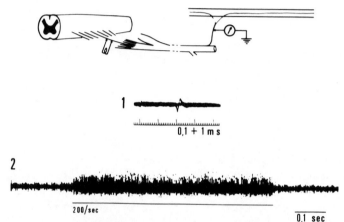

Fig. 1. Persistence of a tenuissimus gamma axon 290 hr after all other motor axons innervating the muscle had been cut. 1 - action potential of the axon recorded from the tenuissimus nerve after stimulation of the intact ventral root filament. Conduction velocity of the axon: 45 m/s. 2 - increase in spindle discharges elicited by repetitive stimulation of the axon (Barker et al., 1973).

The experimental and histological parts of this work were respectively carried out in Toulouse (France) by Emonet-Dénand et al. and in Durham (England) by Barker and Stacey. The experiments were performed in two stages. During the first stage, done under aseptic conditions in adult cats, a ventral root filament containing one gamma axon innervating spindles in a tenuissimus muscle was located and then all the other filaments containing alpha and gamma axons supplying this muscle were cut. The identification of the single gamma axon was made by recording its action potential from the ventral root filament after stimulating the tenuissimus nerve.

The second stage was done 7-12 days later in order to obtain
a complete degeneration of all the endings and terminal branches
of the cut axons. The survival of the preserved single gamma
axons was verified by recording its action potential from the
tenuissimus nerve after stimulation of the intact ventral root
filament and by observing the acceleration of the spindle discharge elicited by its repetitive stimulation (Fig. 1). For technical reasons (see Barker et al., 1970), the function of the surviving gamma axon was determined with a method (Emonet-
Denand et al., 1970) based on the integration of the discharges
of several spindles led from the tenuissimus nerve while the
muscle was sinusoidally stretched (Fig. 2).

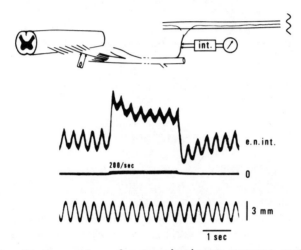

Fig. 2. Static action of a tenuissimus gamma axon in a muscle deprived of all other motor innervation. Conduction velocity of the axon: 35 m/s. Degeneration period: 220 hr.
The distal part of the tenuissimus muscle, 8 cm long, was
sinusoidally stretched; the upper branch of the nerve was cut.
Upper trace - integrated afferent electroneurogram.
Middle trace - stimulation of the axon; this line also indicates
the zero of the integrator. Lower trace - displacement of the
extremity of the distal portion of the muscle. (Barker et al.,
1973)

The morphology and the distribution of the endings of the surviving axon was then ascertained in teased silver preparations.
In the ten successfully prepared muscles the functions of the surviving gamma axon (conduction velocity ranging from 33-48 m/s)

was static. In these preparations extrafusal motor end plates and intrafusal p1 and p2 plates were absent. The spindles not supplied by the surviving gamma axon were devoid of all motor innervation, thus showing that the degeneration period was sufficient to allow the disappearance of the endings and terminal branches of the cut axons. In each preparation, it was observed that the surviving axon supplied several spindles with trail endings.

The distribution of the gamma axon was systematically analyzed in thirty spindles belonging to six preparations selected for the quality of their silver impregnation. It was found that the spindle poles in which single static gamma axons supplied both bag and chain muscle fibres were approximately twice as numerous as the poles in which chain or bag fibres were exclusively innervated: bag and chain fibres in 18 poles, only chain fibres in 10 poles, only bag fibres in 9 poles (Barker et al., 1971, 1973).

IDENTIFICATION OF INTRAFUSAL MUSCLE FIBRES

By Procion Yellow Intracellular Injection

This histophysiological investigation was also made in collaboration between the laboratory of Physiology in Toulouse (Bessou et al.) and the laboratory of Zoology in Durham (Barker and Stacey). The experimental part consisted of impaling intrafusal muscle fibres activated by single axons of identified functions with microelectrodes filled with an aqueous solution of Procion Yellow; this fluorescent dye was injected iontophoretically inside the muscle fibres. No attempt was made to inject Procion Yellow in more than one intrafusal muscle fibre except in one experiment in which two fibres were stained.

The experiments were carried out on tenuissimus spindles. Their nervous connections with ventral and dorsal roots were intact so as to prepare motor and afferent axons supplying these spindles and to identify the function of the single gamma axons. The distal half of the tenuissimus muscle was mounted in a flat transparent chamber, the proximal extremity of which was in contact with the posterior region of the thigh of the cat. With dark field illumination, the layers of extrafusal muscle fibres covering the spindle whose motor innervation had been previously analyzed were excised without damaging the innervation and blood supply of that spindle.

The identification of the nature of the fluorescent muscle fibre
was based not only on its diameter and length but also on its
ultrastructure and equatorial nucleation. In a preliminary communication, Barker et al. (1972) reported that of ten intrafusal
muscle fibres activated by static axons, six were bag fibres and
four chain fibres. In the experiment in which Procion Yellow
was successively injected in two muscle fibres activated by
the same static axon, one of them was a bag fibre, the other a
chain one (Fig. 3). In two experiments dealing with single
dynamic axons the impaled fibres were bag fibres.

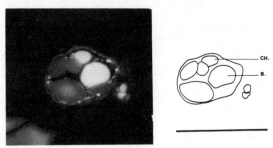

Fig. 3. Transverse section of a cat tenuissimus spindle
showing Procion Yellow fluorescence in a bag fibre (B)
and in a chain fibre (CH) innervated by the same static
gamma axon. (Barker et al., 1972). Bar: 60 μm. The
small fluorescent spots in the capsule wall are due to
cell nuclei; the two medium-size fluorescent spots outside
the capsule are due to erythrocytes inside a small blood
vessel.

By Depletion of Intrafusal Muscle
Fibre Glycogen

Brown and Butler (1973) using the glycogen depletion technique
of Edström and Kugelberg (1968) have recently found that prolonged stimulation of single static axons innervating cat tenuissimus spindles depletes glycogen in both bag and chain muscle
fibres. Their observations were made on muscles fixed in
Rossman's fluid. Similar results were obtained when the
muscles were frozen before fixation (Barker, Emonet-Dénand,
Harker, Jami and Laporte, unpublished observations).

CINEMATOGRAPHY OF THE CONTRACTION OF
INTRAFUSAL MUSCLE FIBRES

Bessou and Pagès (1973) have recently made a cinematographic study of the contraction elicited in intrafusal muscle fibres of tenuissimus spindles by single gamma axons of identified function (38 static and 15 dynamic axons). Intrafusal muscle fibres of a diameter superior to 17μ and extending well beyond the capsule were considered as bag fibres while short fibres mostly intra-capsular and with a diameter of less than 13μ were considered as chain fibres.

Of 38 static axons, 12 elicited the contraction of chain fibres only and 11 the concomitant contraction of chain and bag fibres. The other 15 static axons did produce the contraction of bag fibres. In most cases, it was not tried or it was not possible to determine whether these axons also activated chain fibres: in three cases however, the authors felt certain that the only contracting fibres were bag fibres.

The 11 dynamic axons exclusively elicited the contraction of bag fibres. Bessou and Pagès also made the observation that, in general, static axons supply several intrafusal muscle fibres while dynamic axons often supply only one fibre and frequently only a pole of the fibre.

All these observations conclusively show that many fusimotor static axons do supply both types of intrafusal muscle fibre. The number of spindle poles in which there is a common innervation of bag and chain fibres appears to be high. Barker et al. (1973), by tracing the distribution of single static axons in spindles deprived of any other motor innervation, found common innervation of bag and chain fibres in more than 50% of the poles. Bessou and Pagès (1973) obtained cinematographic evidence that of 38 static axons 11 elicited contraction of both types of muscle fibre. At the beginning of their work these authors focussed their attention on the relation between static axons and bag fibres and did not try to ascertain whether some chain fibres were also contracting; for this reason it is likely that among the 15 other axons whose stimulation elicited contraction of bag fibres, some also supplied chain fibres.

Boyd et al. (1973), in spindles of the abductor digiti quinti muscle of the cat, also observed the contraction of intrafusal muscle fibres produced by the stimulation of single gamma axons

of identified function. Eight static axons were studied; four
elicited local contractions in chain fibres only and the other four
elicited some movement in one of the nuclear bag fibres in addition to the contraction of chain fibres. Four dynamic axons produced local contraction at one pole of bag fibres only.

The demonstration that bag fibres can be activated by static
axons and that common innervation of bag and chain fibres is a
frequent feature of the motor innervation of cat spindles is not
compatible with the simple model originally proposed by Boyd
(1962) and considered by Matthews (1972) as the most satisfactory
basis for explaining the actions of fusimotor axons. According
to this model, bag and chain intrafusal muscle fibres are to a
large extent separately innervated, the bag fibres by dynamic
axons and the chain fibres by static ones. Only that part of the
model concerning dynamic axons should be maintained since
direct evidence that these axons almost exclusively supply bag
fibres is now available (Barker et al., 1972; Bessou and Pagès,
1973; Boyd et al., 1973; however, see Brown and Butler, 1973).
The intrafusal mechanism by which static axons exert their
actions on the primary endings is certainly more complex than
previously believed.

REFERENCES

Barker, D., Bessou, P., Jankowska, E., Pagès, B. and Stacey, M.,
    1972. Distribution des axones fusimoteurs statiques et
    dynamiques aux fibres musculaires intrafusales chez le Chat.
    Compt. Rend. Acad. Sci. Paris. 275, 2527-2530.
Barker, D., Emonet-Dénand, F., Laporte, Y., Proske, U., and
    Stacey, M., 1970. Identification des terminaisons motrices
    des fibres fusimotrices statiques chez le Chat. Compt. Rend.
    Acad. Sci. Paris. 271, 1203-1206.
Barker, D., Emonet-Dénand, F., Laporte, Y., Proske, U. and
    Stacey, M., 1971. Identification of the endings and function
    of cat fusimotor fibres. J. Physiol. 216, 51-52P.
Barker, D., Emonet-Dénand, F., Laporte, Y., Proske, U., and
    Stacey, M., 1973. Morphological identification and intrafusal
    distribution of the endings of static fusimotor axons in the cat.
    J. Physiol. 230, 405-427.
Bessou, P., and Pagès, B., 1973. Nature des fibres musculaires
    fusales activées par des axones fusimoteurs statiques ou
    dynamiques chez le Chat. Compt. Rend. Acad. Sci. Paris.
    In press.

Boyd, I.A., 1962. The structure and innervation of the nuclear bag muscle fibre system and the nuclear chain muscle fibre system in mammalian muscle spindles. Phil. Trans. Roy. Soc. B <u>245</u>, 81-136.

Boyd, I.A., Gladden, M.H., McWilliam, P.N. and Ward, J., 1973. Static and dynamic fusimotor action in isolated cat muscle spindles with intact nerve and blood supply. J. Physiol. <u>230</u>, 29-30P.

Brown, M.C., and Butler, R.L., 1973. Depletion of intrafusal muscle fibre glycogen by stimulation of fusimotor fibres. J. Physiol. <u>229</u>, 25-26P.

Edström, L., and Kugelberg, E., 1968. Histochemical composition, distribution of fibres and fatiguability of single motor units. J. Neurol. Neurosurg. Psychiat. <u>31</u>, 424-433.

Emonet-Dénand, F., Laporte, Y., and Proske, U., 1970. Identification de l'action statique ou dynamique des fibres fusimotrices basée sur les modifications de l'électroneurogramme afférent 'intégré'. Compt. Rend. Acad. Sci. Paris. <u>270</u>, 2480-2482.

Matthews, P.B.C., 1972. Mammalian Muscle Receptors and Their Central Actions. Edward Arnold, Lond.

SYSTEMS APPROACH TO THE STUDY OF MUSCLE SPINDLES

R. E. Poppele

Laboratory of Neurophysiology, University of
Minnesota, Minneapolis, Minnesota

This paper presents an outline of a systems analysis of the
mammalian muscle spindle receptors. Such an analysis is a
systematic and quantitative method of studying the behaviour
of a device for which one can define an input and an output.
The receptor organ is conceptually partitioned into three
compartments: a mechanical filter, transducer and encoder.
The contribution of each of these compartments to overall
receptor behaviour is examined quantitatively. It is found
that the mechanical filter of the intrafusal muscle properties
can account for the slower transients and adaptations exhibited
by spindles while the more rapid dynamics including the velocity and acceleration responses are probably due to properties of the mechanoelectrical transducer. The encoder is a
non-linear oscillator whose operation depends on a time
varying membrane leak, a quantity determined by membrane
conductance and capacitance. The mean value of the leak is
different for primary and secondary endings and results in a
different behaviour of the respective encoders.

It has now been forty years since recordings from single
mammalian muscle spindles were first reported by Matthews
(1933) and there has been a constant probing of the properties of
this receptor since. The past dozen years have seen a particularly
rapid increase of detailed information on the functional and anatomical organization of these complex receptors. Nevertheless,

we are still far from completely understanding the mechanisms
or the purpose of this receptor organ. That understanding ultimately requires a quantitative analysis, which is capable of
effectively distinguishing among various hypotheses. The systems
approach offers such a systematic, quantitative method (see
Terzuolo, 1969). It consists of examining the relationship between
input and output and using that relationship to construct a model
or mathematical replica of the device or to test a mechanistic
hypothesis about its operation (Poppele, 1970).

This paper is an outline of a systems analysis of the mammalian
muscle spindle. In presenting it I wish to acknowledge the help of
Drs. Bowman, Chen, Fohlmeister, Kennedy and Purple, each of
whom contributed significantly to some aspect of this work, and to
thank them for their permissiom to present unpublished data. I
will deal here only with the passive spindle behaviour, although
recently the analysis has been extended to include the effects of
fusimotor activation (Chen and Poppele, 1973).

It is generally accepted that the spindle receptors can be com-
partmentalized according to fundamental processes contributing
to their overall behaviour, and that these compartments may be
considered to be serially arranged and independent of each other
(Houk et al., 1966; see Fig. 1).

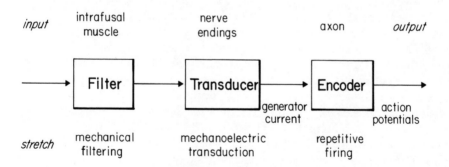

Fig. 1.   Compartmental model of spindle receptor.

This representation is particularly convenient for a linear systems
analysis where it is assumed that each box in the series acts as a
filter producing a characteristic linear transformation of the input
signal to generate an output signal.

In order to apply this approach, it must first be demonstrated that either the system is linear, or its operation can be restricted to a domain in which its behaviour is linear. For the muscle spindle neither condition strictly holds since the output, a train of pulses, is not a linear transformation of the input stretch. Furthermore, even if we consider a parameter of the pulse train, namely its probability density, which is a smooth function that can be related to input stretch, we find that the spindle, in general, exhibits an overall non-linear behaviour. This is because the sensitivity of the spindle (output per unit stretch) is not independent of the magnitude of muscle stretch.

NON-LINEARITIES

In Figs. 2 and 3 the sensitivity of a primary and a secondary ending from the same tenuissimus spindle are shown to be functions of both stretch amplitude (Fig. 2) and of muscle length (Fig. 3). The spindle, located in an isolated segment of muscle, was stimulated by a sinusoidally stretching the muscle at 1 Hz (see Poppele and Bowman, 1970, for method). At this frequency the primary ending was about ten times as sensitive as the secondary for a particular muscle length. The sensitivity of both changed about five-fold as the muscle was pulled from slack to taut or relaxed from taut to slack - a change in total length of this piece of tenuissimus muscle of 18%. When the muscle was held at a fixed length and subject to sinusoidal stretches of increasing amplitudes, both endings showed an initial increase in sensitivity, up to an amplitude of about 10 μ, followed by a monotonic decrease. (Sensitivity continues to decrease for amplitudes greater than the 100μ shown here - see Chen and Poppele, 1973).

The non-linearities depicted in both Figs. 2 and 3 are 'static' because only the sensitivity varies and not receptor dynamics. Thus, with sinusoidal stimulation the phase relation between applied stretch and output impulse density is independent of the amplitude or mean value of the input. Systems containing such static non-linearities can be treated using linear analysis since the response of the system is approximately linear when the input is restricted to 'small' signals. In these cases linear analysis will reveal the dynamics of the system, but not the dependence of sensitivity (or gain) on the magnitude of the input.

The restriction to small signals is still not quite sufficient for

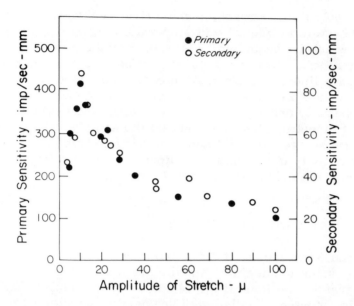

Fig. 2. Non-linear sensitivity of primary and secondary endings from the same tenuissimus spindle as a function of sinusoidal stretch amplitude. Frequency of sinusoidal stretching was 1 Hz. Muscle length was 46 mm for primary data and 52 mm for secondary data.

a linear analysis of the muscle spindle, however, since there are also time dependent non-linearities which can be attributed to the encoding process (and possibly also to the mechanical filter - see Matthews, 1963; Brown et al., 1969; Hasan and Houk, 1972). The encoding non-linearity is manifest as a tendency for output pulses to phase-lock to cyclic inputs (Rescigno et al., 1970) which in turn causes changes in system dynamics that depend on the rate of impulse activity in the spindle. Some understanding of this non-linearity has been obtained from theoretical (Knight, 1972) and model (Stein and French, 1970; Poppele and Chen, 1972) studies which have shown that the transfer function of the entire system is not basically altered by the non-linearity, but merely contains additional terms due to encoder behaviour. Furthermore, these additional terms affect the frequency domain only when the

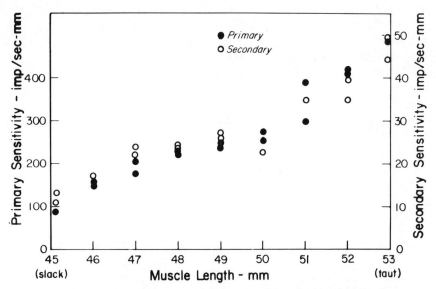

Fig. 3. Non-linear sensitivity of primary and secondary endings from the same tenuissimus spindle as a function of muscle length with sinusoidal stretching at 1 Hz. Amplitude of sinusoidal stretch was 12μ for primary and 47μ for secondary.

input frequency is close to the unmodulated rate of impulses from the receptor. Therefore, by varying that unmodulated rate, it is possible to determine separately the linear dynamics of the receptor and the dynamics due to the encoder.

Models obtained by linear analysis are purely operational in the sense that they do not suggest specific mechanisms for the observed behaviour; they only describe it in a quantitative and general way. The fact that there are also non-linearities does not invalidate this description, it only means that it is incomplete. The observed linear transformations are indeed due to the behaviour of one or more of the three components mentioned above.

LINEAR ANALYSIS

An overall analysis of the muscle spindle receptors within the guidelines outlined above has led to the formulation of a model that

predicts spindle behaviour for any small amplitude stimulus
(Poppele and Bowman, 1969, 1970). There are two forms of the
model, one which describes the linear behaviour of the primary
ending and one of the secondary. Using the familiar Laplace
notation to express these in the frequency domain, they are:

$$H_1(s) = K_1 \frac{s(s + .4)(s + 11)(s + 44)}{(s + .04)(s + .8)} \qquad \text{(1) for the primary}$$

and

$$H_2(s) = K_2 \frac{(s + .4)(s + 11)}{(s + .8)} \qquad \text{(2) for the secondary.}$$

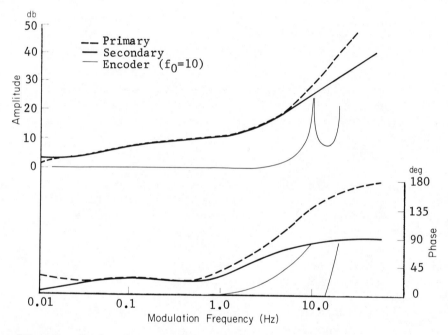

Fig. 4. Bode plots of the model for muscle spindle behaviour.
Absolute value and arguments of equations 1, 2 and 3 are
plotted as amplitude (in db) and phase (in degrees). See text
for details.

When the complex variable $s = j\omega = j\,2\pi f$ (the frequency of sinusoidal stimulation) these expressions describe the amplitude and
phase of spindle response as a function of stimulus frequency.

Fig. 4 is a Bode plot of those quantities. (Transformed into the time domain, the expressions are the solutions to differential equations that govern the system behaviour.) The K's in these equations are constants which denote the static sensitivities. In a complete description these factors are actually functions of stretch magnitude which describe the static non-linearities.

In summary, these expressions imply that there is a close correspondence between the behaviour of primary and secondary endings in that both respond proportionally (or nearly so) to stretch for slow changes in length and both show a response to velocity of applied stretch for signals having frequency components greater than 1.7 Hz (ω = 11 rad/sec)(see also Matthews and Stein, 1969 and Fig. 4). In addition, the behaviour of the primary ending includes dynamic components which lead to a complete or nearly complete adaptation with a long time constant (25 sec = 1/.04) and a response to the acceleration of stretch stimuli that are faster than 7 Hz (ω = 44 rad/sec).

For frequencies above 40 Hz (ω = 260 rad/sec), the applicability of the model is not known since we have no data in that range, although the data of Matthews and Stein (1969) suggest that it is valid to at least 200 Hz. As they are stated, equations 1 and 2 are not physically realizable since they are not bounded for large s; therefore additional high frequency terms are required.

As stated above, this linear analysis gives us only a quantitative description of the behaviour of the spindle; it does not reveal the non-linear behaviour nor does it tell us which component parts of the system are involved. Therefore we have extended our analysis: a) to examine the major non-linearity which is due to the encoder, and b) to determine which behaviour is due to the properties of the mechanical filter and which to the mechano-electric transducer.

ENCODER

A key to understanding the nature of the encoder has been its tendency to phase-lock to cyclic stimuli. This tendency is different for primary and secondary encoders. The primary exhibits phase locking for small input signals only when the stimulation rate is very nearly equal to the firing rate of the receptor and then

it is a one-to-one phase locking. In contrast, the secondary
ending shows phase-locked patterns over a range of frequencies
with very little tendency to lock on a one-to-one basis with the
stimulus. This behaviour led us to consider a physical model
(the leaky integrator or RC encoder) which was shown to have the
same phase locking properties (Stein and French, 1970; Rescigno
et al., 1971) and a similar frequency response (Poppele and Chen,
1972). Moreover, the observed difference in encoder behaviour
can be explained in terms of this model.

The model has a single parameter, γ (membrane leak), which
can be equated to real membrane parameters: $\gamma = 1/R_m C_m$,
where R_m is membrane resistance and C_m is membrane capacitance.* It fires repetitively when subjected to a current input.
Current charges the membrane capacity and then leaks through
the membrane resistance. When the membrane is charged to its
threshold voltage, an action potential is produced and the process
is reset. The interspike interval is determined by the magnitude
of the generator current and the value of the membrane leak.

The transfer function for the model is

$$H(s) = K_3 \frac{s}{(s + \gamma)} \frac{\exp(\gamma/f_0) - \exp(-s/f_0)}{1 - \exp(-s/f_0)} \qquad (3)$$

(Knight, 1972) where f_0 is the unmodulated rate of discharge of
the model and K_3 is its sensitivity expressed as a rate of impulses
per unit input.

While the leaky integrator model accounts for many features
of encoder behaviour, there are two important exceptions: a)
the model exhibits a minimum stable rate of impulses which is
inconsistent with the low rates of firing possible from the spindle
receptor, and b) the value of the "leak" for the spindle (particularly the secondary ending) is a function of its mean rate of firing
such that

$$f_0 = k\gamma \qquad (4)$$

_____

* Formally, the quantity γ is a rate constant with units sec^{-1}.
However, we have chosen a different terminology to emphasize
the fact that γ is not constant but rather a function of both time
and voltage (Fohlmeister, 1973). The term 'leak' is suggested
by the fact that γ is proportional to membrane conductance.

where k is a constant. The latter finding was interpreted to suggest that the membrane leak is changing within the interspike interval, since the mean value of leak is inversely proportional to the interval duration; and further that the variable leak can account for the observed differences between the spindle encoder and the leaky integrator or constant RC model.

To test this suggestion, Drs. Fohlmeister, Purple and I have examined the encoder of the slowly adapting crayfish stretch receptor, which shows a dynamic behaviour similar to that of the spindle encoder (Poppele and Purple, 1971) and which has the advantage of allowing us to excite the encoder directly with intracellularly applied current. A train of action potentials was evoked by constant current and the resulting voltage record was analyzed for membrane leak according to the following expression:

$$\gamma = \frac{-\dot{u} + \sigma}{u} \quad \text{(Knight, 1972)} \tag{5}$$

where γ = membrane leak, σ is proportional to the applied current, u is membrane potential and $-\dot{u}$ is the time derivative of u. The results calculated from this equation are redrawn in Fig. 5 and show that the leak does indeed vary during the interval, being large immediately following the spike, then decreasing to very small values as the interval progresses. If we assume that the large leak following the spike is primarily due to potassium conductance then the initial value of leak accounts for the after-hyperpolarization observed following the spikes. Furthermore, the calculated time course of γ can explain the relationship observed above for the spindle which as expressed in equation 4.

If we define

$$\bar{\gamma} = \frac{1}{T} \int_0^T \gamma(t) \, dt \tag{6}$$

as the mean value of leak in an interval T, then

$$\bar{\gamma}/f_0 = \text{constant (from equation 4)}$$

$$= 1/(T \cdot f_0) \int_0^T \gamma(t) \, dt \tag{7}$$

$$= \int_0^T \gamma(t) \, dt$$

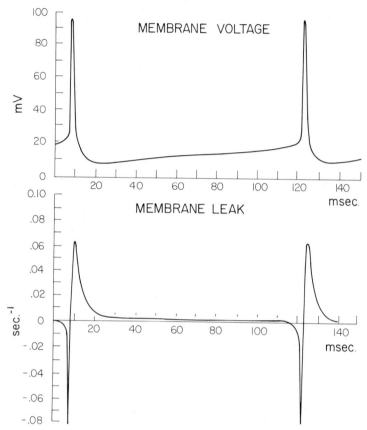

Fig. 5. Membrane leak function for the slowly adapting stretch receptor of the crayfish. See text for details.

From the shape of the γ curve in Fig. 5, it is apparent that the integral of $\gamma(t)$ (Equ. 7) over an interval, T, is nearly constant and independent of the length of the interval, except during the first 15 msec. Moreover, Fohlmeister (1973) has recently shown that a γ-dependency like that calculated for the crayfish is sufficient to account for tonic repetitive firing even at rates as low as those observed for the spindle. Work presently in progress strongly suggests that details of the observed dynamics of both muscle spindle and crayfish encoders can be accounted for by such a leak function.

As for adaptive behaviour that may be due to encoder properties,

I refer again to the crayfish. In this case, it has been shown that even for the slowly adapting receptor, the encoder adapts to a constant current and that the adaptation is due to an accumulative hyperpolarization resulting from an electrogenic Na pump (Nakajima and Takahashi, 1966; Sokolove and Cooke, 1971). This behaviour leads to a slight phase lead (10-15°) and decreased sensitivity to low frequencies (0. 1-0. 3 Hz) of sinusoidal stretch which are readily identified in the Bode plot of crayfish encoder behaviour (Poppele and Purple, 1971). Whether or not a similar process is active in the spindle is uncertain because of the indirect means employed to obtain the Bode plot in that case. Other data, obtained with extracellular current stimulation are also inconclusive on this point (Emonet-Dénand and Houk, 1969).

MECHANICAL FILTER

If we can determine the dynamic properties of the mechanical filter, then we may argue by exclusion that whatever components of equations 1 and 2 have not been accounted for are likely to be due to the mechanoelectrical transducer.

The mechanical filter has two elements, the extrafusal muscle lying in parallel with the receptor, and the intrafusal muscle in series with the sensory endings.

As for the extrafusal muscle, several lines of evidence suggest that its contribution to spindle dynamics is negligible. For one, the properties of spindles in such different muscles as the soleus, gastrocnemius and tenuissimus were found to be nearly identical. Second, we have measured the dynamics of the length-tension relationships of the tenuissimus muscle, which reveal the viscoelastic properties of the extrafusal muscle. We found that this muscle behaves like a simple spring within the range of frequencies where the receptor exhibits complex dynamics (Poppele and Bowman, 1970; see Fig. 8). In addition, we have recently observed the behaviour of isolated muscle spindles with no extrafusal component and found that it is exactly as predicted by equations 1 and 2 (Kennedy and Poppele, 1973 and unpublished observations).

The role of intrafusal muscle in determining spindle dynamics is not so clear. It has been commonly believed, since first suggested by Matthews (1933), that the viscoelastic properties of intrafusal muscle do indeed determine the dynamic behaviour of muscle spindle receptors. Furthermore, it has recently been shown that the transfer characteristics of primary and secondary endings can be fully accounted for if one makes certain ad hoc assumptions about the viscoelastic properties of the intrafusal muscle (e.g. Angers, 1965; Houk and Stark, 1962; Gottlieb et al., 1969; Rudjord, 1970a, b). However, until we have quantitative data about intrafusal muscle dynamics, it is not possible to confirm or deny that the mechanical filter is responsible for receptor dynamics.

Morphologically, we know that the primary and secondary endings are in many cases associated with different classes of intrafusal fibres and also that they are found on identifiably different regions of those fibres (Barker, 1967; Boyd, 1962). These facts may be sufficient to account for the observed differences in dynamics and sensitivity of the two endings, and indeed many investigators have suggested exactly that (see Matthews, 1972 for ref.). Several other lines of evidence based on in vitro observations of isolated spindles and anatomical data, all qualitative in nature, tend to support this hypothesis (Boyd, 1966; Boyd and Ward, 1969; Cooper and Daniel, 1967). However, a quantitative study based on direct cinematography of sensory endings during ramp stretches failed to reveal a consistent phasic component that might account for the dynamic response of primary endings (Beacham et al., 1971). In summary, it is not clear what components of the model discussed above, if any, can be accounted for by intrafusal muscle dynamics. Therefore, Dr. Kennedy and I have applied the systems approach to observations of single isolated tenuissimus muscle spindles using Zeiss Nomarski interference contrast optics and high speed cinematography.

Spindles were dissected free of the extrafusal muscle in oxygenated Krebs Ringer and a fine thread was tied to the extracapsular portion of the intrafusal bundle at each end. One thread was fixed and the other attached to a Pye Ling vibrator controlled by a Hewlett-Packard function generator. Stretches of 10-200µ were applied and the movements of fibres in the equatorial and juxtaequatorial regions were observed and plotted.

Following a step stretch the muscle bundle is seen to creep in a direction opposing the stretch (see also Boyd and Ward, 1969). While these movements are much larger in the equatorial region than in adjacent and more polar areas, they all appear to follow a similar time course. Fig. 6 is a plot of the time course of this adaptation to stretch for two separate spindles and shows that the

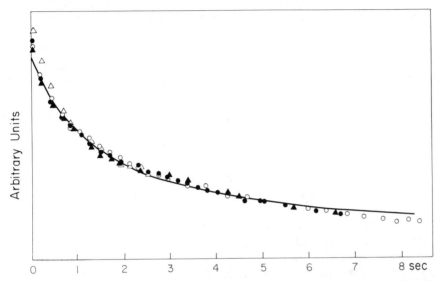

Fig. 6. Time course of intrafusal muscle adaptation following a step stretch. Stretches varied from 50-200 μ and responses are normalized to arbitrary units. Dots (●) are plotted from measurement made in the equatorial region of two spindles. Triangles (△) are plotted from the juxta-equatorial region of the same spindles. Data from two spindles are included; open symbols are from one spindle and filled symbols are from the other. Solid line is a plot of the step response of the spindle model. See text for details.

movement lasts for at least 8 sec. Although it was not possible for us to positively identify bag and chain fibres there was a clear relative movement between fibres, some showing more extensive adaptive movements than others. The solid line drawn in Fig. 6 is a plot of the step response of a system whose transfer function is:

$$H(s) = \frac{s(s + .4)}{(s + .04)(s + .8)} \qquad (8)$$

which may be recognized as the first four terms of equation 1, the transfer function of the primary ending. Therefore, we may conclude that this low frequency behaviour of the primary ending (i. e.

below 0.5 Hz) can be explained <u>quantitatively</u> by the dynamics of
the intrafusal muscle. Supposedly, the difference in adaptation
magnitude observed for equatorial and juxta-equatorial regions
and for different fibres can account for the differences in very
low frequency behaviour between primary and secondary endings.
However, additional quantitative measurements are necessary to
settle the point. This quantitative result agrees with the report
of Boyd and Ward (1969) that relaxation following quick stretches
has a time course similar to spindle discharge adaptation.

In contrast to these findings, many attempts at modelling
spindle behaviour have attributed the more rapid dynamics of
spindle behaviour to intrafusal muscle properties. In fact,
Smith (1966) has observed a rapid but very small component of
adaptation of nuclear bag fibres that might account for some of
the observed high frequency dynamics of these receptors. It is
not clear from data obtained with step stretches, however,
whether the muscle dynamics can quantitatively account for this
behaviour because of the inherent difficulty in resolving rapid
dynamics with a step input. More appropriate for this type of
study are ramp or sinusoidal inputs. When sinusoidal stimuli
are employed, the higher frequency dynamics of the receptor
endings produce a <u>phase lead</u> of output with respect to the input
stretch which exceeds 45° at 4 Hz. If it is indeed responsible for
the dynamic spindle response, the intrafusal muscle should also
show a similar phase lead. This can be determined directly by
observing the relative movement between equatorial and polar
regions of an intrafusal muscle fibre in response to sinusoidal
stretching in the range of 1-10 Hz. Fig. 7 shows the result of one
such experiment.

The data indicate clearly a lack of phase lead at those frequencies where spindle response significantly leads input stretch.
Therefore, the data are consistent with similar data from other
muscles in showing a lack of dynamic behaviour in the range of
1-10 Hz as shown in Fig. 8, and are also consistent with the
previous report of a lack of correspondence between spindle
discharge and intrafusal muscle dynamics. The result is also
consistent with the findings of Ottoson and co-workers for the frog
spindle that indicated no correspondence between the early adaptation of the receptor potential and muscle relaxation after step
stretches (Ottoson and Shepherd, 1970). They also found little
difference in receptor response with constant length and constant
tension stimuli (Husmark and Ottoson, 1971). It should be noted,

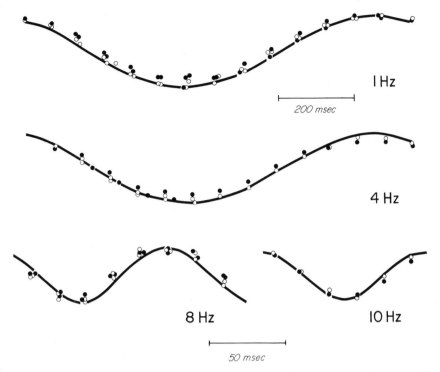

Fig. 7. Response of intrafusal muscle to sinusoidal stretches
of 10 μ. Closed dots (●) are plots of the movement of the spindle
pole as a function of time. Open dots (o) are a plot of the simultaneous movement of sensory endings at the spindle equator.
Solid lines are sine waves drawn for reference. Film speed at
1 Hz was approximately 16 frames/sec and at 4, 8 and 10 Hz,
64 frames/sec. Movement of pole and equator are approximately
in phase at the frequencies tested.

however, that the data reported here for the mammalian spindle
are from a single receptor whose viability was not directly controlled (although the adaptation to step stretches, absent in dead
muscle, was present), and further experimentation is required to
confirm the result. Therefore, we tentatively propose that the
velocity and acceleration responses which are apparently absent
from the responses of the intrafusal muscle must be a property of
the mechanoelectrical transduction.

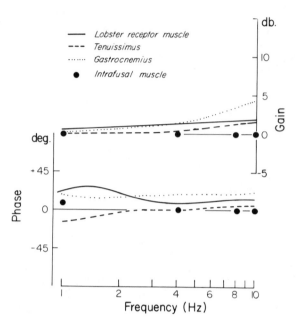

Fig. 8. Dynamics of different muscles in the frequency range
of 1-10 Hz for muscles stretched sinusoidally. Gain and
phase refer to the relationship between length and tension.
Lobster stretch receptor data are replotted from Terzuolo
and Knox (1971), tenuissimus data from Poppele and Bowman
(1970), gastrocnemius data from Rosenthal et al. (1970).
Intrafusal muscle points are plotted from the data in Fig. 7.

SUMMARY

From the systems analysis of the muscle spindle reviewed
above we can now state the following hypothesis about the mechanisms governing the passive behaviour of these receptors (see
Fig. 9):

Filter

A viscoelastic element having components whose arrangement
has been proposed as the basis of a model of spindle behaviour
(see Rudjord, 1970a; Henatch, 1972), but with longer time constants (by an order of magnitude) than previously supposed. This

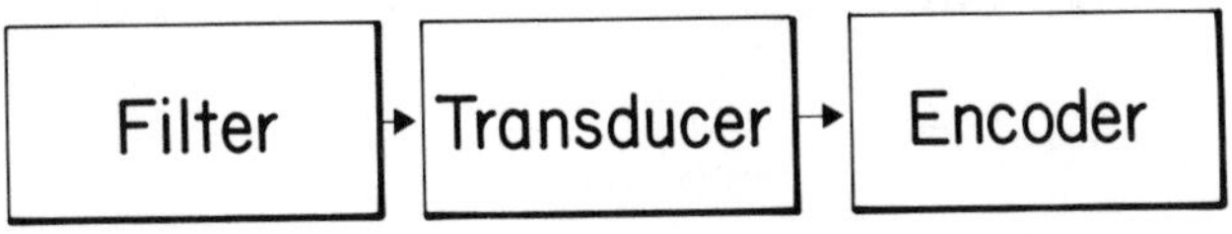

	Filter	Transducer	Encoder
Common Elements	$\dfrac{(s+.4)}{(s+.8)}$	$\dfrac{(s+11)}{(?)}$	$\dfrac{s}{s+\gamma}\left\{\dfrac{e^{\gamma/f_o}-e^{-s/f_o}}{1-e^{-s/f_o}}\right\}$
Primary	$\dfrac{s(s+.4)}{(s+.04)(s+.8)}$	$\dfrac{(s+11)(s+44)}{(?)}$	$\gamma(t)$ small
Secondary	$\dfrac{(s+.4)}{(s+.8)}$	$\dfrac{(s+11)}{(?)}$	$\gamma(t)$ large

Fig. 9. A proposed mathematical model of the mammalian muscle spindle.

element can fully account for the behaviour of the spindle in the range below 0.5 Hz (in the frequency domain) corresponding to time constants 1.25 sec and longer.

Transducer

A basically unknown mechanism which seems to be responsible for the velocity and acceleration responses of the receptor. It accounts for the behaviour of the spindle in the range above 1 Hz (in the frequency domain) with components having time constants shorter than 100 msec. Transducer mechanisms which could exhibit the necessary rapid adaptation have been suggested (Zerbst et al., 1966; Houk, 1969).

Encoder

A non-linear oscillator which tends to phase lock to cyclic inputs. It accounts for the non-linear behaviour when frequencies are applied which are close to the rate of the receptor's discharge and has little effect on non-cyclic inputs such as ramps and steps. The mechanism of repetitive firing depends on a time varying membrane leak, which is different for primary and secondary endings.

Acknowledgment: I am grateful to Drs. J. Bloedel, R. Purple and C. Terzuolo for helpful comments on the manuscript. The experimental work cited in this paper was supported by Public Health Service Grants NB-07421 and EY-00293, and by Grants from the Graduate School, University of Minnesota. IBM 1800 computer facilities were made available from the Air Force Office of Scientific Research (AFSC), AF-AFOSR-1221.

REFFRENCES

Angers, D., 1965. Modèle mécanique de fuseau neuromusculaire dé-éfferente: terminaisons primaries et secondaires. Compt. Rend. Acad. Sci. (Paris) 261, 2255-2258.

Barker, D., 1967. The innervation of mammalian skeletal muscle. In Myotatic, Kinesthetic and Vestibular Mechanisms. Churchill, London. pp. 3-15.

Beachman, W.S., Fukami, Y. and Hunt, C.C., 1971. Displacement of elements within mammalian muscle spindles. Proc. Int. Congr. Physiol. XXV 9, 46.

Boyd, I.A., 1962. The structure and innervation of the nuclear bag muscle fibre system and the nuclear chain muscle fibre system in mammalian muscle spindles. Phil. Trans. Roy. Soc. B245, 81-136.

Boyd, I.A., 1966. The mechanical properties of mammalian intra-fusal fibers. J. Physiol. 187, 10-12P.

Boyd, I.A. and Ward, J., 1969. The response of isolated cat muscle spindles to passive stretch. J. Physiol. 200, 104-105P.

Brown, M.C., Goodwin, G.M. and Matthews, P.B.C., 1969. After-effects of fusimotor stimulation on the response of muscle spindle primary afferent endings. J. Physiol. 205, 677-694.

Chen, W.J. and Poppele, R.E., 1973. Static fusimotor effect on the sensitivity of mammalian muscle spindle. Brain Res. 57, 244-247.

Cooper, S. and Daniel, P.N., 1967. Elastic tissue in muscle spindles of man and cat. J. Physiol. 192, 10-11P.

Emonet-Dénand, F. and Houk, J.C., 1969. Some effects of polarizing current on discharges from muscle spindle receptors. Amer. J. Physiol. 216, 404-406.

Fohlmeister, J., 1973. A model for phasic and tonic repetitively firing neuronal encoders. Kybernetik. In press.

Gottlieb, G., Agarwal, C.G. and Stark, L., 1969. Stretch
receptor models. I. Single efferent, single afferent innervation.
I.E.E.E. Trans. MMS- 10, 17-27.

Hasan, Z. and Houk, J.C., 1972. Nonlinear behavior of primary
spindle receptors in response to small, slow ramp stretches.
Brain Res. 44, 680-683.

Henatsch,H.D., 1972. Structural and functional aspects of fusimotor mechanics in mammalian muscle spindle.In Biocybernetics
IV. Veb.Gustav Fischer Verlag, Leipzig, pp. 170-181.

Houk, J.C., 1969. Rate sensitivity of mechanoreceptors. Ann.
N.Y. Acad. Sci. 156, 901-916.

Houk, J.C., Cornew, R.W. and Stark, L., 1966. A model of
adaptation in amphibian spindle receptors. J. Theor. Biol.
12, 196-215.

Houk, J.C. and Stark, L., 1962. An analytical model of a spindle
receptor for simulation of motor coordination. M.I.T. Res.
Lab. of Electron. Quart. Progr. Rep. 66, 384-389.

Husmark, I. and Ottoson, D., 1971. The contribution of mechanical
factors to the early adaptation of the spindle response.
J. Physiol. 212, 577-592.

Kennedy, W.R. and Poppele, R.E., 1973. Sensory activity of human
muscle spindles. Proc. VIII Int. Congr. of EEG and Clin.
Neurophysiol. In press.

Knight, B.W., 1972. Dynamics of encoding in a population of
neurons. J. Gen. Physiol. 59, 734-766.

Matthews, B.H.C., 1933. Nerve endings in mammalian muscle.
J. Physiol. 78, 1-53.

Matthews, P.B.C., 1963. The response of de-efferented muscle
spindle receptors to stretching at different velocities.
J. Physiol. 168, 660-678.

Matthews, P.B.C., 1972. Mammalian Muscle Receptors and their
Central Actions. William and Wilkins Co., Baltimore, pp. 315-318.

Matthews, P.B.C. and Stein, R.B., 1969. The sensitivity of
muscle spindle afferents to small sinusoidal changes in length.
J. Physiol. 200, 723-745.

Nakajima, S. and Takahashi, K., 1966. Post-tetanic hyperpolarization and electrogenic Na pump in stretch receptor
neurone of crayfish. J. Physiol. 187, 105-127.

Ottoson, D. and Shepherd, G.M., 1970. Length changes within the
frog muscle spindle during and after stretch. J. Physiol.
207, 747-759.

Poppele, R.E., 1970. The system approach to the function of the
nervous system. In Excitatory Synaptic Mechanisms. Universitetsforlaget, Oslo. pp. 259-268.

Poppele, R.E. and Bowman, R.J., 1969. Linear analysis of muscle
spindles. In Systems Analysis in Neurophysiology. Univ.
of Minn., Minneapolis, pp. 128-140.

Poppele, R.E. and Bowman, R.J., 1970. Quantitative description
of the linear behavior of mammalian muscle spindles. J.
Neurophysiol. 33, 59-72.

Poppele, R.E. and Chen, W.J., 1972.   Repetitive firing behavior
  of mammalian muscle spindles.   J. Neurophysiol. 35, 357-364.

Poppele, R.E. and Purple, R.L., 1971.   Repetitive firing in
  receptor neurons.   Proc. Int. Congr. Physiol. XXV 9, 457.

Rescigno, A., Stein, R.B., Purple, R.L. and Poppele, R.E., 1970.
  A neuronal model for the discharge patterns produced by cyclic
  inputs.   Bull. Math. Biophys. 32, 337-353.

Rosenthal, N.P., McKean, T.A., Roberts, W.J. and Terzuolo, C.A.,
  1970.   Frequency analysis of stretch reflex and its main
  sybsystems in triceps surae muscles of the cat.   J. Neurophysiol.
  33, 713-749.

Rudjord, T., 1970a.   A second order mechanical model of muscle
  spindle primary endings.   Kybernetik 6, 205-215.

Rudjord, T., 1970b.   A mechanical model of the secondary endings
  of mammalian muscle spindles.   Kybernetik 7, 122-128.

Smith, R.S., 1966.   Properties of intrafusal muscle fibers.   In
  Muscular Afferents and Motor Control.   Almquist and Wiksell,
  Stockholm.   pp. 69-80.

Sokolove, P.G. and Cooke, I.M., 1971.   Inhibition of impulse
  activity in a sensory neuron by an electrogenic pump.   J. Gen.
  Physiol. 57, 125-163.

Stein, R.B. and French, A.S., 1970.   Models for transmission of
  information by nerve cells.   In Excitatory Synaptic Mechanisms.
  Universitetsforlaget, Oslo.   pp. 247-258.

Terzuolo, C.A., 1969.   Systems Analysis in Neurophysiology,
  Univ. of Minn., Minneapolis   280 pp.

Terzuolo, C.A. and Knox, C.K., 1971.   Static and dynamic behavior
  of the stretch receptor organ of Crustacea.   In Handbook of
  Sensory Physiology, Vol. I.   Springer-Verlag, Berlin. pp. 500-522.

Zerbst, E., Dittberner, K.-H., William, E., 1966.   Ansatze zur
  quantitativen Analyse der Nachrichtenaufnahme und-verarbeitung
  in biologischen Rezeptoren.   Helgolander Wiss.   Meersunters.
  14, 51-71.

NON-LINEAR BEHAVIOUR OF SPINDLE RECEPTORS

J. C. Houk*, D. A. Harris and Z. Hasan*

Department of Physiology, Harvard University
Medical School, Boston, Massachusetts

Non-linear characteristics of primary and secondary spindle receptors were studied in decerebrate cats with and without intact ventral roots. Inputs consisted of slow ramp stretches and releases applied to the soleus muscle. Highly reproducible departures from a smooth change in discharge rate occurred during constant velocity stretching. When the stretch was more rapid, the departures were earlier and resembled initial bursts. Responses of each receptor to a family of ramps of constant duration and variable amplitude were used to construct "linearity plots". These plots demonstrated a transition from a region of high sensitivity to a region of low sensitivity that was evident during the stretch (or release), during adaptation, and in the steady state. Transition in sensitivity was associated with a particular change in length (100-200 µm). The high sensitivity to small changes in length reset after a receptor had adapted to a new length. All of these non-linearities could result from friction in the poles of intrafusal fibres. Non-linear behaviour was most conspicuous for de-efferented primary endings and least for secondary endings that received spontaneous gamma input. Stretch reflexes studied simultaneously reflected in their properties some of the non-linear features of spindle receptors, but the stretch reflex appears not to be a simple additive result of feedback from primary and secondary endings.

---

* Present Address: Department of Physiology, Johns Hopkins University School of Medicine, Baltimore, Maryland

INTRODUCTION

Primary receptors in muscle spindles are very responsive to
small changes in length, but when the applied stretch is greater
than a fraction of a millimiter, the responses do not increase
proportionately (Matthews and Stein, 1969; Poppele and Bowman,
1970; Goodwin and Matthews, 1971; Hasan and Houk, 1972). The
transition to a lower sensitivity is also accompanied by marked
modifications in dynamic properties (Houk, 1972; Matthews,
1972). Both aspects of the transition represent highly non-linear
behaviour. We have attempted to study directly the non-linearity
of spindle receptors by including as inputs ramp stretches and
releases which slowly cross the transitional region. Our earlier
results were restricted to de-efferented primary endings (Hasan
and Houk, 1972). The present study includes responses of secondary endings, in addition to primary endings, studied both in the
absence and in the presence of spontaneous gamma activity.

METHODS

Most of the data were obtained from cats decerebrated under
ether by an intercollicular transection, but the results shown in
Fig. 2 were from anaesthetized cats (pentobarbital). The dissected
soleus muscle was bathed in mineral oil (37° C), the limb was
denervated, and standard procedures were employed to identify
discharges of single primary and secondary endings recorded
from filaments of dorsal root. When spontaneous gamma activity
was to be preserved, a small filament was teased from the otherwise intact dorsal roots. In de-efferented studies, L7 and S1
dorsal and ventral roots were cut soon after the decerebration.

Changes in muscle length were produced by one of two electro-
magnetic pullers controlled by feedback systems. The system
associated with the more powerful puller had some friction which
caused the applied stretch to depart slightly from a ramp waveform
at the beginning of the stretch. The departure was brief (less than
50 msec for a ramp lasting 2 sec) and amounted to less than 4% of
the final amplitude of the ramp. This irregularity probably contributes to the discontinuities marked by dots in Fig. 3, but not to
those marked by arrows since they occurred when the ramp was
perfectly smooth. Ramps delivered by the small system were
smooth throughout.

Muscular force was continuously monitored with a strain gauge transducer and the operating length of the muscle was recorded with reference to maximum physiologic length (Houk et al., 1971). With spontaneous gamma activity, spindles were usually studied at lengths ranging from -16 to -4 mm compared to maximum physiologic length. When the ventral roots were cut it was necessary to stretch the muscle more (-8 to 0 mm) to provide a resting discharge. A PDP-12 computer was used on-line to record length, force and interpulse intervals. Intervals were measured with 1 msec accuracy and recorded sequentially; length and force were sampled at 30 msec intervals. All analysis was done off-line.

Responses of de-efferented spindles were sufficiently free of noise and repeatable (cf. Fig. 2) for making measurements and conclusions from single responses. Standard deviations among the responses ranged from 1.5-3.7 pps and standard deviations for the measurements used in constructing linearity plots ranged from 1-2.8 pps. When the ventral roots were intact, however, spontaneous gamma activity caused a considerable increase in variability both among responses (standard deviation ranged from 3-16 pps) and for the measurements from them (standard deviation ranged from 3-11 pps). This variability and our procedures for dealing with it are illustrated in Fig. 1. Traces A illustrate two responses to an identical stretch of a primary ending in a decerebrate preparation with intact ventral roots. Traces B illustrate the same responses after a certain amount of digital filtering (averaging instantaneous frequency over a certain number of successive intervals). Digital filtering decreases high frequency noise; however, low frequency noise is still apparent in the individual records or in variability between records. Trace D illustrates the result of averaging an ensemble of 14 responses (such as those in traces A). The instantaneous frequencies of each record of the ensemble were sampled every 30 msec; these samples were then averaged and plotted at the appropriate time, producing the ensemble average plot illustrated in trace D. Ensemble averaging over a sufficient number of records reduces noise of both high and low frequencies.

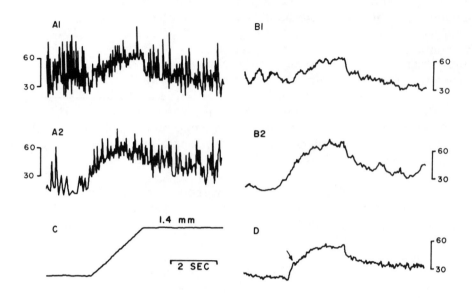

Fig. 1. Response obtained in the presence of spontaneous gamma activity. Traces A illustrate two responses to the ramp stretch shown in trace C; considerable variability is apparent. Traces B show the same responses after digital filtering; low frequency noise is still present as is variability between responses. Trace D is ensemble average of 14 responses (including those in traces A). Ensemble averaging produces clear records from which reliable observations may be made. Arrow points to a discontinuity which occurs at 145 μm. Primary ending, 112 m/sec (conduction velocity); operating length of muscle, -12 mm (with respect to maximal physiologic length).

RESULTS

Discontinuities

Responses of four de-efferented spindle receptors recorded while the soleus muscle was stretched at low velocities are shown in Fig. 2. For each ending one or more departures from a smooth change in discharge rate occurred during the constant velocity phase of the stretch. These departures, which we have

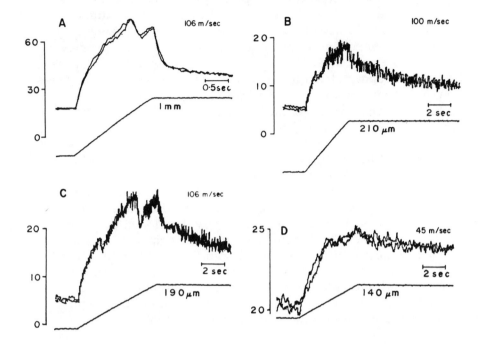

F i g . 2. Comparison of two successive responses to the
same ramp stretch in the case of four de-efferented endings,
three primaries (A, B and C) and one secondary (D). The responses show one or more discontinuities in their slope; superposition of two responses in each case demonstrates the
repeatability of the discontinuities. The period of waiting
between stretches was either 2 or 3 minutes. The discharge
rates (pps) are shown on the ordinate scales. Stretch waveforms and time scales are indicated. The smaller of the two
stretching devices was employed. For A and D, the instantaneous
discharge rates were smoothed by a first order low-pass filter
whose cross-over frequency was 1. 8 Hz. Conduction velocities
of the afferent axons are indicated.

called "discontinuities" (Hasan and Houk, 1972), are quite reproducible as illustrated by the superposition of two responses for
each receptor in Fig. 2. Since the stretch is smoothly applied and
since the discontinuity occurs at different amounts of stretch for
different receptors, the discontinuities are not due to an artifact
created by the stretching device.

Both primary and secondary receptors exhibit discontinuities in their responses (Fig. 2). The point at which the first discontinuity occurs depends mainly on the amount of stretch (typically 50-500 μm), but increases slightly with velocity. In the presence of spontaneous gamma activity, it is usually impossible to determine whether discontinuities are present unless ensemble averages are constructed (arrow in Fig. 1). Two more examples of discontinuities in responses of primary endings with spontaneous gamma activity are illustrated by the ensemble averages in Fig. 3.

The "initial burst" commonly observed when stretching at high velocities appears to be related to the discontinuities seen with slower stretches. Fig. 3 shows, for three primary endings, that as the amplitude of the ramp was increased the discontinuities (arrows) occurred earlier and progressively developed the appearance of initial bursts. This result demonstrates that the initial burst is only coincidentally associated with the acceleration that occurs at the beginning of a stretch. More properly, the initial burst and discontinuities reflect non-linear behaviour. This follows from the observation that the position in time of the discontinuity changes when the ramp is altered by a constant scaling factor.

Linearity Plots

The discontinuities appeared to be associated with the transition from the small-signal region of high sensitivity to the large-signal region of low sensitivity. In most cases the slope of a response following a discontinuity was much less than before (Fig. 3). The change in sensitivity was also evident in those portions of the response which followed termination of the ramp. For example, the adaptation phases of the responses of the first primary ending in Fig. 3 to 0.2 and 2.0 mm ramps are quite similar although the stretch differed by an order of magnitude.

To investigate this transition quantitatively, we have used a particular type of input-output graph which we call a "linearity plot". Its construction requires the responses to any family of inputs which differ from each other by scaling factors. The family that we used consisted of ramp stretches and releases as illustrated in the lower left of Fig. 4. The responses to each of the inputs are superimposed in the upper left. The linearity plot is shown on the right.

Primary Ending (91 m/sec), De-efferented, Single Responses

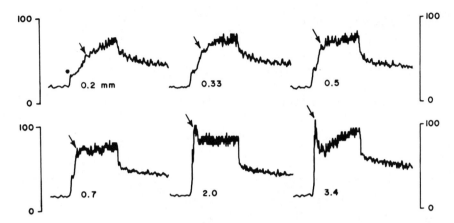

Primary Ending (110 m/sec), Spontaneous γ, Ensemble Averages

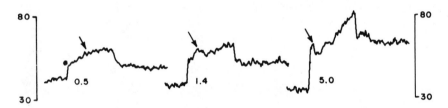

Primary Ending (105 m/sec), Spontaneous γ, Ensemble Averages

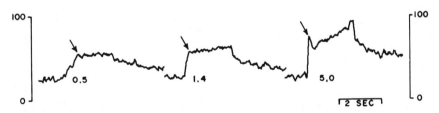

Fig. 3. Responses of three primary endings in two different preparations to ramp stretches of various amplitudes. The amplitude of the stretch (mm) is indicated for each response. The dynamic phase of stretching lasts slightly more than 2 sec in each case. Time calibration (lower right hand corner) applies to all records. Ordinate scales are discharge rates (pps).

Fig. 3, continued: Arrows point to discontinuities in the
responses; for the larger velocities, the discontinuities
appear as initial bursts. The stretch corresponding to points
marked by arrows in the case of the de-efferented ending was
between 70 and 90 μm as determined from an expanded display.
For the other two endings the ranges were 250-350 μm, and
70-100 μm respectively. The second ending shows a progressive
decline in discharge rate which is not an infrequent finding
when large stretches are applied. In many cases there were
initial irregularities (●) caused by one puller (Methods).
Responses for the three endings were obtained at operating
lengths of -4, -8 and -12 mm respectively. The averaged
responses were obtained from ensembles of 8-11 individual
responses.

Each of the plotted points represents, for a single input-response
pair, the difference between the discharge rate at a particular
time (T_1 or T_2) and the initial rate prior to the ramp (at time T_0).
This value is plotted along the ordinate and the change in length at
the same point in time is plotted along the abscissa. Points representing measurements at corresponding times made from other
input-response pairs are joined by straight lines to form the curves
labelled T_1 and T_2. The curve labelled "steady state" is constructed
from comparisons between initial rates prior to release and those
prior to stretch. For a linear system all the curves would be
straight lines through the origin since the input waveforms differ
only by scaling factors. The departures from straight lines
through the origin indicate non-linear behaviour.

The curves illustrate clearly that this secondary ending behaved
non-linearly during the dynamic phase of the stretch (or release),
during the phase of adaptation just after completion of the ramp
and in the steady state. The transitions in sensitivity were quite
pronounced. For example, concerning the adaptation phase the
sensitivity for small changes in length was about 40 pps/mm,
which is the slope near the origin of curve T_2. When stretches
larger than 200 μm were applied, the sensitivity to further change
in length was only 3 pps/mm. The non-linearity associated with
all three phases became pronounced when the stretch exceeded a
transitional amplitude of approximately 200 μm, but some non-
linearity was apparent for smaller stretches. The non-linearity
associated with release appeared to be similar, although its
study for this receptor was hampered because the discharge fell
below threshold.

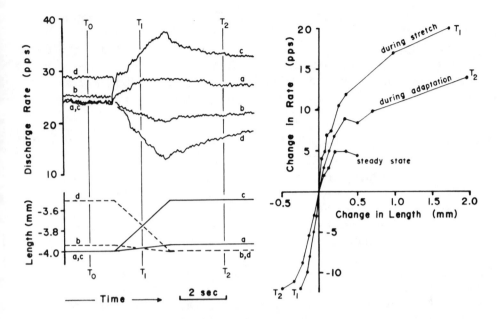

Fig. 4. Construction of Linearity Plot. Part A shows responses of a de-efferented secondary ending (34 m/sec) to two
ramp stretches and two ramp releases. Length is with respect
to maximum physiologic extension. Each input response pair
can be identified by the lower case letters which label the
traces at each end. Linearity plot in B is constructed from
measurements of discharge rate and muscle length at the
discrete times T_0, T_1, T_2. Change in rate, the ordinate in B,
is the difference between discharge rate at time of measurement (T_1 or T_2) and rate prior to stretch or release (T_0); the
abscissa is corresponding change in length. Measurements
from many input response pairs at the corresponding point in
time were joined to obtain curves T_1 and T_2. The curve
labelled steady state was derived from the difference in discharge rate prior to releasing and prior to stretching (at
time T_0). Releases larger than 0.5 mm were not used in this
experiment. Departures from straight lines passing through
the origin indicate non-linearity. This secondary ending
behaved non-linearly during the dynamic phase of stretching
(curve T_1), during adaptation (curve T_2) and in the steady
state.

The linearity plot also illustrates the dynamic sensitivity of
this receptor. Curve T_1 provides a measure of the dynamic

responsiveness that can be compared for different sizes of stretch with the responsiveness during adaptation which, in this case, was computed approximately 2 sec after the termination of the ramp (curve T$_2$). This in turn exceeds the steady stage responsiveness of this secondary ending. Thus, a linearity plot illustrates quite effectively the salient non-linear and dynamical characteristics of a receptor.

Three more linearity plots are shown in Fig. 5. Together with the plot in Fig. 4, they illustrate our typical findings for the four categories: primary and secondary endings with and without spontaneous gamma activity. The greatest departures from linearity were those of de-efferented primary endings and the most linear behaviour occurred with secondary endings when the ventral roots were intact.

An abstraction that is useful in describing and comparing linearity plots is to consider that the curves are constituted in each quadrant by two straight-line segments. One passes through the origin and has a steep slope corresponding to a high sensitivity. The other segment has a shallow slope corresponding to a low sensitivity and, when extrapolated to zero stretch, has an offset in rate. The intersection of the two segments specifies an idealized value for the transitional amplitude whereas the transition actually occurs over a small range of amplitudes. Most linearity plots fit this simple model fairly well, but a few did not. In those cases in which the fit was reasonable (judged by eye), the parameters of the straight lines were tabulated. The averages for some of these parameters are listed for comparison in Table 1.

The high sensitivity to small increases in length of de-efferented primary endings was reduced by spontaneous gamma activity, but it was still considerably greater than the sensitivity to large stretch. A similar trend is evident for secondary endings. Gamma activity also tends to make the characteristics associated with release more like those associated with stretch, as illustrated by the linearity plots but not included in the table. Two indicators of departure from linearity are the offset in rate and the ratio of sensitivity to small and large stretch. Primary receptors depart more from linear behaviour than do secondary endings. Both receptors behave more linearly when there is spontaneous gamma activity. In all cases the transitional amplitudes are similar; our estimate of approximately 100-200 μm agrees well with the results of Matthews and Stein (1969).

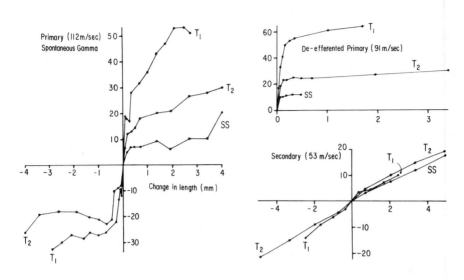

Fig. 5. Linearity plots for two primary and one secondary ending under conditions indicated. In each case the abscissa is the change in length (mm) and the ordinate the change in discharge rate (pps). (cf. legend to Fig. 4.) Departure from linearity is greatest for the de-efferented primary ending and least for the secondary ending with spontaneous fusimotor activity. Averaged responses were used for the construction of plots in the two cases with spontaneous gamma activity, digitally filtered for the primary and ensemble averaged for the secondary. The operating length was -12 mm in these cases and -4 mm for the de-efferented primary. The latter was the same receptor whose responses were shown in the upper part of Fig. 3. Responses of the other primary were illustrated in Fig. 1.

Resetting of the High Sensitivity to Small Changes in Length

The high sensitivity of spindle receptors to small changes in length is not a characteristic feature for a particular length of the muscle nor for a particular rate of discharge. Rather, it re-establishes itself at each operating point. This striking feature of spindle non-linearity is illustrated for a primary ending with spontaneous gamma activity in the upper part of Fig. 6. At each of a succession of steady state operating points, indicated by the

	de-efferented primary (6)	spontaneous γ primary (7)	de-efferented secondary (5)	spontaneous γ secondary (4)
sensitivity to "small" stretches (pps/mm):				
during stretch	293(155)	167(61)	128(90)	22(8)
during adaptation	131(91)	69(39)	98(37)	25(7.5)
amplitude of transition from "small" to "large" stretches (μm):				
during stretch	116(34)	110(34)	134(31)	205(135)
during adaptation	167(53)	182(82)	150(51)	138(16)
"offset" in response to large stretches (pps):				
during stretch	29(17)	16(6)	14(8)	2.5(.5)
during adaptation	17(9)	8.5(4.9)	14(5)	1.7(1.1)
in steady state	10(3)	5.3(3.6)	7.5(2.2)	1.7(1.1)
sensitivity to "large" stretches (pps/mm):				
during stretch	17(8)	13(9)	12(11)	5.2(2.3)
during adaptation	2.4(.6)	3.3(2.4)	3.7(2.5)	4.0(1.2)
in steady state	1.5(.5)	2.2(3.1)	1.7(2.0)	3.5(1.5)

Table 1. Parameters obtained from linearity plots. The captions "during stretch", "during adaptation" and "in steady state" refer to curves T1, T2 and SS respectively. Two straight line segments are fit to each curve by eye, the one for "small" stretches goes through the origin and the other one, for "large" stretches, has a y-intercept referred to as "offset". The numbers in the table are averages; the standard deviations of the sample are given in parentheses after each average. The number of examples are in parentheses after each category.

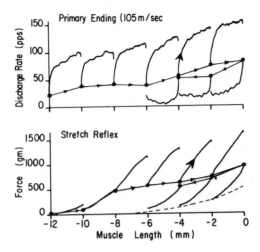

Fig. 6. Above - discharge rates of a primary ending in response to 2 mm ramp stretches and releases (at 1 mm/sec)
applied at different muscle lengths. The abscissa is the muscle
length measured with respect to the maximum physiologic length.
The ordinate is the discharge rate of the primary ending in a
decerebrate preparation with spontaneous fusimotor activity.
Points denote average discharge rates in the steady state.
The responses of the ending are plotted during the dynamic
phase of stretch (or release) as a function of instantaneous
muscle length (e. g. the large arrowhead). At each operating
length, from 6 to 9 responses to the same change in length
were obtained waiting 20 sec between the records. The records
of the responses were ensemble averaged and plotted after a
small amount of time averaging (over 150 msec) to reduce the
high frequency noise. The operating lengths were increased
from -12 mm to 0 in 2 mm steps and then decreased as indicated by the small arrows. Below - muscle force as a function
of instantaneous muscle length in the same decerebrate preparation. Points denote average forces in the steady state. Ensemble
averaged responses of the forces (e. g. the large arrowhead) to
2 mm ramp stretches and releases (at 1 mm/sec) are shown at
different operating lengths. The records of force from which
the ensemble averages were computed were obtained simultaneously with the records of the responses of the spindle
ending depicted above. The dashed line shows the (passive)
force recorded from the tendon after the muscle nerve was cut.

filled circles, a series of 2 mm ramp changes in length were applied at a velocity of 1 mm/sec. The ensemble averages of each series were calculated and then plotted as trajectories on a graph of discharge rate versus muscle length. The force responses of the muscle recorded simultaneously are plotted in a similar manner in the lower part of Fig. 6, but will not be referred to again until the Discussion.

The large arrow in Fig. 6 (upper part) shows the direction of the change in rate and length for one trajectory. It consists of a steeply rising portion that corresponds with the region of high sensitivity. The flattening of the trajectory accompanying further stretch reflects the transition to a lower sensitivity. The vertically descending portion corresponds to the first portion of the adaptation to the new length. All of the trajectories in response to stretch are basically similar. Those to release also show an initial high sensitivity that later flattens. This resetting phenomenon thus consists of an adaptation to any operating length following which a spindle receptor will respond with high sensitivity to small changes in length about that operating point (also see Matthews, 1972). Interestingly, a similar phenomenon has been shown to occur in certain vertebrate visual receptors (Werblin, 1973).

DISCUSSION

The Hypothesis for Friction in Intrafusal Fibres

Certain after-effects of gamma stimulation studied by Brown et al. (1969) suggested to them that intrafusal muscle fibres possessed a frictional property which they called stiction. This property, they argued, was responsible for the initial burst in responses of primary endings to rapid stretch. The hypothesis for friction was subsequently elaborated as an explanation for the small signal region of high sensitivity for primary endings and for resetting (Matthews, 1970, 1972; Houk, 1972; Hasan and Houk, 1972). The arguments can be summarized as follows.

The striated regions of intrafusal fibres possess friction, probably as a result of resting bonds between actin and myosin (cf. Hill, 1968). Friction in the poles of bag fibres results in greater initial rigidity which allows the sparsely striated equatorial region, including primary endings, to stretch disproportionately.

The high sensitivity that results gives way to much lower sensitivity
when the friction in the poles ruptures. The subsequent resetting
of high sensitivity occurs when the intrafusal fibre adapts to a
new length allowing the friction to re-establish intself. The discontinuities, and the initial bursts, capture the moments of
rupture.

The present results lend support to this hypothesis in several
ways. First, they demonstrate a close relationship between discontinuities and initial bursts permitting a single explanation for
the two. Second, they demonstrate that the transition in sensitivity
for all phases (dynamic, adaptation and steady state) occurs at a
certain amount of stretch or release. Matthews and Stein (1969)
had suggested earlier that the transition corresponded to a certain
modulation in rate which might be explained as resulting from
non-linear properties of transduction rather than mechanical
friction. Third, our results indicate an approximate correspondence between the transitional amplitude and the amplitudes
at which discontinuities occur, although the latter appear to occupy
a broader range.

The non-linear behaviour of de-efferented secondary receptors
was unexpected. Chain fibres, upon which secondary endings lie,
would not cause mechanical amplification of the sort postulated for
the bag fibre if friction were distributed uniformly along their
lengths. The rather uniform distribution of striations along chain
fibres may not, however, reflect accurately the distribution of
contractile activity and friction. The well known fact that secondary
receptors increase their rates of discharge when static gamma
fibres are stimulated implies a greater contraction of the poles of
chain fibres than of regions beneath a secondary ending. We
therefore propose that a distribution of friction favouring the poles
of chain fibres causes mechanical amplification that is responsible
for the high sensitivity region of de-efferented secondary endings.
Their more linear behaviour with spontaneous gamma activity
may be analogous to the melting of friction during contraction of
extrafusal muscle fibres reported by Hill (1968).

Effects of Spindle Non-Linearity on Reflex Contractions

When spindles receive the spontaneous gamma activity present
in decerebrate cats, secondary endings behave nearly linearly
whereas primary endings present a complex behaviour including a

transition in sensitivity and non-linear adaptation. If the stretch reflex depends on feedback from primary and secondary receptors, it should reflect in its properties the characteristics of these receptors. Matthews (1969) has described a transition in the stiffness of the stretch reflex which may correspond to the transition in sensitivity of primary endings. In one case in which a primary ending and the stretch reflex were studied simultaneously, we compared the linearity of the two. The linearity of the stretch reflex exceeded greatly the linearity of this and other primary endings. One might explain this result as due to a dominance of feedback from secondary receptors. However, the stretch reflex showed an appreciable adaptation over a period of many seconds which secondary endings did not. Since this is typical behaviour for primary receptors, the opposite conclusion, that primary receptors dominate the stretch reflex, might be drawn. These speculations neglect feedback from tendon organs (Houk et al., 1970) and the inherent mechanical stiffness of the muscle (Grillner, 1972).

The resetting feature of the high sensitivity region of spindle receptors is also shown by the stretch reflex. Simultaneous comparisons of the trajectories followed by muscular force and the discharge rate of a primary ending were illustrated in Fig. 6 for 2 mm stretches and releases applied at 1 mm/sec. Even at this slow velocity of stretch, which is often taken to yield a "tonic" stretch reflex, there remains a very considerable adaptation to each operating length, which is probably equivalent to the plasticity of the reflex described by Sherrington (1909). Again we have the paradox that the adaptation of primary endings could explain that of the reflex, but left unexplained is the different shape of the trajectories during the applications of stretch. Those of primary endings are typically flattened while those of the reflex are more linear. Perhaps a more quantitative consideration of muscular properties and force feedback from tendon organs, in addition to feedback from primary and secondary spindle receptors, will lead to a more adequate explanation of the stretch reflex. But, the possibility of complex interactions within the central nervous system should not be neglected.

REFERENCES

Brown, M.C., Goodwin, G.M. and Matthews, P.B.C., 1969. After-
effects of fusimotor stimulation on the response of muscle
spindle primary afferent endings. J. Physiol. 205,
677-694.

Goodwin, G.M. and Matthews, P.B.C., 1971. Effects of fusimotor
stimulation on the sensitivity of muscle spindle endings to
small-amplitude sinusoidal stretching. J. Physiol.
218, 56-58P.

Grillner, S., 1972. The role of muscle stiffness in meeting the
changing postural and locomotor requirements for force development by the ankle extensors. Acta Physiol. Scand. 86, 92-108.

Hasan, Z. and Houk, J.C., 1972. Nonlinear behavior of primary
spindle receptors in response to small, slow ramp stretches.
Brain Res. 44, 680-683.

Hill, D.K., 1968. Tension due to interaction between the sliding
filaments in resting striated muscle. The effect of stimulation.
J. Physiol. 199, 637-684.

Houk, J.C., 1972. A comment on paradoxical properties of primary
and secondary endings. In Research Concepts in Muscle Development and the Muscle Spindle. (Ed. Banker, B. et al.) Excerpta
Medica, Amsterdam. pp. 337-340.

Houk, J.C., Singer, J.J. and Goldman, M.R., 1970. An evaluation
of length and force feedback to soleus muscles of decerebrate
cats. J. Neurophysiol. 33, 784-811.

Houk, J.C., Singer, J.J. and Henneman, E., 1971. Adequate stimulus for tendon organs with observations on mechanics of ankle
joint. J. Neurophysiol. 34, 1051-1065.

Matthews, P.B.C., 1969. Evidence that the secondary as well as
the primary endings of the muscle spindles may be responsible
for the tonic stretch reflex of the decerebrate cat. J.
Physiol. 204, 365-394.

Matthews, P.B.C., 1970. The origin and functional significance
of the stretch reflex. In Excitatory Synaptic Mechanisms.
(Ed. Andersen, P. and Jansen, J.K.S.) Oslo Universitetsforlaget,
pp. 301-315.

Matthews, P.B.C., 1972. Mammalian Muscle Receptors and Their
Central Actions. Williams and Wilkins Co., Baltimore.

Matthews, P.B.C. and Stein, R.B., 1969. The sensitivity of muscle
spindle afferents to small sinusoidal changes in length. J.
Physiol. 200, 723-743.

Poppele, R.E. and Bowman, R.J., 1970. Quantitative description of
linear behavior of mammalian muscle spindles. J. Neurophysiol.
33, 59-72.

Sherrington, C.S., 1909. On plastic tonus and proprioceptive
reflexes. Quart. J. Exp. Physiol. 2, 109-156.

Werblin, F.S., 1973. The control of sensitivity in the retina.
Sci. Amer. 228(1), 70-79.

DISCUSSION SUMMARY

R. Granit

Nobel Institute for Neurophysiology, Karolinska
Institutet, Stockholm, Sweden

The papers by Kernell, by Burke et al., by Wyman, and
Stephens et al. initiated a discussion along two main lines:
(1) the order of the recruitment of neurones into activity, and
(2) the general validity of the classification of motoneurones
by the indices applied by Burke et al. A sideline was introduced by Wyman in taking up the problem of how nerve fibres
find their way to the next synaptic station. Wyman introduced
a hypothesis based on their successive occupation of nuclei
according to a somatotopic or 'place' principle. However, an
array of arguments in favour of the generally accepted notion
of 'specificity' followed from the floor. In particular, it was
pointed out that microelectrode recordings of cells only
100 μm apart could reveal entirely different sets of connections
and properties.

To (1) above, the order of recruitment in Kernell's work
was statistically speaking according to spike amplitude, but
exceptions were common. The order, however, was never
completely reversed to a recruitment beginning with large and
ending with small spikes. Wyman, when asked whether or not
his results agreed with the size principle, could only maintain
that the order of recruitment in his pairs was variable but that
this technique was not relevant to the main issue of spike
size. Burke reminded the participants of the physical reasons
for the lower threshold of the smaller cells of an ensemble and
regarded the "size principle" as a useful general concept holding
together a large body of information. However, he also pointed
out that in intracellular studies one finds many neurones of
different size excited by a stimulus causing actual firing in the

165

subgroup of fibres to which work at the split filament or split
nerve level is restricted. Basmajian's experience also was that
generally neurones are recruited in the order of increasing
spike size but that by training, a subject can make any unit fire
at will. In passing, it was pointed out that there are published
papers showing reversal of the order of recruitment according
to spike size.

To (2), Dr. V. G. Edgerton (U. C. L. A., Los Angeles)
summarized his comments on the papers by Burke and Stephens
as follows:

"The wide range of motor units in terms of the fatigue
index pointed out by Dr. Stephens but seen only rarely by
Dr. Burke would seem to be contradictory to some degree.
Since the histochemical enzyme and substrate profiles
have been shown repeatedly to reflect the dynamic as well
as the fatigue properties (oxidative enzymes and blood
supply) one would expect a more frequent appearance of
motor units that would be 'unclassified' or fall between
the extremes of the FR and FF units with respect to
fatigue properties as Dr. Stephens has demonstrated in
'Arizona' cats. The histochemistry of the cat medial
gastrocnemius shows a wide range of oxidative enzyme
activities (NADH-D) among the fast-twitch fibres. A
logical explanation for the difference is the history and
prior care of the cat. For example, it has been shown
that in rats and guinea pigs several weeks of physical
endurance training results in a shift from fast-twitch,
low oxidative, high glycolytic fibres (FF) to fast-twitch,
high oxidative, high glycolytic fibres (FR) and that this
shift is accompanied by a greater resistance to fatigue.
Similar histochemical results have been found in human
muscle. Therefore, the difference in the population
distribution with respect to the fatigue index as seen by
Drs. Burke and Stephens could very well be reflecting the
condition of the cat with regards to physical activity, or
inactivity."

Burke did not see any fundamental difference of opinion between
himself and Stephens. A classification based on fatigue index
was valuable although it is likely to be dependent on the history
of the animal. His own data on the medial gastrocnemius could
not be directly transposed to muscles differently composed, but

because this muscle had a broad range of fibre types it would show up a large spectrum of fibre properties.

A brief discussion of human motor units followed upon the paper of Stein and Milner-Brown. This work re-excited the discussion of recruitment orders by the observation that after accidental severance of a nerve and subsequent regeneration, the original recruitment of units according to increasing twitch tensions was lost. The point was raised that the effect might have been due to permanent loss of spindles. However, it is known from earlier work and was emphasized by Laporte that the evidence is all in favour of regeneration of spindle function. Dr. McComas was unable to attend the conference due to pressing family problems. His manuscript has been included and Drs. W.F. Brown (University of Western Ontario, London, Canada) and R.G. Lee (Toronto Western Hospital and University of Toronto) presented studies related to those of Dr. McComas.

Brown described work which critically assessed electro-myographic techniques used for estimating the number of motor units in the thenar muscles of man. These methods have been developed by McComas et al. and by Brown's group for estimating the number of motor units in human foot and hand muscles. Healthy humans less than age 60 have thenar motor unit estimates of 275 $\pm$ 75 S.D. (range 193 - 586). Older subjects often showed a substantial drop in the number of functioning motor units. The estimates are obtained by dividing the maximum compound muscle action potential by an average of the first several motor unit potential steps, as activated to threshold value by a graded electrical stimulus to the motor nerve. The methods, though simple in concept, involve a number of assumptions including:

(1) the order of activation of motor axons is constant during the repeated changes in the stimulus intensity that are necessary to demonstrate superimposition of individual unit potential steps.

(2) The position of the recording electrode does not favour motor units of equivalent anatomical size but closer proximity to the recording electrode, or, if so, that the order of activation of motor units of varying distances from the electrode is random.

(3) That the first few motor unit potentials are representative of the whole motor unit population. Individual
motor unit potentials cannot be separated reliably above
the first 10 - 20 successive unit step potentials. This
means, that in healthy subjects, the motor unit estimate
may be based on as few as 2 - 10% of the estimated
motor unit population. Motor unit potentials with higher
stimulus thresholds may, however, be sampled by
studying the size of single recurrent (F) motor unit
potential discharges appearing at stimulus intensities
from threshold to supramaximal for the direct response.
Only motor unit potentials of identical bi- or triphasic
configuration and constant latency (variation in
latency <500 μsec) were considered to be single motor
unit discharges.

In controls and pathological nerves, single motor unit
recurrent discharges, appearing at stimulus intensities well
above that of the first several unit potentials, may be many
times the size of the average unit potential used to estimate the
number of motor units. For example, in one control subject
with an average thenar unit potential size of 47 μV (control
53 ± 11 μV; mean ± S. D.) there were four single recurrent
motor unit discharges were twenty times the average
unit potential size. This suggests,that there may be a mixed
population of small and large motor units in the thenar muscles.
Motor unit estimates, biased by an average unit potential size
based on a population of small motor units, may be misleadingly
high.

An apparent loss of motor units in pathologically altered
nerve may result not only from motor axon loss, but may also
be due to conduction block in remaining motor axons. In human
neuropathies, known to be associated with substantial demyelin-
ation, cooling and warming the forearm has shown a reversible
conduction block in many thenar muscle motor axons.

Dr. Lee described two lines of work. The first, done in
collaboration with Dr. A. J. Aguayo (Montreal) provided anatomical
evidence which was consistent with Brown's physiological estimates of the number of motor units in thenar muscles. The
second, done in collaboration with Dr. Ashby (Toronto Western
Hospital) used the averaging techniques described by Stein to
obtain the contributions of single motor units to the surface EMG.

These could then be used to reconstruct thè compound action potential obtained by nerve stimulation, and also provided another method of determining the number of motor units in a muscle.

DISCUSSION SUMMARY

P. B. C. Matthews

University Laboratory of Physiology
Oxford, England

The discussion of this session was largely concerned with matters of detail following individual papers; these lose interest outside their original context and will not be related. The two initial papers on crustacean and amphibian motor units by Drs. Atwood and Smith, respectively, evoked a special interest by providing models of motor organization which may be more applicable to the mammalian muscle spindle than are the motor units of the cat gastrocnemius. Two points which received emphasis were that a single motor axon may supply muscle fibres of quite different contractile properties, and that when a single muscle fibre is activated by two different axons it appears to respond similarly provided that the synaptic potentials are matched in size. Dr. Laporte's paper was supplemented later in the afternoon by a film of isolated muscle spindles prepared by Bessou and Pagès which showed the intrafusal contraction elicited by stimulating individual fusimotor fibres. Static fibres frequently caused contraction of both bag and chain intrafusal muscle fibres, whereas dynamic fibres affected only the bag intrafusal muscle fibres and not the chain fibres. In the discussion it seemed agreed that the controversies of the last ten years should now be laid to rest with honour for all parties, as all had been vindicated to some degree. The motor innervation still appears to show a degree of specificity with regard to intrafusal type, but not the simple arrangement with the bag and chain fibres each receiving an entirely private motor supply. The papers by Abrahams and by Fetz widened the perspective of the afternoon by emphasizing that the fascination of unravelling the internal working of the muscle spindle should not be allowed to distract attention from the problem of its

171

functional role in motor performance and the action of the spindle projections to higher levels of the nervous system. These points were returned to by several speakers after the papers by Poppele and by Houk, who both rebutted the charge that the stimuli they used were too small to be of significance for normal motor control. They emphasized that postural regulation demands very fine control of the muscles. On the other hand, the spindle can also be expected to be contributing to the control of large movements so that interest attaches equally to the study of their small linear range, their larger non-linear range and to the transitions between them.

A THIRD MODE OF REPETITIVE FIRING: SELF-REGENERATIVE FIRING DUE TO LARGE DELAYED DEPOLARIZATIONS

W. H. Calvin

Department of Neurological Surgery, University of Washington School of Medicine, Seattle, Washington

One may distinguish three modes of repetitive firing, each with a characteristic input-output relation: 1) an occasional spike mode; 2) a rhythmic firing mode; and 3) a self-regenerative firing mode where large depolarizing after-potentials may rise through the falling threshold several milliseconds after a spike, causing an extra spike. This extra spike may similarly produce an additional extra spike, etc. This self-regenerative behaviour produces spike timing patterns similar to those in the stereotyped high frequency bursts of epileptic and experimentally deafferented CNS neurones.

Fifteen years of intracellular studies into the repetitive firing properties of spinal motoneurones (e.g. Kolmodin and Skoglund, 1958; Kernell, 1965; Granit et al., 1966; Calvin and Schwindt, 1972) have suggested that there are two distinct modes of repetitive firing, which will be summarized here as 1) an occasional spike mode where synaptic depolarizations only occasionally cross threshold (at times long compared to spike after-potential durations), and 2) a rhythmic firing mode where prolonged depolarizing currents would produce a membrane potential above threshold were it not for the spike after-hyperpolarization. The large after-hyperpolarization interacts with the prolonged depolarizing currents to produce a subthreshold membrane potential

trajectory which intersects threshold at a predictable time after
the previous spike, i.e. rhythmic firing. Due to the way in
which this trajectory changes with current (Schwindt and Calvin,
1972; Schwindt, 1973), a rather linear relation between the current (injected through the recording microelectrode) and the
rhythmic firing rate (Kernell, 1965) is produced. This linear
input-output relation in the rhythmic firing mode is quite different from the conspiracy-to-cross-threshold type of input-output
relation seen in the occasional spike mode. We have further
shown (Schwindt and Calvin, 1973), by extending the work of
Kernell (1969), that prolonged synaptic inputs which change the
resting input resistance of the cat spinal motoneurone have
remarkably different effects on the two modes: While membrane
potential may be the "adequate stimulus" in the occasional spike
mode (more current is needed with a reduced input resistance to
reach a fixed voltage threshold) it is apparent that current is
the important parameter once it exceeds rheobasic levels and
the rhythmic firing mode is engaged.

One may additionally distinguish a third mode of repetitive
firing: a self-regenerative firing mode where depolarizing spike
after-potentials rise to intersect the falling threshold near the
end of the relative refractory period. Thus a normal spike
evoked by either the occasional or rhythmic mode may be followed
by an extra spike shortly thereafter. This mode was first seen
in crustacean stretch receptors (Eyzaguirre and Kuffler, 1955)
and in hippocampal pyramidal cells (Kandel and Spencer, 1961);
we have noted it during rhythmic firing of motoneurones (Calvin
and Schwindt, 1972). Here I describe some of the characteristics
of this self-regenerative cycle which may result in a burst of
spikes rather than a mere doublet (Calvin, in preparation).

Fig. 1A shows the rhythmic discharge resulting from a step
of injected current (top trace). The delayed depolarizations
(Kernell, 1964; Nelson and Burke, 1967; Calvin and Schwindt,
1972) following each rhythmic spike are exceptionally large in
this cat spinal motoneurone (cf. Fig. 4 in Calvin and Schwindt,
1972) but become less prominent with each successive spike
following the second rhythmic spike. Extra spikes often appear
after the second rhythmic spike (Fig. 1B) at slightly higher
current levels. Since threshold has typically recovered to normal levels by the time of the peak in the delayed depolarizations
(Calvin, in preparation), the delayed depolarizations in this case
would appear to have straddled threshold, often eliciting an extra

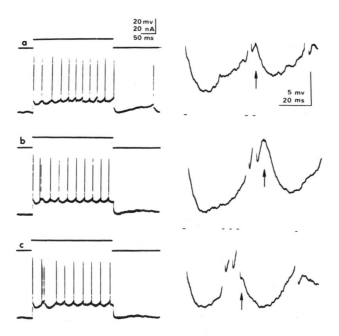

Fig. 1. Extra spikes arising from delayed depolarizations crossing the falling threshold. All records from a single motoneurone. A - Trial where no extra spikes occurred; note large hump-type delayed depolarizations starting with second spike but declining with later spikes. Left column shows injected current (upper) and membrane potential response (lower trace). Right column shows magnified versions (Calvin, 1973) of the early portions of the spike trains in the left column. B - Trial in which one extra spike is seen after second rhythmic spike. Note large delayed depolarizations following extra spike (arrow). C - Two extra spikes are seen following second rhythmic spike. Note smaller delayed depolarization after second extra spike (arrow). Threshold-straddling behaviour seen comparing A, B and C suggest delayed depolarizations cause a self-regenerative cycle to produce burst firing.

spike. Fig. 1B (arrow) indicates that the extra spike itself produces a large delayed depolarization ; Fig. 1C indicates that it sometimes evoked another extra spike, i.e. a self-regenerative cycle repeated twice to give three spikes where only one spike would have otherwise appeared.

The declining size of the delayed depolarization with successive spikes in the rhythmic train (cf. Fig. 6A in Calvin and Schwindt, 1972) may be sufficient to explain the termination of the self-regenerative cycle in such cells; the extra spikes might merely contribute to this "adaptation of the delayed depolarizations", thus shutting off the burst (Fig. 1C, arrow).

The input-output relation of the self-regenerative mode is essentially a multiplication factor atop the input-output relation of whatever mode is eliciting the normal spikes which trigger the self-regenerative cycle.

This self-regenerative mode of repetitive firing causes characteristic spike timing patterns, e.g. a stereotyped burst with interspike intervals shorter than the duration of the delayed depolarization. Neurones of the lateral cuneate nucleus often exhibit doublet and triplet firing patterns similar to those infrequently displayed by the motoneurones we have studied; when chronically deafferented (Kjerulf et al., 1973) they exhibit stereotyped high-frequency bursts. While such extracellular studies cannot determine the role of the delayed depolarizations, one may hypothesize that deafferentation exaggerates a normally active self-regenerative mode so that many more extra spikes are produced before shutoff.

Because delayed depolarizations are often seen in CNS neurones (for cortical PT cells, see Fig. 7 in Koike et al., 1970), the self-regenerative mode may be a latent property of many types of neurones. A striking characteristic of neurones in chronic epileptogenic foci is that some fire in high-frequency bursts (Calvin et al., 1968, 1973) whose stereotyped interspike intervals fit the self-regenerative pattern very well.

Acknowledgement: Supported in part by research grants NS 09677 and NS 04053 from the National Institutes of Health.

REFERENCES

Calvin, W.H., 1973. Computer-based "kymograph" for photographing raw neurophysiological data. J. Appl. Physiol. 34, 133-135.

Calvin, W.H., Ojemann, G.A. and Ward, A.A. Jr., 1973. Human cortical neurons in epileptogenic foci: comparison of inter-ictal firing patterns to those of 'epileptic' neurons in animals. Electroencephlogr. Clin. Neurophysiol. 34, 337-351.

Calvin, W.H. and Schwindt, P.C., 1972. Steps in production of motoneuron spikes during rhythmic firing. J. Neurophysiol. 35, 297-310.

Calvin, W.H., Sypert, G.W. and Ward, A.A. Jr., 1968. Structured timing patterns within bursts from epileptic neurons in un-drugged monkey cortex. Exp. Neurol. 21, 535-549.

Eyzaguirre, C. and Kuffler, S.W., 1955. Further study of soma, dendrite, and axon excitation in single neurons. J. Gen. Physiol. 39, 121-153.

Granit, R., Kernell, D. and Lamarre, Y., 1966. Algebraical summation in synaptic activation of motoneurons firing within the 'primary range' to injected currents. J. Physiol. 187, 379-399.

Kandel, E.R. and Spencer, W.A., 1961. Electrophysiology of hippocampal neurons. II. Afterpotentials and repetitive firing. J. Neurophysiol. 24, 243-259.

Kernell, D., 1964. The delayed depolarization in cat and rat motoneurons. Progr. Brain Res. 12, 42-55.

Kernell, D., 1965. The adaptation and the relation between dis-charge frequency and current strength of cat lumbosacral moto-neurons stimulated by long-lasting injected currents. Acta Physiol. Scand. 65, 65-73.

Kernell, D., 1969. Synaptic conductance changes and the repeti-tive impulse discharge of spinal motoneurons. Brain Res. 15, 291-294.

Kjerulf, T.D., O'Neal, J.T., Calvin, W.H., Loeser, J.D. and Westrum, L.E., 1973. Deafferentation effects in lateral cun-eate nucleus of the cat: correlation of structural alterations with firing pattern changes. Exp. Neurol. 39, 86-102.

Koike, H., Mano, N., Okada, Y. and Oshima, T., 1970. Repetitive impulses generated in fast and slow pyramidal tract cells by intracellularly applied current steps. Exp. Brain Res. 11, 263-281.

Kolmodin, G.M. and Skoglund, C.R., 1958. Slow membrane potential changes accompanying excitation and inhibition in spinal moto- and interneurons in the cat during natural activation. Acta Physiol. Scand. 44, 11-54.

Nelson, P.G. and Burke, R.E., 1967. Delayed depolarization in cat spinal motoneurons. Exp. Neurol. 17, 16-26.

Schwindt, P.C., 1973. Membrane potential trajectories underlying motoneuron rhythmic firing at high rates. J. Neurophysiol. 36, 434-449.

Schwindt, P.C. and Calvin, W.H., 1972. Membrane potential tra-jectories between spikes underlying motoneuron firing rates. J. Neurophysiol. 35, 311-325.

Schwindt, P.C. and Calvin, W.H., 1973. Equivalence of synaptic
   and injected current in determining the membrane potential trajectory during motoneuron rhythmic firing. Brain Res. 59,
   389-394.

FATIGABILITY OF MEDIAL GASTROCNEMIUS MOTOR UNITS IN THE CAT

J. A. Stephens*, R. L. Gerlach, R. M. Reinking
and D. G. Stuart

Department of Physiology, College of Medicine,
University of Arizona, Tuscon, Arizona

The physiological properties of motor units in cat medial
gastrocnemius have been studied with particular reference
to fatigue. A broad range of fatigability was encountered,
particularly within the fast twitch group. These findings
were consistent with the vascular and histochemical profile
of this muscle.

In a recent report, Burke et al. (1971) have presented evidence
which suggests that motor units of medial gastrocnemius of the
cat may be classified into three non-overlapping groups: type FF,
fast contracting, fast fatigue; type FR, fast contracting, fatigue
resistant; and type S, slowly contracting, fatigue resistant. It
was further found that each of these groups of motor units had a
characteristic histochemical profile and this was considered to
be consistent with the mechanical properties of the group. In our
laboratory we have used this classification scheme to show that
a single Golgi tendon organ will respond to contractions of different types of motor unit. During the course of these experiments
we encountered, however, many motor units (28 out of a total of
86 in 7 cats) whose fatigue profiles could not be classified into
either the S or FR categories (<25% fatigue in 2 mins) or the FF
(>75% fatigue in 2 mins) category. The stimulation procedure
used in this study for estimating the fatigability of a motor unit

---

* Home Address: Sherrington School of Physiology,
St. Thomas's Hospital Medical School, London, England

was identical to that suggested by Burke et al. (1971) except that
the muscle was held at the optimum length for tetanus of each
motor unit rather than a length corresponding to a passive tension of 80-100 gms for the whole muscle.

Fig. 1A shows fatigue test force profiles for typical fast fatigable and fatigue resistant motor units as reported by Burke et al.

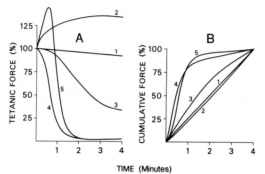

TIME (Minutes)

Fig. 1. Normalization of a motor unit fatigue test. A shows
the tetanic force developed by five different motor units (1 to
5) as a function of time during a 4 min fatigue test. Units were
stimulated at 40 pps for 330 msec of each second. The force
developed during the first tetanus is denoted as 100%. B shows
the same data displayed in the form of cumulative force profiles. The total force developed by each unit for all tetani
over a 4 min period is denoted as 100%.

(1971) together with three other profiles commonly encountered
in this study which: first potentiate then fatigue rapidly; display
gradual potentiation over a 4 min period; or, fatigue more than
25% but less than 75% after 2 mins stimulation. In order to compare such a broad array of responses, the cumulative force developed by each motor unit has been plotted, integrating over either
a 2 or 4 min period. In each case the total force developed has
been normalized to 100%. Fig. 1B shows how this procedure
results in a 45° line for fatigue resistant units, lines becoming
increasingly more concave to the time axis for units showing increased fatigability including those with limited periods of potentiation, and a line convex to the time axis for slowly potentiating
units.

Fig. 2 presents cumulative force profiles for 20 motor units
from a single experiment, 4 of which would be classified as type

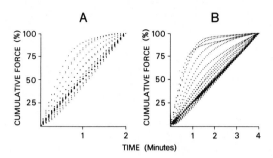

Fig. 2. Cumulative force profiles for 20 motor units studied
during a single experiment. In A, cumulative force profiles
are shown for the first 2 mins of stimulation, while in B the
integration period has been extended to include the force developed over the entire 4 mins of stimulation.

S by Burke et al. (1971) while the remaining 16 would be classified as fast units on the basis of contraction time and the "sag"
test (see Burke et al., 1971). For both the 2 and 4 min integration
periods this fast contracting population displays a broad spectrum
of cumulative fatigue profiles from fatigue resistant to highly
fatigable behaviour.

In order to quantitate these cumulative force profiles, the percentage accumulative force developed at 1 min for the 2 min integration period and 2 mins for the 4 min integration period was
noted. Such a fatigue index would be near 50% for a fatigue resistant unit and near 100% for a highly fatigable unit. Fig. 3 shows
the distribution of such fatigue indices for 86 motor units (seven
experiments), 15 of which are cross-hatched and correspond to
Burke et al.'s (1971) type S units (no "sag" and contraction
times from 39-83 msec). Note that the values for the type S
population are in the range 46-55% for both integration periods.
In contrast, the remaining 71 units (contraction times from 23-69
msec, and 65 with "sag" during unfused tetanus) exhibited a
broad range of values for the fatigue index. In particular, the
behaviour of these units cannot be classified into two distinct
populations on the basis of their cumulative fatigue profiles
taken over a 2 min period (see Fig. 3A). Rather, they have a
continuous distribution of fatigability over this time period. On
the other hand, if the cumulative sum is formed over a 4 min
period (Fig. 3B), the distribution of fatigue indices then becomes
concentrated at both ends of the fatigue scale. The type FR and

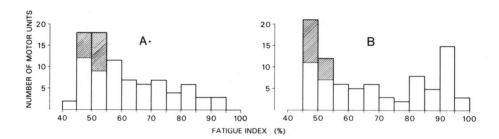

Fig. 3. Distribution of fatigability index based on cumulative force profiles. Each of 86 motor units (seven experiments) is assigned a fatigability index which in A is based on the percentage cumulative force developed at 1 min for a 2 min period of integration and in B at 2 mins for a 4 min integration period. Cross-hatching marks units which would be described as type S according to the Burke et al. (1971) nomenclature. All other units are fast contracting.

type FF units of Burke et al. (1971) fall into fatigue index bins 46-60% and 76-100% respectively. The remaining 28 units which could not be classified in this way have fatigue indices in the range 51-95% but are largely concentrated in the range 61-85 (21 out of 28), corresponding to an intermediate degree of fatigability.

The relative importance of contractile element fatigue in contrast to possible neuromuscular transmission failure during the fatigue test used in this study remains uncertain. Table 1 presents the average change in EMG amplitude associated with motor units falling into the fatigue index bins of Fig. 3. In general fatigue resistant units exhibited less reduction in EMG amplitude after both 2 and 4 min stimulation. Type S units showed similar EMG changes to fast contracting units in the same fatigue index range. However, there was a progressive reduction in EMG amplitude for the more fatigable fast contracting units. This contrast became more pronounced after 4 min stimulation. These findings differ from those of Burke et al. (1971) who found "usually little change" in EMG amplitude with fatigue. The reductions in EMG amplitude observed in this study might be expected for two reasons. First, the rapid loss of contractility observed

Fatigue Index (%)

Integration Period		41-45	46-50	51-55	56-60	61-65	66-70	71-75	76-80	81-85	86-90	91-95	96-100
2 Minutes	X̄	100	96	93	65	77	60	60	49	50	44	64	-
	Range	-	100-67	100-69	100-17	100-25	88-21	89-11	63-30	95-24	83-17	92-36	-
4 Minutes	X̄	-	84	72	84	44	66	40	37	40	26	38	14
	Range	-	100-67	100-30	100-73	62-14	93-35	56-13	43-30	100-2	50-15	83-11	20-9

Table 1: Changes in EMG amplitude of motor units during fatigue. Same bins and motor units as in Fig. 3B. X̄ is the average motor unit EMG amplitude at the end of each integration period expressed as a percentage of the initial value for motor units grouped according to their fatigability.

in fast fatiguing units must reflect profound changes in the internal metabolism of these muscle fibres which may in turn also affect the action potential producing mechanisms. Such an interdependence between contractile failure and muscle action potential fatigue has been observed in frog muscle (Lüttgau, 1965) and could account for the graded reduction in motor unit EMG amplitude with fatigue. Second, it is also known that fast fatiguing muscle fibres have few surrounding capillaries (Romanul, 1965). In particular the neuromuscular junctions of these units may have a relatively poor blood supply (Romanul, 1965), and hence be susceptible to failure, again leading to a reduction in EMG amplitude, especially at a stimulation rate of 40 pps (Krnjević and Miledi, 1958). On the basis of these arguments, non-fatiguing muscle fibres which are well supplied by capillaries, would not be expected to show such changes in EMG amplitude.

Despite these uncertainties, it should be emphasized that the fatigue test procedures used in this study indicate a broad spectrum of fatigability for fast contracting motor units. This finding is in keeping with the histochemical evidence in the medial gastrocnemius of both cat (Burke and Tsairis, 1973) and guinea pig (Edgerton et al., 1970) that fibres which stain for myosin ATPase have a broad rather than double-peaked spectrum of staining density for oxidative enzymes.

Acknowledgements: Supported in part by USPHS Grant NS 07888 and the General Research Support Fund of the University of Arizona College of Medicine.

REFERENCES

Burke, R.E., Levine, D.N., Zajac, F.E., Tsairis, P., and Engel, W.K., 1971. Mammalian motor units: physiological-histochemical correlation in three types in cat gastrocnemius. Science 174, 709-712.
Burke, R.E., and Tsairis, P., 1973. The correlation of physiological properties with histochemical characteristics in single muscle units. Ann. N.Y. Acad. Sci. In press.
Edgerton, V.R., Barnard, R.J., Peter, J.B., Simpson, D.R., and Gillespie, C.A., 1970. Response of muscle glycogen and phosphorylase to electrical stimulation in trained and non-trained guinea pigs. Exp. Neurol. 27, 46-56.
Krnjević, K., and Mildei, R., 1958. Failure of neuromuscular propagation in rats. J. Physiol. 140, 440-461.

Lüttgau, H.C., 1965. The effect of metabolic inhibitors on the
    fatigue of the action potential in single muscle fibres. J.
    Physiol. 178, 45-67.
Romanul, F.C.A., 1965. Capillary supply and metabolism of muscle
    fibers. Arch. Neurol. 12, 497-509.

MOTOR FIELDS OF PRECENTRAL CELLS ELICITED BY OPERANT REINFORCEMENT OF UNIT ACTIVITY

E. E. Fetz, D. V. Finocchio and M. A. Baker

Regional Primate Research Centre and Departments of
Physiology and Biophysics and Neurological Surgery,
University of Washington, School of Medicine, Seattle,
Washington

Motor responses in which a given motor cortex cell may play
a functional role can be elicited by operantly reinforcing bursts
of cell activity and observing the correlated behavioural responses. Under isometric conditions, operant bursts were often
repeatedly correlated with EMG bursts in specific contralateral
arm muscles. These EMG bursts broadly coincided with the
operant unit bursts, but their onset and peak usually followed
the onset and peak of the precentral unit burst. One may refer
to the set of muscles co-activated with operant bursts of a motor
cortex cell as the cell's "motor field". Under isometric conditions the motor field of a given cell generally remained stable
over many bursts, not only with respect to the set of co-activated
muscles, but also with respect to the relative intensity of their
activation. Different units in the same cortical region could
have quite different motor fields. Many of the unit-muscle
correlations observed when the unit was reinforced were repli-
cated during other reinforced response patterns.

To study relations between activity of motor cortex cells and
movements, one may train the animal to make specific motor responses and study correlated cell activity (Evarts, 1968; Humphrey
et al., 1970; Luschei et al., 1971; Porter et al., 1971); an alternative strategy is to reinforce cell activity and determine the

187

correlated motor responses (Fetz and Baker, 1973). The former
approach offers advantages in that the reinforced movement may
be standardized and quantified with respect to variables like
position and force; however, its fruitfulness depends on the
experimenter's accuracy in anticipating which responses would
engage the cells of interest and his skill in isolating cells related
to the pretrained responses. Usually only a proportion of the cells
in a given area have been strongly related to a given movement.
If the object is to determine for each cell the movements with which
it may be optimally involved, a more direct approach would be to
train the animal to activate that cell and determine the correlated
movements.

To this end we operantly reinforced bursts of precentral cortex
cells and observed correlated motor responses. Under conditions
of relatively free limb movement operant bursts of different precentral cortex cells were observed to be correlated with different
types of motor activity: bursts of some cells were associated with
generalized and variable movements; other cells were repeatedly
associated with simple movements of specific joints; some cells
were driven in bursts with no observable movements. To better
quantify the muscle activity associated with operant bursts of a
cell, we recorded isometric activity of four representative arm
muscles with permanently implanted electrodes (Fetz and Finocchio,
1971). With the arm held semiprone in a cast operant bursts of
different precentral cells were reliably correlated with bursts of
EMG activity in specific sets of muscles. The four units in Fig. 1
were located within 3 mm of each other in the precentral gyrus of
one monkey. In each case, reinforcement was made contingent
only on bursts of unit activity, and not on any muscle activity.
Bursts of cell A were repeatedly associated with bursts of EMG
activity in biceps and both wrist muscles; cell B was predominantly
correlated with triceps and biceps; cell C with triceps and wrist
muscles; and cell D fired in bursts without any correlated EMG
activity. Thus the relative amount of EMG activity in each arm
muscle was different for each cell. Although the unit and muscle
bursts overlapped to a great extent, the beginning and peak of
average unit activity preceded the beginning and peak EMG activity,
respectively.

It proves convenient to call the set of muscles which are co-
activated with operant bursts the "motor field" of the cell. Fig. 1
indicates that different cells in the same area of motor cortex had
different motor fields. The fact that correlated muscle bursts were

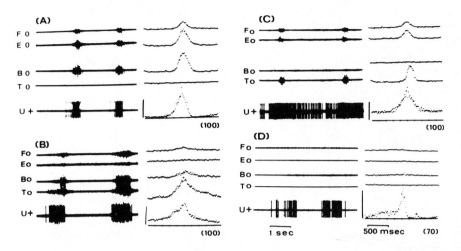

Fig. 1. Isometric muscle responses correlated with operant
bursts of four precentral cortex cells in the same monkey.
Sampled muscles include flexor carpi radialis (F), extensor
carpi radialis (E), biceps (B) and triceps (T); U+ indicates
that bursts of unit were reinforced. Sample of two successive
responses is shown in 5 sec sweep at left; average at right was
compiled over a number of responses in parentheses (vertical
bar = 50 impulses/sec). Units B, C and D were identified as
pyramidal tract cells.

usually temporally delayed with respect to operant unit bursts
suggests that the motor field may represent an efferent analog of
a sensory receptive field: it represents the loci of peripheral
elements (muscles rather than receptors) whose activity is correlated with activity of the cell. However, insofar as it involves a
behavioural response, the operational definition of motor field
differs from that of a sensory receptive field. Whereas stimulating
in a receptive field provides relatively secure evidence for a
functional pathway from receptors to responding cells, the observation that certain muscles are consistently co-activated with a
unit provides only suggestive evidence for a functional connection.
A closer motor analog of a receptive field would be the set of
muscles whose motoneurones a given motor cortex cell may
synaptically affect. This set, which might be called the cell's
"muscle field", could be determined experimentally by stimulating
the cell in isolation and recording postsynaptic responses in

appropriate motoneurones. While this procedure is prohibitively
complex, a practical approximation may be Asanuma's microstimulation technique which activates a local population of cortical
cells (Asanuma and Rosen, 1972). The relation between the
behaviourally determined motor field and the physiologically
determined muscle field of a cell would be of considerable experimental interest.

Acknowledgement: Supported in part by NIH grants RR 00166,
NB 5082-13, NS 04053 and NS 11, 072.

REFERENCES

Asanuma, H., and Rosen, I., 1972. Topographical organization of
    cortical efferent zones projecting to distal forelimb muscles
    in the monkey. Exp. Brain Res. 14, 243-256.
Evarts, E.V., 1968. Relation of pyramidal tract activity to force
    exerted during voluntary movement. J. Neurophysiol. 31, 14-27.
Fetz, E.E., and Baker, M.A., 1973. Operantly conditioned patterns
    of precentral unit activity and correlated responses in adjacent
    cells and contralateral muscles. J. Neurophysiol. 36, 179-204.
Fetz, E.E., and Finocchio, D.V., 1971. Operant conditioning of
    specific patterns of neural and muscular activity. Science
    174, 431-435.
Humphrey, D.R., Schmidt, E.M., and Thompson, W.D., 1970. Predicting
    measures of motor performance from multiple cortical spike trains.
    Science 170, 758-762.
Jasper, H., Ricci, G. and Doane, B., 1960. Microelectrode analysis
    of cortical cell discharge during avoidance conditioning in the
    monkey. Electroenceph. clin. Neurophysiol., Suppl. XIII, 137-155.
Luschei, E.S., Garthwaite, C.R., and Armstrong, M.E., 1971. Relation-
    ship of firing patterns of units in face area of monkey pre-
    central cortex to conditioned jaw movements. J. Neurophysiol. 34,
    552-561.
Porter, R., Lewis, M., and Horne, M., 1971. Analysis of patterns
    of natural activity of neurons in the precentral gyrus of conscious
    monkeys. Brain Res. 34, 99-113.

NECK MUSCLE AND EXTRAOCULAR RECEPTORS AND THEIR RELATIONSHIP TO THE TECTO-SPINAL TRACT

V. C. Abrahams, F. Rancier and P. K. Rose

Department of Physiology, Queen's University at Kingston, Kingston, Ontario

Afferents from extraocular and neck muscles constitute the richest projection to the superior colliculus. Sixty percent of cells of origin of the tectospinal tract within the superior colliculus are excited by this muscle afferent input. The superior colliculus thus constitutes a site where a variety of influences can be brought to bear on the regulation of head movement.

The regulation of head movement constitutes a special case of postural control, for head movement must be integrated with eye movement. Evidence has been obtained by Bizzi, Kalil and Tagliasco (1971) that some combined head and eye movements are integrated in such a way as to suggest that a central mechanism develops patterned motor output simultaneously to neck muscles and extraocular muscles, minimally controlled and corrected during the execution of the movement. We now provide evidence of connections within the superior colliculus that suggest that the organization of such combined head and eye movement might be a collicular function.

The extraocular muscles of the cat's eye are well provided with receptors giving information about muscle length and load (Bach-y-Rita and Ito, 1966). There has been little concrete evidence as to what use might be made of such information by the brain. There is no stretch reflex in extraocular muscles and

most theories propose that these receptors are involved in
"subconscious nervous control of muscle contraction" (Bach-y-
Rita, 1971). The neck muscles of the cat are rich in muscle
spindles. In our own examination of rectus capitis major (one of
the dorsal muscles of the neck) spindle densities exceeding 57/gm
have been found, a density only exceeded in the interossei. Originally assigned only a minor role in the regulation of posture,
evidence has been accumulating for more than a century that neck
muscle receptors may play a more important role, for damage
or interference with neck muscles or their nerves can lead to
widespread postural deficiencies extending beyond interference
with head movement (for review, see Abrahams, 1972a).

In experiments on anaesthetized cats we have found that neck
muscle afferents relay to the superior colliculus and constitute
the single richest relay to this structure. More units in the
superior colliculus can be activated by stimulation of neck muscle
nerves than by a wide variety of visual stimuli (Abrahams and
Rose, 1972). We have further found that the projection of extraocular muscle afferents to the superior colliculus is also particularly rich, and such connections are as abundant as neck muscle
projections (Rose and Abrahams, 1973). The evidence that these
projections play a role in the organization of head movement comes
from an examination of the afferent connections of those units to
cells of origin of the tectospinal tract.

Anderson, Yoshida and Wilson (1971) identified two pathways
from the superior colliculus to the motoneurones of the neck, the
tectospinal pathway terminating on interneurones in the ventral
cervical cord, and the tectoreticulospinal which terminates
directly on motoneurones after synapsing in reticular nuclei.
Both pathways are disynaptic. Using the usual criteria of antidromic invasion we have identified cells of origin of the tectospinal tract within the superior colliculi. We have found that
about 60% of these cells can be fired by neck muscle or extraocular muscle afferents. These experiments demonstrate that
at the level of the superior colliculus eye and head muscle afferent activity can influence output to neck motoneurones via the
tectospinal pathway. What information concerning the head and
the eyes is conveyed to the superior colliculus is as yet unknown,
but we have found the projection to the superior colliculus from
neck muscles to be exclusively from afferents conducting with a
group II velocity.

Vestibulospinal connections to neck motoneurones are mono-synaptic (Wilson and Yoshida, 1969), and thus might appear to be pre-emptive. Receptors in neck muscles can inhibit or excite vestibulospinal output at cervical levels (Gernandt and Gilman, 1959; Gernandt and Proler, 1965) and can suppress vestibulospinal output at lumbosacral levels for several hundred msec. (Abrahams, 1972b). A central organization thus exists which could suspend the dominant control of head position by labyrinthine structures and allow the systems taking origin in extraocular and neck muscle afferents to exert an extensive role in the control of head movement.

Acknowledgement: Work supported by grants from the Medical Research Council of Canada and Queen's University.

REFERENCES

Abrahams, V.C., 1972a. Neck muscle proprioceptors and a role of the cerebral cortex in postural reflexes in subprimates. Rev. Can. Biol. 31, Suppl., 115-130.

Abrahams, V.C., 1972b. Neck muscle proprioceptors and vestibulo-spinal outflow at lumbosacral levels. Can. J. Physiol. Pharmacol. 50, 17-21.

Abrahams, V.C., and Rose, P.K., 1972. Proprioceptive connections to the superior colliculi of the cat. Fed. Proc. 31, 383.

Anderson, M.E., Yoshida, M., and Wilson, V.J., 1971. Influence of superior colliculus on cat neck motoneurones. J. Neurophysiol. 34, 898-907.

Bach-y-Rita, P., 1971. Neurophysiology of Eye Movements. In The Control of Eye Movements. Academic Press, N.Y., pp. 7-45.

Bach-y-Rita, P., and Ito, S., 1966. Properties of stretch receptors in cat extraocular muscles. J. Physiol. 186, 663-688.

Bizzi, E., Kalil, R.E., and Tagliasco, V., 1971. Eye-head co-ordination in monkeys; evidence for centrally patterned organization. Science 173, 452-454.

Gernandt, B.E., and Gilman, S., 1959. Differential supraspinal control of spinal centers. Exp. Neurol. 3, 307-324.

Gernandt, B.E., and Proler, M.L., 1965. Medullary and spinal accessory nerve responses to vestibular stimulation. Exp. Neurol. 11, 27-37.

Rose, P.K., and Abrahams, V.C., 1973. Extraocular muscle proprio-ceptive projections to the superior colliculus in the cat. Fed. Proc. 32, 698.

Wilson, V.J., and Yoshida, M., 1969. Bilateral connections between labyrinths and neck motoneurons. Brain Res. 13, 603-607.

PART II: CONTROL OF POSTURE

POSTURAL ADAPTATION. THE NATURE OF ADAPTIVE MECHANISMS IN THE HUMAN MOTOR SYSTEM

G. L. Gottlieb and G. C. Agarwal

Department of Biomedical Engineering,
Rush-Presbyterian-St. Luke's Medical Centre,
Chicago, Illinois and School of Engineering, University
of Chicago Circle, Chicago, Illinois

Postural adaptation implies a change in motor system parameters in response to certain types of stimuli. In the peripheral limb of the motor control system there are two sites at which such changes might occur; at the muscle and at the muscle spindle. Intimately related to these forms of adaptation are changes in the gain of the stretch reflex loop within the spinal cord.

This paper will consider evidence for adaptive control at these sites and the implications such mechanisms would have on motor system performance.

Adaptation is a process whereby an organism changes to better conform to the demands of its environment. The purpose of this paper is to discuss the motor control system as an adaptive mechanism for maintaining a stable posture and consider by what means its parameters can be controlled and changed and what effects those changes might have on the system's performance.

Consider first the simple, general feedback system shown in Fig. 1. Signals originate in the controller (the central nervous system) causing the plant (the skeletal muscles) to generate

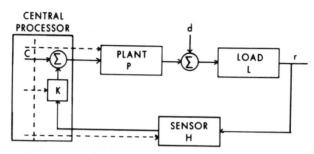

Fig. 1. A simple adaptive feedback system with driving signals (solid lines) which produce proportional outputs and adaptive signals (broken lines) which modify block parameters. The transfer function for a linear system of this configuration is:

$$r = \frac{PL}{1 + KPLH} C + \frac{L}{1 + KPLH} d. \tag{1}$$

when KPLH >> 1, this reduces to

$$r \approx \frac{1}{KH} C + \frac{1}{KPH} d. \tag{2}$$

Only the plant, the feedback sensor and the feedback gain are shown with adaptive inputs. The load is considered external and inaccessible to direct influence of the central controller.

forces which, when summed with disturbing forces from the external world act on the load (the body) to produce some output or response (body position). Sensors monitor this output and the controller is informed thereby of the consequences of its original commands.

The behaviour of the system in Fig. 1 is described by equation 1 of the caption. If the gain of this closed loop is high ($|KPLH|$ >> 1), the approximation of equation 2 shows that the performance of this system is not dependent on the load (L). If $|KPH|$ >> 1, it is also relatively immune to external disturbances.

However, biological feedback systems in general and motor systems in particular have a rather low loop gain (Granit, 1970) and cannot take advantage of this principle. Given such a situation, we can note three "problems" a nonadaptive system would have in performing adequately.

1. If the dynamic characteristics of the load (L) or the plant (P) change significantly, these changes would be directly felt in overall system performance.

2. If the character of the external disturbance (d) changes the system itself may no longer be suited to its task of regulating the controlled variable r in spite of d.

3. If the definition of adequate performance is changed, then what might have been a well designed system may no longer be one.

A system which cannot alter its own parameters has no way of responding to any of these situations. Each of these is a real situation with which the postural motor system must cope. The motor system plants or effectors, skeletal muscle, are subject to fatigue and other sources of inherent lability. Perhaps of greater importance, is that the body loads which must be stabilized are inertial and exert torques at each joint which depend on the joint angle. Damping of these continuously varying loads is accomplished solely by the active intervention of postural control mechanisms.

The second problem, dealing with changes in the nature of external disturbances will not be discussed at any length here because the mechanisms involved are unknown, but this is a real problem experienced, for example, when going from standing on a dock to standing on the deck of a small boat. The adapted individual can do both with little conscious effort. The period of adaptation is sometimes subjectively unpleasant though.

Concerning the third problem of changing performance criteria, we are handicapped by our lack of knowledge of the "design criteria" which were important in the evolution of the motor system. The Designer has certainly not taken us into His confidence. Nevertheless, it seems intuitively clear that during relaxed standing and standing while sighting a rifle, we are asking rather different things of the postural control system.

We will now consider some specific examples of adaptive mechanisms within the motor system. At the periphery of the

motor system we can distinguish three sites where this may
occur: at the plant, at the feedback sensor and at the controller.
Depending both on the site and nature of the adaptive process, the
consequences will differ.

ADAPTIVE MECHANISMS

Adaptation of the Plant

The plant or effector organ of all motor mechanisms is made
up of the skeletal muscles. It might first appear that muscle cannot be an adaptive organ because there is but one final common
pathway, the alpha motor neurone, by which it can be controlled.
It lacks any separate path for adjusting its parameters independently. A closer inspection reveals, however, that this is no real
obstacle to adaptive behaviour.

As an example, consider the simple, non-linear input-output
relation in Fig. 2A. This sort of non-linearity with the rate at

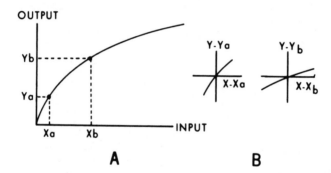

A   **B**

Fig. 2. A. An example of adaptation of the small signal gain
by shifting the operating point on a non-linear gain curve.
B. For small variations of the input about two different operating points X_a and X_b, the effective gain of the system varies
greatly.

which the output increases diminishing as the absolute level of the
output grows large is a commonly observed phenomenon. When the
dynamic range of some particular input covers only a portion of
the range of all possible inputs, this system becomes adaptive in

the following manner.

Consider two inputs whose tonic values are X_a and X_b. Small phasic or transient changes in the inputs about these operating points will cause different changes in the corresponding outputs as shown in Fig. 2B. This trick for altering the gain of a system according to the average level of its input has been frequently exploited in the design of such ordinary devices as AM radio receivers. Strong signals, which would be received when the transmitter is near, cause the operating point to shift to the right on the curve, reducing the gain. Weaker signals from a distant transmitter place the operating point at the left, high gain region. As a result, both signals are heard with almost equal loudness.

The adjustment of system parameters over a short time interval according to the average input over a somewhat longer time interval need not be limited to the system gain nor to a single parameter. In Fig. 3, we have drawn a relationship between

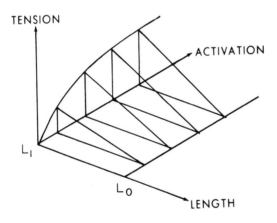

Fig. 3. With more than two variables, a variety of adaptive forms are possible. Here it is illustrated how the effective elastic stiffness of the muscle can change by altering the level of contraction. Length is considered to be increasing in the direction from L_1 to L_0 where L_0 is the resting length. Observe that for any given length between L_1 and L_0, as tension is increased by increasing activation, the slope of the length-tension curve (i.e. elastic stiffness) is also increased.

muscle activation, length and tension. The length-tension curve steepens as it moves to the right, to higher levels of muscle activation. The steepness of this curve is the measure of the muscle's elastic stiffness which is thus controlled by the level of neural activation.

There is an abundance of experimental evidence, from both animals and man, to show that processes such as these are indeed at work in mammalian muscle. One example is illustrated in Fig. 4. These data, derived from Wilkie (1950), show how the

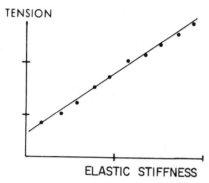

TENSION

ELASTIC STIFFNESS

Fig. 4.   An example of how the effective elastic stiffness increases with the level of muscle contraction. Data redrawn from Wilkie (1950) for the human biceps.

elastic stiffness of the muscle is altered by contraction. A similar increase occurs in the viscous stiffness. The result is that, with increasing active force of contraction, there is also a sharp increase in the mechanical impedance with which the muscle resists forcible extension. One way this property is exploited may be by the co-contraction of antagonist muscle groups. The effect is to fix the position of a joint without the production of any net torque.

Adaptation of the Sensory Receptor

Let us turn now to how the properties of the spindle can also be recruited to adapt the motor system to changing requirements. Feedback systems are generally very sensitive to the parameters of the feedback path.

The two fusimotor pathways to the spindle provide distinct adaptive controls. The static fusimotor nerves appear to be able to drive the spindle in parallel with the extrafusal muscle (Vallbo, 1971). One way of looking at the spindle in this mode of operation, is as a model for the muscle as shown in Fig. 5. Here the intrafusal spindle fibres mimic the behaviour of the extrafusal fibres

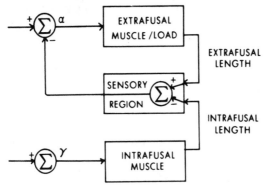

Fig. 5. A conditional feedback system in which, when the gamma driven intrafusal fibres contract at the same rate as the alpha driven muscle/load, no deformation of the spindle sensory endings occurs and there is no change in the afferent signal. The fusimotor system functions as a model of the skeletomotor system and if that model is in error, reflex compensation for the skeletomotor system is generated.

and to the extent that the spindle model is an accurate representation of the muscle-load system; no error signal is generated (Houk, 1971). Should the two sets of fibres contract at different rates, however, the reflex arc provides rapid compensation.

This scheme, as described thus far, is not adaptive in that no explicit means of altering system dynamics has been suggested. Additional effects of static fusimotor stimulation are to moderately enhance the length sensitivity (Lennerstrand and Thoden, 1968), and reduce the velocity sensitivity (Crowe and Matthews, 1964) of the primary afferents. Both of these factors tend to reduce the effective damping of the loop. This is an adaptive effect which might aid in rapid movement.

The task of postural adaptation, however, is more one of stabilizing the body. This is an extremely complex problem because the dynamics of erect standing, for example, are labile

and depend strongly on such variables as limb position and the
location of the body's centre of mass with respect to the point of
balance. These dynamics are also characterized by a large, un-
damped inertial load.

In order to stabilize such a system, postural mechanisms must
not only generate balancing forces to counteract gravity, but must
also provide adequate damping to minimize postural sway. One
good mechanism to provide this damping is afforded by dynamic
fusimotor control of the primary spindle afferents. The dominant
effect of this efferent pathway is exercised over the velocity sensitivity of the spindle as shown in Fig. 6. The result, in terms of
system dynamics, is to control the damping of the stretch reflex
loop.

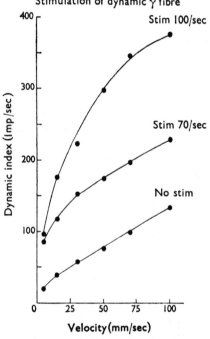

Fig. 6. The effects of dynamic fusimotor activity on the
velocity sensitivity of the primary spindle endings from Crowe
and Matthews (1964).

Adaptation of the Controller

The central nervous system, in the course of processing
afferent signals and generating efferent ones, is, of course, the

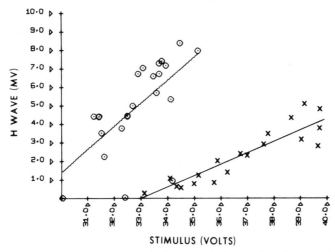

Fig. 7. The lower curve (X) shows the stimulus-response curve for a Hoffman reflex in a relaxed soleus muscle. No reflex is elicited with stimulus voltages less than 33 volts and the effective "gain" of this component of the reflex arc is 0.74 mv/volt. The upper curve (O) was generated by triggering the stimulator on the rising phase of the electromyogram produced by vigorous soleus contraction. The threshold has dropped to less than 29 volts and the gain has approximately doubled (Gottlieb, unpublished data).

ultimate effector of all adaptive processes. The adaptation which goes on within supraspinal centres is beyond the scope of this paper. What we would like to consider here is the nature of those adaptive processes which go on within the cord which are so closely intertwined with the peripheral forms of adaptation already discussed.

In principle, by controlling the order of recruitment of individual motor neurones from within the pool serving each muscle, slower or faster units could be selected as an independent means of adaptive control. However, on the contrary, recruitment seems to be determined by Henneman's size principle (Henneman et al., 1965) and appears unaffected by whether units are activated reflexively or voluntarily (Ashworth et al., 1967; but see also the chapter by Wyman in this volume). Whether the dynamic adaptive effects attributable to a heterogeneous motor unit population can

be separated out from those already discussed in terms of the
muscle itself remains controversial.

Another adaptive mechanism, for which there is good evidence,
can be described as control of the reflex loop gain (Gottlieb et al.,
1970). Fig. 7, showing the stimulus-response curve of the Hoffman
reflex in the soleus muscle under conditions of rest (lower curve)
and contraction (upper curve) illustrates how both the slope and the
threshold of the reflex arc may be modified. The effects of
elevating the loop gain are to enhance the speed of the system
response but also to reduce the effective damping and therefore
the stability of the affected loops.

DISCUSSION

The problems encountered in investigating adaptive systems
such as we have described are formidable. The questions that
are raised concern, not only what the system does, but in identifying what, in fact, is the system. Some specific examples for
adaptation of system components have been described already.
We will now consider how the behaviour of the entire system is
affected by such changes in its components. Studies of the whole
system cannot usually specify the site at which adaptation occurs
but they are vital in learning which of the extremely large range
of all possible adaptive responses actually occur.

Stark (1968) asked subjects to rotate a handle using their wrist
and forearm. He then applied sudden, impulsive rotational disturbances to that handle and observed the resulting motion. A
simple, linear second-order differential equation was used to
model the motion that was produced. He noted that asking his
subjects to vary the level of tension in their forearm produced a
systematic variation in the solutions of his differential equation
paradigm. The variations of those solutions are shown graphically
in Fig. 8.

Increasing voluntary tension causes the poles of the system to
migrate away from the origin in a manner indicating that the
overall control system is becoming stiffer and faster but less
stable. These results are, in part, due to changes in muscle dynamics produced by voluntary shifts in the contractile operating
point. Changes in other parts of the system are also expected
but cannot be separated out.

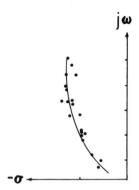

Fig. 8. A plot of the real (σ) and imaginary (jω) parts of the
poles of a second-order model of the wrist rotation control
system from Stark (1968). A line drawn from the origin to a
data point gives a vectorial representation of the solution of
the differential equation describing a single stimulus response.
The length of the vector may be considered representative of
the speed or bandwidth of the system response. The angle of
the vector makes with the -σ axis is a measure of the stability
of the system, small angles being very stable, large angles
indicating an oscillatory response.
Increasing forearm tension results in solutions further from
the origin and more oscillatory. One may conveniently think
of the poles migrating along the solid line as a function of
voluntary tension.

Studying the dynamics of quiet standing in man, Nashner (1970)
observed that the gain of the ankle reflex loop was only about one-
third of that necessary for postural stability. This gain increased
when body sway exceeded a certain threshold, however. Whether
this is mediated by fusimotor or spinal mechanisms is not known.

Marsden et al. (1972) have recorded electromyograms of muscles controlling the thumb when its movement was suddenly im-
peded. One conclusion was that voluntary movement was associated with an increase in the gain of the stretch reflex loop.

Experiments in our own laboratory concur with this. Using both
Hoffman reflexes and the Achilles tendon jerk reflex, we have
seen that the effective gain of this loop is elevated by contraction
of remote muscles (Gottlieb and Agarwal, 1973). Evidence impli-
cating both fusimotor and intraspinal mechanisms is discussed in
that paper.

Common to all three forms of adaptation described here is an
effective stiffening of the affected reflex loops. Each increases
the resistance of postural motor mechanisms to external forces.
In contrast with this, their effects on postural stability differ.

The characteristics induced by altering the operating point of
the muscles by tonic activation of the alpha motor nerves will
depend on the relative changes in viscous and elastic parameters.
If the viscous element dominates, which seems likely, the dynamic response of the loop will become slower and more stable
while if the elastic element dominates, just the reverse will
ensue.

Dynamic fusimotor activity will clearly increase system
stability and slow its dynamic response. Static fusimotor
activity, by reducing the dynamic index, will tend to counteract
this but the net result of joint activity in the two pathways probably
favours the dynamic effect.

Increasing the loop gain will tend to speed the dynamic response
of a system and reduce its stability. Any negative feedback system
of more than trivial complexity will, in fact, become unstable
if its gain becomes excessively large.

In light of these adaptive processes, it is interesting to consider some common motor pathologies. Clonus for example is
the expected consequence of elevated gain of the stretch reflex
loop. The intentional tremor and past-pointing of some cerebellar
disease could be caused by a failure of the dynamic fusimotor
system to properly damp the movement. (It is interesting that the
facial muscles which work with relatively constant and non-inertial
loads are poorly supplied with muscle spindles.) Slowness of
movement in Parkinsonism may be the result of increased muscle
viscous damping. In each case, the failure of the system is not
so much that the muscles are not sent the right controlling signals as that the adaptive mechanisms have failed to make the
system controllable.

Accepting the fact that components of the motor system do alter their dynamic characteristics according to specific inputs from the central nervous system, we are still far from understanding how these characteristics are exploited by postural control mechanisms. Perhaps the most crucial question concerns the degree of independent control exercised over these adaptive processes. The observation that the human operator behaves in a highly adaptive fashion is an old one (Tustin, 1944). The degree to which this adaptation may be localized in the periphery of the motor system has yet to be established.

Acknowledgement: This work was partially supported by the National Science Foundation.

REFERENCES

Ashworth, B., Grimby, L., and Kugelberg, E., 1967. Comparison of voluntary and reflex activation of motor units. J. Neurol. Neurosurg. Psychiat. 30, 91-98.

Crowe, A., and Matthews, P., 1964. The effects of stimulation of static and dynamic fusimotor fibres on the response to stretching of the primary endings of muscle spindles. J. Physiol. 174, 109-131.

Gottlieb, G., Agarwal, G., and Stark, L., 1970. Interaction between voluntary and postural mechanisms of the human motor system. J. Neurophysiol. 33, 365-381.

Gottlieb, G., and Agarwal, G., 1973. Modulation of postural reflexes by voluntary movement: II Modulation at an inactive joint. J. Neurol. Neurosurg. Psychiat. In press.

Granit, R., 1970. The Basis of Motor Control. Academic Press, Lond. Chap. 12.

Henneman, E., Somjen, G., and Carpenter, D., 1965. Functional significance of cell size in spinal motoneurons. J. Neurophysiol. 28, 560-580.

Houk, J., 1971. The phylogeny of muscular control configurations. III Symposium of Biocybernetics, Leipzig.

Lennerstrand, G., and Thoden, U., 1968. Position and velocity sensitivity of muscle spindles in the cat. III Static fusimotor single-fibre activation of primary and secondary endings. Acta Physiol. Scand. 74, 30-49.

Marsden, C., Merton, P., and Morton, H. 1972. Servo action in human voluntary movement. Nature 128, 140-143.

Nashner, L., 1970. Sensory feedback in human posture control. Sc.D. Thesis, MIT.

Stark, L., 1968. Neurological Control Systems: Studies in Bio-Engineering. Plenum Press, N.Y.

Tustin, A., 1944. An Investigation of the Operator's Response
  In Manual Control of a Power Driven Gun. Memo #169, Metropolitan-
  Vickers Electrical Co.
Vallbo, Å., 1971. Muscle spindle responses at the onset of
  isometric contractions in man: time difference between fusimotor
  and skeletomotor effects, J. Physiol. <u>218</u>, 405-431.
Wilkie, D., 1950. The relation between force and velocity in
  human muscle. J. Physiol. <u>110</u>, 249-280.

THE SIGNIFICANCE OF INTRAMUSCULAR RECEPTORS IN LOAD COMPENSATION DURING VOLUNTARY CONTRACTIONS IN MAN

Å. B. Vallbo

Department of Physiology, Biological Institute
University of Umeå, Sweden

Muscle spindle afferent discharge was analysed in single unit recordings from the median nerve of awake human subjects. Impulse frequency from spindle in the antebrachial finger flexor muscles was related to metacarpo-phalangeal joint angle when the muscles were relaxed, and to active torque at the same joint during isometric voluntary contractions. The steady state impulse frequency was varied linearly with joint angle within the range of study. The average position sensitivity, defined as impulses per second per degree joint movement (ips/deg), was 0.18 ips/deg for the spindle primary endings and 0.14 ips/deg for the secondaries. It was estimated that the maximal position sensitivity during muscle contraction, would be 0.9 ips/deg for the primaries and 0.7 ips/deg for the secondaries. In isometric voluntary contractions the spindle discharge increased, due to the fusimotor outflow running parallel with the skeletomotor outflow. The relation was found to be approximately linear, and the average slope was 32.8 ips/Nm (metre-Newton) for the primaries and 22.8 ips/Nm for the secondaries. From these data the muscle stiffness accounted for by the intramuscular receptors may be deduced, if some additional assumptions are adopted, the most crucial one being that the central effects of the muscular afferents are the same in isometric voluntary contractions and in load carrying contractions. The stiffness of the contracting muscles accounted for by the intramuscular receptor, as calculated in this way, was found to be as low as 0.03 Nm/deg for the finger flexor muscles at the metacarpo-phalangeal joint. The findings suggest that the muscle spindles do not constitute a very powerful load compensating mechanism with regard to muscle length.

When a human subject performs a voluntary contraction the fusimotor system as well as the skeletomotor system is activated. This is evident from the finding that the discharges in single spindle afferents rise during isometric contractions in spite of the mechanical unloading effect (Hagbarth and Vallbo, 1968; Vallbo, 1970a, b). The power of the fusimotor outflow is illustrated by the fact that practically all the spindle endings in the muscle respond in this way even in weak contractions. In spatial distribution, the fusimotor activity is strictly limited to the contracting muscle or even to the particular portion of a larger muscle which is active in a contraction (Vallbo, 1970a, b). It has further been shown that the skeletomotor outflow is launched from the spinal cord slightly before the arrival of the increased spindle afferent discharge at the onset of a contraction, indicating that the contraction is initiated by descending activity from supraspinal structures onto the skeletomotor neurones (Vallbo, 1971). Hence the principle of control is in accord with alpha-gamma linkage rather than the follow-up length servo hypothesis (Merton, 1951, 1953; Granit, 1955).

A fundamental question in relation to the functional role of the muscle spindles and the fusimotor system is how strong are the central effects exerted by the muscle spindle afferent activity. This may be expressed as the amount of muscle stiffness accounted for by the muscle spindle afferent activity, i.e. the amount of change in muscle force for a change in muscle length.

The present study is an attempt to analyse to what extent the intramuscular receptors and their central connections account for an appreciable muscle stiffness. The analysis is based upon information on spindle position sensitivity and spindle afferent activity as a function of contraction intensity in human finger flexor muscles. The findings suggest that the muscle spindle system does not account for the major stiffness of the muscle.

METHODS

Activity from 64 spindle afferents were studied in 22 experiments on 20 awake human subjects. Single unit impulses were recorded from the median nerve approximately 10 cm above the elbow. The recording method has been described in detail in earlier reports (Vallbo and Hagbarth, 1968; Vallbo, 1970a, 1972). Fine tungsten needle electrodes, insulated to the tip, were inserted percutaneously into the nerve and they were manipulated with a pair of forceps all through the experiment. No anaesthesia was employed. Most of the endings were located in the antebrachial finger flexor muscles and they were identified as spindle endings according to the principles described in previous reports (Vallbo, 1970a, 1973a). The fingers were fixed to a device which kept them extended to $180°$ at the interphalangeal joints but allowed controlled movements at the metacarpophalangeal joints. It also included equipment for continuous measurement of the metacarpo-phalangeal joint angles and the torque around these joints. In most of the experiments, the wrist joint was slightly dorsiflexed as it was kept at $165°$. The experimental data were recorded on tape and processed afterwards. In order to define the steady state discharge as a function of joint angle, the impulse frequency was measured 15 sec after a passive joint movement. Recordings from isometric contractions were analysed by counting the number of nerve impulses and measuring the average torque due to active contraction, every other second over one second, by means of electronic counters appropriately gated. The total number of observations of this type was 1,854 extracted from 33 afferents.

RESULTS

The findings will be described in relation to a schematic diagram of neuronal and mechanical events involved in voluntary contractions (Fig. 1). The skeletomotor neurones are assumed to receive excitatory synaptic activity of two origins. Muscle spindles provide excitation through spinal circuits and possibly also through supraspinal ones. Skeletomotor excitation originates also from other sources, mainly central structures. This activity which is indicated by alpha in the diagram, is assumed to be independent of the muscle spindle afferent activity. Thus, the supraspinal centres have access to the skeletomotor neurones through two routes marked alpha and gamma respectively

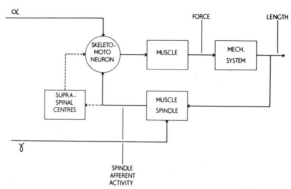

Fig. 1. Schematic diagram of neuronal and mechanical events involved in voluntary contractions. The skeleto-motor neurones are assumed to receive excitation largely from two sources. Intramuscular receptors give rise to excitation through spinal connections and possibly also through supraspinal circuits, represented in the diagram by the two routes from the spindle to the skeletomotor neurones. Skeletomotor excitation is assumed to originate also from central structures independently of muscular afferent inflow. This activity is represented by the arrow marked alpha in the diagram. The arrow marked gamma represents pathways from any relevant motor centres to the intrafusal muscle fibres.

in the diagram, in conformity with well established concepts on motor control (cf. Granit, 1955, 1970; Matthews, 1972). The skeletomotor neurone impulses give rise to a muscle force which acts upon a mechanical system. The force may cause a position change of the system elements and this change, in turn, is measured by the muscle spindles as a change in muscle length.

The purpose of the present study was to determine the amount of muscle force accounted for by the spindle afferent activity when the muscle length is altered by external forces. Two experimental findings form the basis of the analysis. First, the steady state response of muscle spindles to muscle length, or rather joint angle was analysed. Second, the relation between muscle spindle afferent activity and muscle force was studied during isometric conditions. These two sets of data constitute measures of the input-output relations across some of the elements of the loop in Fig. 1 and ideally they may be combined to deduce the change in force as a function of the change in muscle length. More extensive accounts of the experimental findings are given in other reports (Vallbo, 1973a, b).

Muscle Spindle Position Response

The steady state impulse frequency of a spindle afferent as a function of muscle length has been termed position response. For de-afferented mammalian spindles this response is roughly linear with muscle length. The slope of the curve of impulse frequency versus muscle length provides a measure of the steady state sensitivity which has been termed position sensitivity (Lennerstrand, 1968a; Lennerstrand and Thoden, 1968). A basic question is to what extent similar relations are present in the intact organism, between spindle afferent impulse frequency and muscle length, or whether this simple relation is offset by the normally functioning fusimotor system. In Fig. 2

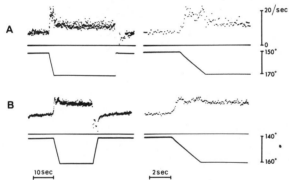

Fig. 2. Spindle afferent responses to passive joint movements in relaxed muscles. Upper traces: instantaneous impulse frequency. Lower traces: metacarpo-phalangeal joint angles. A and B show discharges from two separate spindle afferents, both related to the fourth finger. To the right, the stretch phases are displayed on an expanded time scale (from Acta Physiol. Scand., Vallbo, 1973a).

are shown the responses of two spindle endings from the antebrachial finger flexor muscles to passive extensions of the appropriate metacarpo-phalangeal joint angle by 20°. The same test runs are illustrated on different time scales to the left and right. It may be seen that the impulse frequency from the spin-

dles increased with muscle length and further, that the discharge
rate declined slowly after the stretch phase to attain a steady
frequency within 5-15 sec. This frequency was maintained as
long as the discharge was observed, which was up to 10 min for
some of the units. The unit illustrated in A was classified as a
primary ending on the basis of its high dynamic index whereas
the unit in B was classified as a secondary ending (Crowe and
Matthews, 1964). For most of the units a similar classification
was unequivocal, although a minority was grouped somewhat
more arbitrarily as the dynamic index was intermediate. The
primary and secondary endings will be described separately in
the following.

Plots of the steady state impulse frequency versus metacarpo-
phalangeal joint angle suggested a linear relation for most of the
units. Data from six sample endings are illustrated in Fig. 3

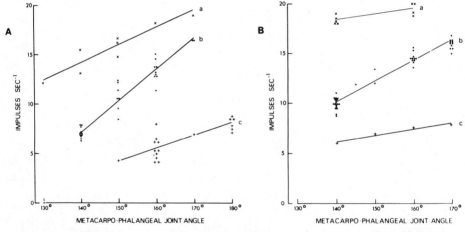

Fig. 3. Steady state impulse frequency of six spindle afferents as a function of joint angle in relaxed muscles. Data from
three primaries are shown in A and data from three secondaries in B. The symbols represent the experimental data
whereas the fulldrawn lines represent linear equations fitted
to the data by means of the method of least squares. The regression coefficients (k) and the correlation coefficients (r)
were as follows: A - a:k=0.18, r=0.93; b:k=0.32, r=0.95;
c:k=0.13, r=0.82. B - a:k=0.06, r=0.76; b:k=0.21, r=0.97;
c:k=0.06, r=0.98. The one observation at zero ips in A was
not included in the calculation. (From Acta Physiol. Scand.,
Vallbo, 1973a).

where the symbols represent experimental findings and the straight lines represent linear equations fitted by the method of least squares. The illustrated data are representative with regard to the scatter of the observations, the slope of the lines and the absolute frequencies which did not exceed 20 ips (impulses per sec) for any of the units at the joint angles tested. It should be pointed out, however, that the muscles were not stretched to their maximal length as the wrist joint angle was some 30° short of full extension.

The correlation coefficient between joint angle and spindle frequency was statistically significant for 70% of the 33 units studied on this point. Non-significant correlations were found largely when very few observations were available for anyone unit, whereas the correlations were, in fact, significant for 90% of the units from which 10 observations or more were available. From these findings it was concluded that linear equations provided adequate descriptions of the relation between spindle frequency and joint angle. Thus, it seems justified to employ concepts similar to position response and position sensitivity also in the intact human subjects, although in the present study the spindle response was related to joint angle rather than muscle length which is commonly measured in animal experiments. The slopes of the lines in Fig. 3 represent the position sensitivity as defined above.

Adequate data for an analysis of the position sensitivity were available from 11 primary endings and 11 secondary endings. The mean figure was 0.184 ips/deg for the primaries and 0.143 ips/deg for the secondaries and the range was 0.05-0.35 ips/deg. The difference between the two samples was not statistically significant (P> 0.05, Komolgorov-Smirnov test).

In addition to the 33 units considered, a number of spindle afferents were encountered which did not give a maintained discharge at any of the joint angles tested. The percentage of active spindle afferents from the muscle at various joint angles was estimated on the basis of the sample studied. Linear equations, fitted to the data from the active units, were extrapolated downwards to 3 ips on the assumption that, on the average, this would be the minimal frequency before the firing stopped   altogether. The histograms shown in Fig. 4 were constructed from these data and from data on the number of non-discharging units encountered at any joint angle. The per-

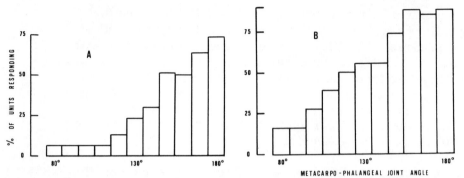

<u>Fig. 4.</u>   Histograms showing the percentage of units which
were continuously discharging in the steady state as a
function of the metacarpo-phalangeal joint angle. Data from
the primaries are displayed in A and data from the secondaries in B. The diagrams were constructed on the basis of
linear equations fitted to the experimental data and extrapolated down to 3 ips and data concerning the number of non-
discharging units encountered at any joint angle. (From Acta
Physiol. Scand., Vallbo, 1973a).

centage of active afferents of   34 primaries is shown in Fig.
4A and of 19 secondaries in B which altogether constitute the
total sample studied under uniform conditions. It should be
pointed out that the histograms very likely give maximal figures
for the percentage of active units at any joint angle, as the
recording method probably involved some bias in favour of discharging units. This selection was clearly more pronounced for
the secondaries as they were, to a large extent, identified as
spindle afferents against Golgi tendon organs on the basis of
their steady state discharge in relaxed muscles. It is difficult
to appreciate the quantitative significance of this selection but
it seems important to stress that the data shown in Fig. 4 represent the upper limit for the percentage of active spindle afferents
at any joint angle. Similarly the difference between the two
histograms may be accounted for by sampling bias. It seems
striking that very few units are active in the steady state at
intermediate muscle lengths. A metacarpo-phalangeal joint
angle of 110° in these experiments probably corresponds to the
comfortable resting position of the human hand with regard to
the muscle lengths. The present findings indicate that less than
10% of the primaries are continuously firing at a comfortable
resting position when the muscles are relaxed.

Amplitude Relations Between Skeletomotor Contraction
Intensity and Spindle Afferent Discharge Rate

When a subject activates his muscles and the finger is held
against a fixed resistance in order to achieve isometric conditions, the afferent discharge from the spindles increases due
to an increase of the fusimotor outflow. A basic question is to
what extent there was a simple and reproduceable relation
between skeletomotor contraction intensity, measured as the
twisting force, and impulse frequency in single spindle afferents
under isometric conditions. A comparison of these two variables
would give some indication of the relation between the fusimotor
and the skeletomotor outflows and thereby define the basic properties of the motor outflow during voluntary contractions.

In Fig. 5 an example is shown of how spindle frequency
varies with contraction intensity during a long lasting voluntary

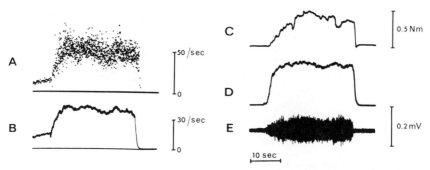

Fig. 5.   Afferent activity from a muscle spindle primary
ending located in the long finger flexor muscles during an
isometric voluntary contraction. The subject flexed his
fourth finger against a fixed resistance. A - instantaneous
impulse frequency of the spindle afferent. B - an analogue
display of the discharge in A produced by means of a filter
circuit with a decay time constant of 0.33 sec. C - torque
due to active contraction. D - the electromyographic activity
of record E rectified and converted into analogue form as in
B. E - electromyographic activity recorded with surface
electrodes over the contracting muscles. (From Acta
Physiol. Scand., Vallbo, 1973b).

contraction. The spindle discharge is displayed as instantaneous impulse frequency in A. Incidentally, it may be seen
that the interspike interval irregularity is high suggesting
static fusimotor outflow to the spindle. In order to facilitate a
visual comparison with other analogue signals the spindle
frequency is displayed in an analogue form in B. The skeletomotor contraction intensity is illustrated as the torque in C and
as the electromyographic activity in E whereas the record
marked D represents an analogue signal of the electromyographic activity. It may be seen that there is a close relation
between spindle frequency and skeletomotor contraction intensity whether this is measured as torque or estimated from the
electromyographic activity. Similar data from all the units
studied were quantified by measuring the number of impulses
per sec and the average torque over 1 sec sampling periods.
Plots of spindle frequency versus torque from 3 units are
shown in Fig. 6 where it may be seen that there was a positive

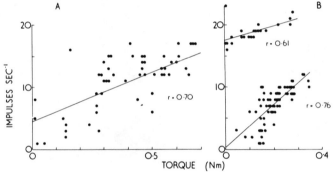

Fig. 6. Impulse frequencies from a muscle spindle primary
ending in A, and two secondary endings in B, plotted against
the torque due to isometric voluntary contractions of the index finger flexor muscles. The points represent the experimental data and the lines represent linear equations fitted by
the method of least squares. The correlation coefficients (r)
are given in the diagrams. Sampling period length was 1.0
sec and sampling interval 2.0 sec. (From Acta Physiol.
Scand., Vallbo, 1973b).

relation between the two variables. The scatter was considerable but statistically significant correlations (P< 0.05) were
found for 88% of the units studied. The plots suggested roughly
linear relations between the two variables although a more

complex function cannot be excluded. Linear equations were
fitted to the data and the regression coefficient of spindle frequency on torque was calculated for the individual unit. The
mean regression coefficient was 32.8 ips/Nm (ips per metre-
Newton) for the primaries and 22.8 ips/Nm for the secondaries
and the range was 3.75-70 ips/Nm.

DISCUSSION

The present study is an attempt to define the amount of
muscle stiffness accounted for by the reflex effects from the
intramuscular receptors in waking human subjects. The outcome of the analysis is not a conclusive answer, largely because
some uncertain assumptions are involved, but the analysis
defines the alternatives which are consistent with the experimental findings obtained from the intact organism.

Related problems have been studied in several investigations,
mostly on the hind limb extensor muscles of decerebrate cats.
The main factors accounting for the total muscle stiffness have
been most comprehensively analysed by Houk et al. (1970). The
length-tension properties of the contracting muscle fibres
account for one component of the total muscle stiffness. This
component is highly dependent upon muscle length as well as the
characteristics of the actual activation pattern, and it may
account for a considerable stiffness as emphasized by Grillner
(1972; see also Rack and Westbury, 1969). In addition, active
resistance to muscle stretch may be the result of the reflex
actions from intramuscular receptors. In several studies it
has been found that these mechanisms may also account for a
considerable muscle stiffness (Houk et al., 1970; Matthews,
1969).

When an active muscle with intact innervation is stretched by
external forces the afferent inflow from the three main types of
intramuscular sense organs rises. The spindle responses increase due to elongation of the muscle and the Golgi tendon
organ response increases due to the rise in active tension
associated with muscle stretch, whether accounted for by the
length tension properties of the muscle fibres alone, or by
additional muscle activation as well (Jansen and Rudjord, 1964;
Alnaes, 1967; Houk and Henneman, 1967). Also in isometric
voluntary contractions the afferent activity from the same types

of receptors rises. The tendon organ discharge clearly rises
with active tension and, as was demonstrated in the present
study, there is a close relation between spindle frequency and
contraction intensity; the spindle frequency rises approximately
linearly with muscle force due to the fusimotor outflow running
parallel with the skeletomotor outflow.

A fraction of the skeletomotor excitation is accounted for by
spindle afferents during isometric voluntary contractions. Its
magnitude is unknown in relation to the excitation due to other
mechanisms, but for the following argument it will be assumed
that the spindle afferent activity was the exclusive source of
skeletomotor excitation. In relation to the diagram of Fig. 1
this would imply that the skeletomotor neurones received no
excitation through the pathway marked alpha. Obviously this is
an extreme assumption, and it is not very likely to be true
(Koeze et al., 1968; Vallbo, 1971), but the assumption is useful.
to deduce an upper limit for the reflex stiffness. On this
assumption an average afferent inflow of 32.8 ips from the
primaries and 22.8 ips from the secondaries together would
give rise to an increase of the skeletomotor activation equivalent to a torque of 1 Nm - in face of the effects from the
simultaneous rise of Golgi tendon organ discharge. These
figures will be employed to deduce the reflex effect when the
active muscle is stretched.

It was shown in the results section that an extension at the
metacarpo-phalangeal joint by 1° resulted in an average spindle
response of 0.18 ips for the primaries and 0.17 ips for the
secondaries. These figures were obtained from relaxed muscles.
It is known that the fusimotor outflow to contracting muscles is
larger and presumably the position sensitivity is larger as well.
Exact data are not available on this point but the order of magnitude of spindle position sensitivity in contracting muscles may
be inferred on the basis of data from animal experiments and
from relaxed human muscles. It seems that an average increase
of the position sensitivity by a factor of five from the de-efferented
spindle position sensitivity is a maximum which may be obtained
by strong fusimotor activation in the cat hind limb muscle
spindles (Jansen and Matthews, 1962; Lennerstrand, 1968b;
Lennerstrand and Thoden, 1968; Brown et al., 1969). It will be
assumed that a factor of five is an upper limit also for human
finger flexor muscle spindles. Thus, the average position
sensitivity would increase to 0.9 ips/deg for the primaries and

to 0.7 ips/deg for the secondaries when the antebrachial finger flexor muscles are contracting forcefully.

If it is assumed that the central effects of the muscular afferent activity are qualitatively and quantitatively similar in the two situations when the subject performs a contraction against a fixed resistance and when he holds a load, it follows that the spindle response to an extension of 1°, i.e. 0.9 ips for the primaries and 0.7 ips for the secondaries, would give rise to an increase of the skeletomotor activity corresponding to a torque of approximately 0.03 Nm. Obviously the relevant figure is the ratio between the position sensitivity and the regression coefficient of spindle frequency on active torque. More exactly this figure is 0.027 Nm/deg for the primaries and 0.031 Nm/deg for the secondaries. Thus, the intramuscular receptors would account for a muscle stiffness not exceeding approximately 0.03 Nm/deg in the steady state. The Golgi tendon organ discharge does not complicate the issue as they provide a background activity which is independent of muscle length: the input from the tendon organs would be similarly altered for a change in muscle force regardless of this being due to higher skeletomotor output alone, as in isometric contractions, or muscle stretch as well, as in the postulated case of the load being changed.

This calculation of the stiffness accounted for by the muscle afferents is independent of whether the secondaries give rise to excitation or inhibition as the ratio between position sensitivity and the regression coefficient of spindle frequency on active torque is the same for the primaries and the secondaries (cf. Matthews, 1969). It is also independent of the reflex effects being mediated through spinal loops exclusively or through supraspinal mechanisms as well (Koeze et al., 1968; Phillips, 1969; Marsden et al., 1972, 1973). However, it is highly dependent upon whether the central effects of the afferent inflow from the intramuscular receptors are the same when the muscle is contracting against a fixed resistance, as in the present investigation, and when the load on the muscle may vary.

The muscle stiffness accounted for by the intramuscular receptors, as found in the present investigation, is obviously not sufficient to hold the muscle at nearly constant length as the load varies. For instance, if a load equivalent to a torque of 1 Nm - which is approximately 25% of the maximal contraction

intensity for the index finger - were added, this would give rise
to a movement of at least 35°. There are also direct observations from human subjects suggesting a low stiffness - a load
equivalent to 15-20% of the maximal contraction intensity of the
extensor muscles causes a flexion excursion of the index finger
by 30-40 mm (Tardieu et al., 1968).

On the basis of the present findings it seems unlikely that the
muscle spindles and the fusimotor system constitute the main
mechanism for load compensation with regard to muscle length.
The evidence on this point is not conclusive, but it seems that a
drastic change of the central effects of the muscular afferent
activity is required, from isometric contractions to load
carrying contractions, if the weak spindle afferent response to
muscle length would account for a considerable load compensation.

REFERENCES

Alnaes, E., 1967. Static and dynamic properties of Golgi tendon
     organs in the anterior tibial and soleus muscles of the cat.
     Acta Physiol. Scand. 70, 176-187.
Brown, M.C., Lawrence D.G. and Matthews, P.B.C., 1969. Static
     fusimotor fibres and the position-sensitivity of muscle
     spindle receptors. Brain Res. 14, 173-187.
Crowe, A. and Matthews, P.B.C., 1964. The effects of stimulation
     of static and dynamic fusimotor fibres on the response to
     stretching of the primary endings of muscle spindles.
     J. Physiol. 174, 109-131.
Granit, R., 1955. Receptors and Sensory Perception. Yale
     Univ. Press, New Haven. pp. 369.
Granit, R., 1970. The Basis of Motor Control. Academic Press,
     Lond. N.Y. pp. 346.
Grillner, A., 1972. The role of muscle stiffness in meeting
     the changing postural and locomotor requirements for
     force development by the ankle extensors. Acta Physiol.
     Scand. 86. 92-108.
Hagbarth, K.-E. and Vallbo, Å.B., 1968. Discharge characteris-
     tics of human muscle afferents during muscle stretch and
     contraction. Exp· Neurol. 22. 674-694.
Houk, J. and Henneman, E., 1967. Responses of Golgi tendon
     organs to active contractions of the soleus muscle of the
     cat. J. Neurophysiol. 30. 466-489.
Houk, J.C., Singer, J.J. and Goldman, M.R., 1970. An evaluation
     of length and force feedback to soleus muscles of decerebrate
     cats. J. Neurophysiol. 33, 784-811.

Jansen, J.K.S. and Matthews, P.B.C., 1962. The effects of
    fusimotor activity on the static responsiveness of primary
    and secondary endings of muscle spindles in the decerbrate
    cat. Acta Physiol. Scand. 55, 376-386.
Jansen, J.K.S. and Rudjord, T., 1964. On the silent period and
    Golgi tendon organs of the soleus muscle of the cat. Acta
    Physiol. Scand. 62, 364-379.
Koeze, T.H., Phillips, C.G. and Sheridan, J.D., 1968. Thresholds
    of cortical activation of muscle spindles and motoneurons
    of the baboon's hand. J. Physiol. 195, 419-449.
Lennerstrand, G., 1968a. Position and velocity sensitivity of
    muscle spindles in the cat. I. Primary and secondary endings
    deprived of fusimotor activation. Acta Physiol. Scand. 73,
    281-299.
Lennerstrand, G., 1968b. Position and velocity sensitivity of
    muscle spindles in the cat. IV. Interaction between two
    fusimotor fibres converging on the same spindle ending.
    Acta Physiol. Scand. 74, 257-273.
Lennerstrand, G. and Thoden, U., 1968. Position and velocity
    sensitivity of muscle spindles in the cat. III. Static
    fusimotor single-fibre activation of primary and secondary
    endings. Acta Physiol. Scand. 74, 30-49.
Marsden, C.D., Merton, P.A. and Morton, H.B., 1972. Servo
    action in human voluntary movement. Nature. 238, 140-143.
Marsden, C.D., Merton, P.A. and Morton, H.B., 1973. Latency
    measurements compatible with a cortical pathway for the
    stretch reflex in man. J. Physiol. 230, 58-59P
Matthews, P.B.C., 1969. Evidence that the secondary as well as
    the primary endings of the muscle spindles may be responsible
    for the tonic stretch reflex of the decerebrate cat. J.
    Physiol. 204, 365-393.
Matthews, P.B.C., 1972. Mammalian muscle receptors and their
    central actions. Edward Arnold, Lond., 630 pp.
Merton, P.A., 1951. The silent period in a muscle of the human
    hand. J. Physiol. 114, 183-198.
Merton, P.A., 1953. Speculations on the servo-control of
    movement. In The Spinal Cord. Ciba Foundation Symp.(Ed.
    Malcolm J.A. and Gray, J.A.B.) pp. 247-260.
Phillips, C.G., 1969. Motor apparatus of the baboon's hand.
    Proc. Roy. Soc. B. 173, 183-198.
Rack, P.M.H. and Westbury, D.R., 1969. The effects of length
    and stimulus rate on tension in the isometric cat soleus muscle.
    J. Physiol. 204, 343-360.
Tardieu, C., Tabary, J.C. and Tardieu, G., 1968. Étude
    mechanique et electromyographique des réponses à différentes
    pertuberations du maintien postural. J. Physiol. (Paris)
    60, 243-259.
Vallbo, Å.B., 1970a. Slowly adapting muscle receptors in man.
    Acta Physiol. Scand. 78, 315-333.

Vallbo, Å.B., 1970b. Discharge patterns in human muscle spindle
    afferents during isometric voluntary contractions. Acta
    Physiol. Scand. 80, 552-566.
Vallbo, Å.B., 1971. Muscle spindle response at the onset of
    isometric voluntary contractions in man. Time difference
    between fusimotor and skeletomotor effects. J. Physiol.
    218, 405-431.
Vallbo, Å.B., 1972. Single unit recording from human peripheral
    nerves: muscle receptor discharge in resting muscles and
    during voluntary contractions. In Neurophysiology Studied
    in Man. (Ed. Şomjen, G.G.) Excerpta Medica, Amsterdam.
    pp. 281-295.
Vallbo, Å.B., 1973a. Afferent discharge from human muscle
    spindles in non-contracting muscles. Steady state impulse
    frequency as a function of joint angle. Acta Physiol. Scand.
    In press.
Vallbo, Å.B., 1973b. Human muscle spindle discharge during
    isometric voluntary contractions. Amplitude relations
    between spindle frequency and torque. Acta Physiol. Scand.
    In press.
Vallbo, Å.B. and Hagbarth, K.-E., 1968. Activity from skin
    mechanoreceptors recorded percutaneously in awake human
    subjects. Exp. Neurol. 21, 270-289.

A CRITIQUE OF THE HYPOTHESIS THAT THE SPINDLE SECONDARY ENDINGS CONTRIBUTE EXCITATION TO THE STRETCH REFLEX

P. B. C. Matthews

University Laboratory of Physiology, Oxford, England

In 1969 I suggested, on indirect evidence, that in the decerebrate cat the group II afferents from the spindle secondary endings contribute excitation to the stretch reflex rather than the classically believed inhibition. This hypothesis has since been vigorously attacked in certain quarters and a variety of alternative explanations offered for the original findings. The present essay reviews the current state of the controversy and concludes that the hypothesis still provides a satisfactory unitary interpretation of a range of experimental findings which would otherwise require a series of ad hoc explanations. The postulated group II autogenetic excitation is, however, unlikely to be mediated by direct action on the motoneurones.

The spinal reflex action of the secondary endings of the muscle spindles has long been an enigma. Since Lloyd's (1943) classical work, investigators employing electrical stimulation of bared nerves have united in agreeing that the addition of a group II volley to a group I volley evokes weak flexor actions, with excitation of flexor motoneurones and inhibition of extensor motoneurones, irrespective of the origin of the excited afferent fibres; this has been shown both by monosynaptic testing and by intracellular recording (reviewed in Matthews, 1972). Thus, the group II fibres from the spindle secondary endings are often included in a non-specific system of flexor reflex afferents (FRA; Holmqvist and Lundberg, 1961), though this has been without

prejudice as to whether they might not also have some more
specific but as yet uncharted supraspinal action. As long recog-
nised, the weakness of this case is that electrical stimulation
activates fibres of a particular size rather than of a particular
function and so is unlikely to elicit a physiologically pure afferent input to the cord. The great majority of muscle group II
fibres may certainly be taken to supply spindle secondary endings,
yet the admixture of a few fibres from pressure-pain receptors
might lead to the proper spinal actions of the spindle group II
afferents being overwhelmed by a prepotent nociceptive response.

The acceptance of a non-specific reflex action for the spindle
secondary endings has always been an unsatisfactory state of
affairs, since an end-organ as highly developed as the muscle
spindle seems unlikely to expend so significant a part of itself
on such a non-specific purpose. The contrast between the specificity of the end-organ and the apparent non-specificity of its
spinal action has become ever sharper as the message transmitted by the spindle group II fibres has been progressively
appreciated to have a high information content and to provide a
better measure of the absolute length of a muscle than that
supplied by the Ia fibres from the spindle primary endings. The
acuteness of the problem has, to some extent, been obscured by
the finding that in the decerebrate preparation many flexor actions
are in abeyance as a result of a tonic inhibition of the relevant
spinal interneurones by activity descending from higher centres,
and it has been suggested that the flexor actions of the spindle
secondary endings could likewise be eliminated if not wanted
during locomotor and other normal activity (Eccles and Lundberg,
1959). This would virtually relegate the spindle secondary endings to being without significant spinal reflex action, which seems
implausible. However, the recent finding that the group II fibres
may penetrate deep into the ventral horn, even as far as the
motoneurones themselves (Fu and Schomburg, 1973), again
speaks against their function being simply to mediate a non-
specific flexor reflex.

In 1969, Matthews suggested on indirect evidence that in the
decerebrate cat the spindle secondary endings in extensor muscles
contribute positively rather than negatively to the tonic stretch
reflex by producing autogenetic excitation rather than the classically believed autogenetic inhibition. Whether this was the result
of a direct action upon the motoneurone or the result of the group
II fibres acting indirectly via some other system was left com-

pletely open. Several groups promptly attacked the new hypothesis vigorously and a variety of alternatives have been offered
to explain away the original findings. In my view, the hypothesis
continues to provide the most satisfactory explanation for a number of experimental observations which would otherwise require
a series of individual ad hoc explanations. The various strands
of evidence will be reviewed here so that external observers of
the controversy can form their own view. At least, the hypothesis would appear to have enough life left in it to encourage
further work directed towards seeking out a physiologically
meaningful reflex action for the spindle secondary endings.

THE ORIGINAL EVIDENCE

The original experiments consisted of a comparison of the
relative strengths and the mode of interaction within a single
preparation of the myographically recorded reflex responses to
stretch and to high frequency vibration of the soleus muscle in
the decerebrate cat. Stretch was found to be a relatively more
potent stimulus than vibration, although vibration is a much
more effective stimulus for the Ia fibres. Moreover, the reflex
elicited by stretch failed to occlude that produced by vibration
in the manner expected if they both depended in their entirety
upon the same afferent pathways. Fig. 1 illustrates these points.

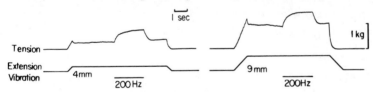

Fig. 1. Myographic records of the reflex responses to
stretch and to vibration of the soleus muscle of the decerebrate cat to show the type of response upon which the group
II hypothesis was originally based. The passive tensions
elicited by the stretches may be neglected. (From Matthews,
1969)

First, increasing the stretch by 5 mm produced a larger increase in tension than did vibration at 200 Hz although the latter
may have been presumed to have driven all the soleus Ia fibres
at 200/sec. Second, the increased stretch reflex showed no
tendency to diminish the response to vibration. Such findings

were earlier analysed in some detail (Matthews, 1969). They
were attributed to the stretch exciting some additional set of
afferent fibres which were not significantly excited by vibration
and which had an autogenetic excitatory action, though not necessarily by means of a direct synaptic action upon motoneurones.
The secondary endings of the muscle spindle were suggested to
be the responsible receptors, since these were well suited to
fill the role and no other group of afferent fibres would appear
to be available to do so.

THE DIFFICULTIES IN INTERPRETATION CREATED BY THE LENGTH-TENSION PROPERTIES OF MUSCLE

Increasing extension of soleus has long been known to increase
its contractile strength, particularly when it is contracting in an
unfused tetanus (Granit, 1958; Matthews, 1959a). The 1969
experiments included various controls for this property and it
did not invalidate the suggestion that the secondary endings contribute excitation to the stretch reflex. Since then, Grillner has
consistently argued that the length-tension properties of muscle
had been wrongfully dismissed and that when they are allowed
for there is nothing left to require the invention of a novel reflex
pathway. Thus in 1970 he denied the conclusions from the earlier
experiments and in 1972 he stated that 'it bears particular emphasis, however, that all the experimental findings are consistent
with a single excitatory system (i.e. the primary endings of
muscle spindles)'.

Fig. 2 illustrates the basis for this view by showing the
length-tension curves for low frequency tetanic contractions of
soleus as obtained by Rack and Westbury and more recently by
Grillner himself. As recognized over a decade ago (Granit,
1958; Matthews, 1959a, 1967), part of the increase in tension
seen in the stretch reflex must be related to an increase in the
strength of the muscle rather than to an increase in the alpha
motor discharge, since the curves are far from flat throughout
their length. The magnitude of this effect will depend crucially
upon the precise range of lengths over which the stretch reflex
is studied and upon the precise frequencies of firing of the motor
units. On Rack and Westbury's figures the effect would be small
over the last 6-7 mm of the physiological range of lengths, which
is where the reflexes were studied in 1969, and for the physiologically important frequencies of 5-10/sec. On Grillner's rather

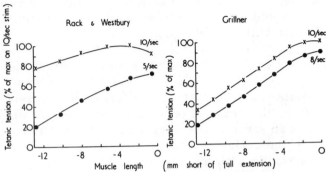

Fig. 2. The tension developed by tetanic muscle contractions
at various lengths of the soleus as described by Rack and
Westbury (1969) and Grillner (1972). In both cases the overall
contraction of the muscle was smoothed by using 'distributed
stimulation' for which five different ventral root filaments
were stimulated out of phase with each other. The frequency
of stimulation shown to the right was that for the individual
filaments. Data redrawn from the original.

different figures the effect would still be large near the physiological maximum length, including for firing at 8/sec which was
found to be the mean frequency of firing in his preparations
(Grillner and Udo, 1971a). Under some conditions the slope of
the tension-length relation in both sets of curves for a fixed frequency approaches that of the stretch reflex (100 g increase in
tension per mm stretching). But such a value only applies to a
maximal tetanic contraction; partial contractions would have
values scaled down in proportion to the number of motor units
involved. In contrast, the stretch reflex may retain a high value
of stiffness when it is involving only a fraction of the motor units,
and the stiffness shows no regular diminution when the length of
the muscle is close to physiological maximum (cf. Matthews,
1959a, b). Thus, many stretch reflexes must obtain a good measure of their strength from an increasing neural discharge.
However, large reflexes, occurring at relatively short lengths
of the muscle, will depend significantly upon muscle properties.
In conformity with the latter view, Grillner and Udo (1971a, b)
found little or no recruitment of new motor units, or increase in
firing of those already active, when applying further stretch to
an already large stretch reflex. If considered in isolation under
the worst conditions, the line of argument based on the excess of
strength of the stretch reflex in relation to the vibration reflex

loses force in the face of the newer findings; in some cases the discrepancy clearly could be related to an increasing contractile strength of the muscle with its extension.

But the slope of the individual length-tension curves cannot alone immediately explain the constancy of the reflex response to a vibration superimposed upon stretch reflexes of different size as in Fig. 1 (i.e. the absence of mutual occlusion between the reflex responses to stretch and to vibration). If the tension developed in the stretch reflex is attributed largely to an increase in muscle strength with muscle length then the additional tension elicited by the vibration, over and above that of the stretch reflex, should increase pari passu with the stretch reflex as the muscle length is increased (any extra motor units excited by the vibration must also increase in strength with muscle elongation). Grillner avoids this difficulty by implying that the extra motor firing elicited by vibration does not depend at all upon the recruitment of new motor units (each with its own tension-length curve) but solely upon an increase in the frequency of firing of those which have already been activated by stretch. Since he found that the tension-length curve for 10/sec stimulation might be simply displaced upwards from that for 8/sec stimulation, without change of slope (cf. Fig. 2), a failure to find occlusion would then be explained. It would, however, be remarkable if vibration should fail regularly to recruit additional motor units. Furthermore, it seems improbable that the tension-length curves should always conveniently run parallel so as to fit in with the numerous conditions under which an absence of occlusion was found. Thus, rather great demands must be made upon the precise form of the tension-length curves of muscle to account for the reflex findings obtained at a variety of muscle lengths, sizes or reflexes and frequencies of vibration (Matthews, 1969, 1970).

SUBORDINATION OF MUSCLE PROPERTIES BY INHIBITORY FEEDBACK

A much more interesting and far-reaching point is that there is no necessity for the tension-length relation of the stretch reflex as a whole to slavishly reflect the tension-length curves of its constituent motor units. This results from the negative feedback loop provided by the Golgi tendon organs, as illustrated in Fig. 3. Any increase in muscle strength with extension in

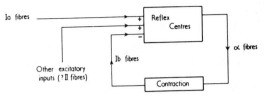

<u>Fig. 3.</u>   The negative feedback of tension provided by the
Golgi tendon organs drawn so as to show how it might free
the reflex centres from being dominated by the length-
tension properties of muscle.

such a system must automatically tend to reduce alpha motor
discharges below what they would have been, for a given
spindle input, had the muscle not increased in strength. All the
components of the system are well known, so the question simply
concerns its effectiveness at over-riding the peripheral length-
tension properties of muscle. Its continuous operation in the
decerebrate cat is shown by the ingenious experiments of Houk
et al. (1970). It would also appear to be partly responsible for
Nichols and Houk's (1973) findings that the change in tension
evoked by applying a ramp stretch to a muscle with a stretch
reflex is quite different in its size and time course from that
evoked by applying the same stretch to a muscle contracting in
response to appropriate motor stimulation. In addition, the contribution of some inhibitory process to the stretch reflex is shown
by the regular observation of a mixture of hyperpolarizing and
depolarizing 'noise' potentials on recording intracellularly from
motoneurones during muscle stretch (Granit et al., 1964).

If the gain of the negative tension feedback is reasonably high,
and this could usefully bear further study, then the muscle properties become largely immaterial in determining the behaviour
of the tonic stretch reflex. In effect, a given quantity of Ia
excitation then simply leads to that quantity of motor firing
which is required to produce a contraction that elicits just
the right quantity of Ib inhibition to balance the Ia excitation.
'Indeed, in some cases the efferent discharge might not even
increase at all as soleus was extended, and the increase in
tension might depend upon the peripheral properties of soleus,
and yet and contraction could remain reflexly controlled'
(Matthews, 1959a). Such tension feedback could well be the
explanation for Grillner and Udo's (1971b) finding that there may
be little or no recruitment of new motor units on applying further

stretch to an already large stretch reflex, although the extra extension must be presumed to be eliciting a greater amount of Ia excitation. Similarly, it can also explain how the 'pseudo stretch reflex' (the increase in tension found on stretching in the presence of a constant motor discharge after cutting the dorsal roots) may sometimes so closely resemble that of the true stretch reflex seen with the dorsal roots intact. (This is the effect which has been nick-named Pompeiano's paradox, see Pompeiano, 1960; Matthews, 1967, 1972; Grillner and Udo, 1971a). If there is an effective negative feedback of tension, then the contractile properties of muscle also become immaterial to the argument as to whether stretch reflexly evokes more exci- tation than vibration. As may be judged from Fig. 3, extra excitation provided by the group II fibres, like that provided by the Ia fibres, leads to just that quantity of contractile tension which is required by the spinal centres to balance the excitation by inhibition. Thus, to write off Matthews' 1969 findings as necessarily due to muscle properties is to treat the stretch reflex with far less respect than it deserves, and to divert attention from one of its potentially most interesting features. Even taken on their own, the two anomolous relations between the reflex responses to stretch and to vibration still seem at least as likely to be due to group II autogenetic exci- tation as to the tension-length properties of muscle.

INTRACELLULAR RECORDING

Westbury's (1972) experiments provide an independent line of evidence against the view that the reflex findings should be attributed to the peripheral properties of skeletal muscle. Westbury recorded synaptic potentials intracellularly from gastrocnemius-soleus motoneurones on stretching and/or vi- brating the muscle in the anaesthetized preparation in which no significant motor discharge occurred. His chief results entirely confirmed those previously described with myographic recording, namely that stretch is a remarkably potent stimulus relative to vibration, and that the excitatory actions of the two modes of stimulation fail to occlude each other in the manner to be ex- pected if both were to depend solely upon the Ia pathway. Considerable advantages were obtained by demonstrating this by intracellular recording rather than by myography. Firstly, of course, the contractile properties of muscle become complet- ely immaterial to the argument. Secondly, because of the anaesthetic, the security of one-to-one driving by the vibration would not have been interferred with either by excess of fusimotor activity or by maintained muscle contraction. Against these, however, must be set the greater difficulty of guaranteeing secure driving of gastrocnemius as compared with soleus primary spindle endings, with the amplitudes of vibration employed (cf. Brown et al., 1967). Westbury's experiments are also interesting in suggesting that the spindle secondary endings may produce a degree of autogenetic excitation in the normal but anaesthetized preparation, as well as in the decerebrate. They also contain a hint of complex integrative processes at work since the amplitude of each individual wave of depolarization elicited by each cycle of stretch would appear to be increased by muscle stretch.

THE EFFECT OF FUSIMOTOR PARALYSIS ON THE VIBRATION REFLEX

Further evidence supporting the hypothesis that the secondary endings should be allocated an autogenetic excitatory action has recently been obtained by studying the effect on the vibration reflex of local paralysis of the gamma efferents by applying procaine to the nerve to the muscle studied (the soleus, McGrath and Matthews, 1970, 1973). Fig. 4 illustrates the rationale of the method. Earlier work (Matthews and Rushworth, 1957a, b) has shown that the ordinary stretch reflex, elicited by stretch alone, is paralysed in separate early and late stages by procaine. The early phase is attributable to an early paralysis of the smaller gamma efferents, and the later phase to a later paralysis of the main reflex pathways consisting of the Ia afferents and the alpha motor fibres. The fusimotor paralysis was originally presumed to reduce the stretch reflex by isolating the muscle spindles from the spontaneous fusimotor firing of the decerebrate preparation, thereby reducing the Ia firing elicited by a stretch; no account was taken of the group II fibres. If that was the whole of the matter the early phase of paralysis should not be found when the reflex was elicited by stretch combined with vibration, since the vibration would then maintain a constant Ia input irrespective of the presence or absence of fusimotor paralysis by causing one-to-one driving, with one spike per cycle of vibration (Brown et al., 1967). On the other hand, if the spindle group II fibres also contribute excitation to the stretch reflex then the early phase of reflex paralysis should

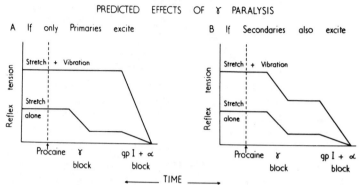

Fig. 4. Diagram of the action to be expected upon the tonic
reflex responses to stretch on its own and to stretch combined with vibration on paralysing the muscle nerve with
procaine. A - if the group I afferents from the primary endings are entirely responsible for the stretch reflex, or
B - if the stimulation by stretch of the group II afferents from
the secondary endings also contributes excitation to the reflex
responses. Procaine paralyses the gamma efferents appreciably before influencing the group I afferents and the alpha
motor fibres, which are paralysed at about the same time.
(From McGrath and Matthews, 1973).

occur during vibration. The secondary endings are largely in-
sensitive to the vibration and so would still decrease their
firing on fusimotor paralysis. Moreover, some of the group II
fibres themselves might be expected to be paralysed relatively
early by procaine. Thus, if the secondary endings make no contribution to the stretch reflex the response to the combined stimuli of stretch and vibration would be as on the left of Fig. 4. If
the secondary endings contribute excitation the result shown on
the right of Fig. 4 should be obtained. Fig. 5 shows an example
of the regular experimental result, namely that the response to
the combined stimuli is greatly reduced at the time of presumed
fusimotor paralysis. The progression of the paralysis is shown
independently of the reflexes by recording the contraction elicited
by stimulating the alpha motor fibres central to the anaesthetized
region of the nerve. Various controls made it very unlikely that
the early diminution in the response should be attributed to any
other factor, such as the Wedensky inhibition of Ia fibres or the
conversion of the pattern of Ia firing from two spikes per cycle
of vibration to one spike. On fusimotor paralysis the background

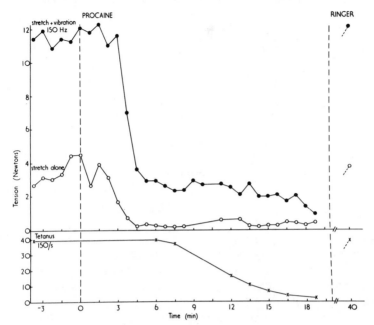

Fig. 5. The early diminution by procaine of the reflex response to the combined stimuli of stretch and vibration occurring at the time of presumed fusimotor paralysis. The top
graphs show active reflex tension over and above the passive
tension produced by the stretching. The bottom graph shows
the muscle contraction elicited by stimulating the nerve central to the anaesthetized region and provides a guide as to
the degree of alpha motor paralysis. (From McGrath and
Matthews, 1973).

firing of the Ia fibres, in the absence of stretch and vibration
will be somewhat reduced. However, it is unlikely that this
would grossly reduce the excitability of the spinal centres and
with it the response to vibration, since the spinal excitability
should have been amply maintained by the regular central
injection of the high frequency discharges elicited by vibration
(usually at 150 Hz for 3-5 sec every 15 sec).

Unfortunately, as with all the other supporting evidence, the
allocation of an excitatory effect to the spindle group II fibres
rests upon argument by exclusion, since they are the only known
group of afferents with the right properties to provide the missing

excitation. If they were not to be allocated this role, it would remain to find another group of afferent fibres which are excited by stretch over a range of muscle lengths, which produce significant autogenetic excitation, and which are rapidly inactivated by procaine.

SPREAD OF VIBRATION

Cook and Duncan (1971) suggested that the earlier findings might have been due to a spread of vibration from the vibrated muscle to the main body of the cat. Some slight spread of vibration did, indeed, occur in many of the experiments which support the group II hypothesis (Matthews, 1969; McGrath and Matthews, 1973), but would not appear to be capable of explaining the results observed under two crucial sets of conditions. First, the spread of vibration should have been the same before and after fusimotor paralysis. Thus, any resulting reflex actions upon the alpha motoneurones should have remained the same and cannot explain the effects illustrated in Fig. 5. Second, spread of vibration will not explain the failure to find the occlusion between the stretch and vibration reflexes which would be expected if they both depended solely upon the Ia pathway (Matthews, 1969). Spread of vibration is certainly potentially able to explain the relative weakness of the vibration reflex in relation to the simple stretch reflex, for this could result from receptors excited by the spread having an inhibitory action on the soleus motoneurones which increased pari passu with the frequency of vibration. But this on its own is insufficient to disprove the present hypothesis. Moreover, it seems unlikely that those receptors which are notably sensitive to vibration (Pacinian corpuscles and other primary endings) would have powerful flexor reflex actions.

SYNCHRONIZED VERSUS UNSYNCHRONIZED AFFERENT VOLLEYS

Thoden et al. (1972) suggested that presynaptic inhibition of Ia fibres may be preferentially elicited by muscle vibration as compared with muscle stretch and that this may be 'at least in part' the explanation for the findings taken to favour the group II hypothesis. This view was based upon a careful study of the presynaptic inhibitory processes which were elicited by static muscle

stretch and by muscle vibration in the decerebrate cat in which
the ventral roots had been cut. Stretch in their experiments was
ineffective at eliciting presynaptic inhibition, whereas vibration
did so. Since vibration produces firing of the various Ia fibres
in synchrony whereas simple stretch excites them to discharge
randomly with regard to each other, they suggested that the stretch
reflex was relatively the stronger because it did not elicit so much
presynaptic inhibition of its own afferent input. However, there
seems little possibility that static stretch within the physiological
range could have excited the primary endings anywhere as near
as powerfully as did vibration at 250-300 Hz of up to 300 μm amplitude (Thoden et al. made no afferent recordings). The experiments, therefore, hardly throw light on the interesting problem
as to whether or not the high degree of synchrony of the Ia discharges elicited by vibration is a feature of importance for their
central action. Moreover, even if highly synchronized volleys
were to be found to have a different action from unsynchronized
ones, this would still fail to explain either the lack of occlusion
between the stretch and vibration reflexes or the effects of fusimotor paralysis. The Ia discharges should have remained fully
synchronized with the vibration irrespective of the degree of
stretch or whether the gamma efferents were functioning, so
their central action should therefore have remained unchanged.

FAILURE OF GROUP II DISCHARGES TO ELICIT A
STRETCH REFLEX WHEN ACTING ALONE

There have now been three separate investigations involving
selective blocking of large fibres in the periphery in the decerebrate without finding any sign of a stretch reflex after the Ia
fibres have been largely inactivated. Cook and Duncan (1971)
compressed the gastrocnemius-soleus nerve and found that they
could thereby eliminate 90% of the myographically recorded
stretch reflex before influencing the motor fibres, as judged by
the twitch contraction elicited by stimulating the nerve above the
block. Control recordings of compound action potentials showed
that the compression abolished conduction in about half the group I
afferents before interfering with the alpha and gamma efferents
or the group II afferents. Emonet-Dénand et al. (1972) selectively
blocked the group I fibres along with other large afferent fibres
running in a dorsal root. This was done by stimulating a dorsal
root for a short period with very strong shocks at a rather high
frequency, which is a form of insult that is better withstood by

small fibres than by large ones. Paralysis of the group I fibres
with preservation of most of the group II fibres, abolished the
tonic stretch reflex recorded electromyographically from the
gastrocnemius-soleus muscle. Cangiano and Lutzemberger (1972)
applied a polarization block to the gastrocnemius-soleus nerve
while recording intracellularly from motoneurones which were
normally excited by muscle stretch, as shown by their depolarization. After eliminating group I activity the stretch elicited a
weak hyperpolarization (inhibition) of each of the eleven cells
studied, and none showed excitation.

Thus, selective blocking of large fibres has entirely failed to
provide the evidence in support of the group II excitatory hypothesis which could reasonably have been hoped for on the basis
of the original experiments. However, such blocking experiments
can never disprove the group II hypothesis, since they can only
strictly show that the group II fibres do not have a direct excitatory action upon motoneurones. Combining the evidence from all
types of experiments, the group II fibres appear to produce an
autogenetic excitatory action indirectly, by virtue of modulating
the reflex effects of some other group of afferent fibres. This
view is favoured by the finding in some of the procaine experiments (McGrath and Matthews, 1973) that the additional reflex
response elicited by increasing the frequency of vibration from
100 Hz to 150 Hz was diminished on fusimotor paralysis, thus
apparently indicating a reduction in central gain for a Ia input.

The complexity of the spinal cord offers numerous possibilities
for indirect action (cf. Andersen and Jansen, 1970). Some possibilities are the interference with Ib autogenetic inhibition, the
interference with Renshaw inhibition of the motoneurone, the
facilitation of possible Ia polysynaptic pathways, and the removal
of presynaptic inhibition from the Ia fibres - whether generated
by the Ia fibres themselves or from some other source. In considering all such possibilities it should be remembered that the
myographic work has been concerned with tonic stretch reflexes,
and the measurements were made after the system has reached
approximate equilibrium so there was ample time for integrative
actions of considerable complexity. However, it seems likely
that these processes largely take place in the spinal cord itself
rather than in higher centres since several of the findings
originally made on the decerebrate preparation have now been
extended to the acute spinal preparation which was temporarily
manifesting a tonic stretch reflex by virtue of being treated with

DOPA (Goodwin et al., 1973).

In conclusion, there is as yet no reason to jettison the hypothesis that the spindle group II fibres cause autogenetic excitation in the decerebrate preparation since this provides a satisfactory unitary interpretation of a range of experimental results which would otherwise require a series of ad hoc special explanations. Further probing of the problem should be welcomed by all, since it would be complacent to believe that the reflex action of the spindle group II fibres can simply be a non-specific flexor reflex just like that elicited by nociceptive afferents.

REFERENCES

Andersen, P., and Jansen, J.K.S., 1970. Excitatory Synaptic Mechanisms. Universitetsforlaget, Oslo, pp. 323-325.

Brown, M.C., Engberg, I.E., and Matthews, P.B.C., 1967. The relative sensitivity to vibration of muscle receptors of the cat. J. Physiol. 192, 773-800.

Cangiano, A., and Lutzemberger, L., 1972. The action of selectively activated group II muscle afferent fibers on extensor motoneurons. Brain Res. 41, 475-478.

Cook, W.A., and Duncan, C.C., 1971. Contribution of group I afferents to the tonic stretch reflex of the decerebrate cat. Brain Res. 33, 509-513.

Eccles, R.M., and Lundberg, A., 1959. Supraspinal control of interneurones mediating spinal reflexes. J. Physiol. 147, 565-584.

Emonet-Dénand, F., Jami, L., Joffroy, M., and Laporte, Y., 1972. Absence de réflexe myotatique après blocage de la conduction dans les fibres du groupe I.   Compt. Rend. Acad. Sci. (Paris) 274, 1542-1545.

Fu, T.C., and Schomburg, E.D., 1973. Intraspinal branching of functionally identified group II muscle spindle afferents. Pflugers Arch. Ges. Physiol. 339, R73.

Goodwin, G.M., McGrath, G.J., and Matthews, P.B.C., 1973. The tonic vibration reflex seen in the acute spinal cat after treatment with DOPA. Brain Res. 49, 463-466.

Granit, R., 1958. Neuromuscular interaction in postural tone of the cat's isometric soleus muscle. J. Physiol. 143, 387-402.

Granit, R., Kellerth, J.-O., and Williams, T.D., 1964. Intracellular aspects of stimulating motoneurones by muscle stretch. J. Physiol. 174, 453-472.

Grillner, S., 1970. Is the tonic stretch reflex dependent upon group II excitation? Acta Physiol. Scand. 78, 431-432.

Grillner, S., 1972. The role of muscle stiffness in meeting the
    changing postural and locomotor requirements for force develop-
    ment by the ankle extensors. Acta Physiol. Scand. 86, 92-108.
Grillner, S., and Udo, M., 1971a. Motor unit activity and stiff-
    ness of the contracting muscle fibres in the tonic stretch reflex.
    Acta Physiol. Scand. 81, 422-424.
Grillner, S., and Udo, M., 1971b. Recruitment in the tonic stretch
    reflex. Acta Physiol. Scand. 81, 571-573.
Holmqvist, B., and Lundberg, A., 1961. Differential supraspinal
    control of synaptic actions evoked by volleys in the flexion
    reflex afferents in alpha motoneurones. Acta Physiol. Scand.
    54, Suppl. 186, 1-51.
Houk, J.C., Singer, J.J., and Goldman, M.R., 1970. An evaluation
    of length and force feedback to soleus muscles of decerebrate
    cats. J. Neurophysiol. 33, 784-811.
Lloyd, D.P.C., 1943. Neuron patterns controlling transmission of
    ipsilateral hind limb reflexes in cat. J. Neurophysiol. 6,
    293-315.
McGrath, G.J., and Matthews, P.B.C., 1970. Support for an auto-
    genetic excitatory reflex action of the spindle secondaries from
    the effect of gamma blockade by procaine. J. Physiol. 210,
    176-177P.
McGrath, G.J., and Matthews, P.B.C., 1973. Evidence from the use
    of procaine during procaine nerve block that the spindle group
    II fibres contribute excitation to the tonic stretch reflex of
    the decerebrate cat. J. Physiol. In press.
Matthews, P.B.C., 1959a. The dependence of tension upon extension
    in the stretch reflex of the soleus muscle of the decerebrate
    cat. J. Physiol. 147, 521-546.
Matthews, P.B.C., 1959b. A study of certain factors influencing
    the stretch reflex of the decerebrate cat. J. Physiol. 147,
    547-564.
Matthews, P.B.C., 1967. Vibration and the stretch reflex. In:
    Myotatic, Kinesthetic and Vestibular Mechanisms,(ed. de Reuck,
    A.V.S. and Knight, J) Churchill, London, pp. 40-50.
Matthews, P.B.C., 1969. Evidence that the secondary as well as
    the primary endings of the muscle spindles may be responsible
    for the tonic stretch reflex of the decerebrate cat. J. Physiol.
    204, 365-393.
Matthews, P.B.C., 1970. A reply to criticism of the hypothesis
    that the group II afferents contribute excitation to the stretch
    reflex. Acta Physiol. Scand. 79, 431-433.
Matthews, P.B.C., 1972. Mammalian Muscle Receptors and their
    Central Actions. Arnold, London.
Matthews, P.B.C., and Rushworth, G. 1957a. The selective effect
    of procaine on the stretch reflex and tendon jerk of soleus
    muscle when applied to its nerve. J. Physiol. 135, 245-262.
Matthews, P.B.C., and Rushworth, G., 1957b. The relative sensiti-
    vity of muscle nerve fibres to procaine. J. Physiol. 135,
    263-269.

Nichols, T.R., and Houk, J., 1973. Regulation of muscle contraction by autogenetic reflexes. Science 181, 182-184.

Pompeiano, O., 1960. Alpha types of 'release' studied in tension-extension diagrams from cat's forelimb triceps muscle. Arch. Ital. Biol. 98, 92-117.

Rack, P.M.H., and Westbury, D.R., 1969. The effects of length and stimulus rate on tension in the isometric cat soleus muscle. J. Physiol. 204, 443-460.

Thoden, U., Magherini, P.C., and Pompeiano, O., 1972. Evidence that presynaptic inhibition may decrease the autogenetic excitation caused by vibration of extensor muscles. Arch. Ital. Biol. 110, 90-116.

Westbury, D.R., 1972. A study of stretch and vibration reflexes of the cat by intracellular recording from motoneurones. J. Physiol. 226, 37-56.

THE STRETCH REFLEX RESPONSE TO MOVEMENT

OF HUMAN ELBOW JOINT

P. M. H. Rack

Department of Physiology, Birmingham University
Birmingham, Great Britain

Measurements were made of the resistance of the human
elbow joint to imposed movements. The forearm was driven
through sinusoidally alternating flexion-extension movements
of different frequencies and amplitudes while the subject maintained a steady flexing effort.

Although the subject was able to keep the mean force constant,
the force still increased and decreased during each cycle of
movement in an approximately sinusoidal way. These force
fluctuations were usually so timed that they tended to oppose
the movement, as they would in any passive mechanical system
that showed some friction. There was, however, a range of
frequencies around 10 Hz in which the force was sometimes so
timed that the limb exerted a greater flexing force when it was
actually flexing than when it was being pulled into extension.
Such a force implies a reflex excitation of the flexor muscles
of the elbow joint which was greatest when the muscle was
shortening. This reflex activity was seen when the amplitude
of movement was small and the subject exerted a large flexing
force. The frequency range in which it appeared suggests that
it was due to a fast reflex pathway, perhaps the same pathway
that serves the tendon jerk.

While it is possible to study many aspects of the stretch reflex
in spinal, decerebrate, or anaesthetized preparations, the over-

all response of a normal limb to a sudden displacement can only
be satisfactorily investigated in the conscious animal. In practice,
some co-operation is needed for experiments of this sort and they
can most easily be carried out on human subjects. This paper
describes the forces that develop at the normal human elbow joint
when it is driven through sinusoidally alternating flexion-extension
movements.

A mere record of the force with which a limb resists movement
gives little indication of the reflex activity, since much of the
force is expended in accelerating its mass, and in overcoming
elastic and frictional resistance of soft tissues that is quite independent of reflex activity. In a simple mechanical system it
might be possible to calculate the force required to overcome
these 'passive' elements and then arrive at the reflex force by a
process of subtraction; in a limb, however, no such simple calculation is possible since the effective mass is difficult to measure
with sufficient accuracy, and the resistance offered by muscles
and other soft tissues follows no simple pattern.

SINUSOIDAL ANALYSIS

The problem becomes somewhat simpler when sinusoidal
movements are used. The force developed can then be resolved
into two components, a component in phase with the movement,
and a component that is $90°$ out of phase, or 'in quadrature' to the
movement.

Sinusoidal movement of a mass is associated with a sinusoidal
force that reaches its maximum at the limit of the movement where
its direction reverses. Sinusoidal movement of an elastic element
is also associated with a sinusoidally varying force and this too
reaches its maximum at the limit of the movement when the elastic material is fully extended. Both mass and elastic components
thus resist with a force that is in phase with the movement, though
these forces are opposite in direction.

Any friction within the limb, and this includes the 'viscous'
properties of the muscles, meets the movement with a force
that is greatest during movement, becoming zero when the limb
is momentarily at rest at either end. This force is in phase with
the velocity of movement and $90°$ in advance of the limb position;
it is described as a positive quadrature component of force. The

direction of this force component is such that it always opposes
the movement and work has to be done on the limb to overcome
it and maintain the movement.

It is important to note that whereas a passive limb responds
to movement with forces in phase with the movement which may
act in either direction, the quadrature components of force act
in one direction only, and that is the direction that opposes the
movement; this is still true if the muscles within the limb are
contracting, so long as they are contracting steadily, their rate
of activation being unchanged through the movement cycle.

Any muscle contraction that occurs as a reflex response to
the movement will occur at some time in the cycle that is determined by the properties of the sensory receptors and the time
delay in the reflex pathway. This reflex force will add to the
forces that have already been described. If, for example, the
afferent signal arises during muscle lengthening and the reflex
delay is very short compared with the cycle time, then the
resulting muscle contraction will also occur during lengthening
and add to the positive quadrature component of force opposing
the movement; its effect will then be the same as the effect of
extra friction. If, on the other hand, the delay is so long, or the
frequency of movement so rapid that the reflex muscle contraction
occurs during the subsequent shortening movement, there will
be an opposite effect and the reflex changes in force will tend to
offset the effect of friction in the limb and may appear as a force
that is greater during shortening than during lengthening.

The reflex response will also contribute to the components in
phase with sinusoidal movement and may resemble the effect of
any of the passive elements within the limb. However, if suitably
timed, it contributes a negative quadrature force which amounts
to a higher tension in the muscles during shortening than during
lengthening. Such a force tends to assist and sustain the movement and when it is present the limb actually does work on the
driving mechanism; its effect can be regarded as equivalent to a
'negative friction'.

Whenever an analysis of the forces developed during sinusoidal
movement reveals that the quadrature component of force is negative, i.e. the force rises higher during shortening than during
lengthening, one can confidently assume that the muscles concerned
are subject to intermittent excitation. If this negative quadrature

force recurs in repeated cycles of a movement which is faster than the subject can voluntarily sustain, then it can further be assumed that it arises from a reflex response to the movement.

EXPERIMENTAL METHOD

In a series of experiments on normal human subjects, the left forearm and hand were fixed in a mould which was mounted on bearings that allowed only a flexion-extension movement of the elbow joint. The forearm was then driven through sinusoidally alternating flexion-extension movements by a crank and rotating fly-wheel (Fig. 1). In each sequence of movements the fly-wheel

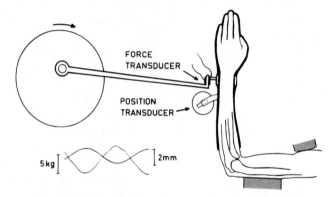

Fig. 1. The experimental arrangement. A mould enclosing the forearm and hand is coupled through a crank to a fly-wheel. Rotation of the fly-wheel generates a sinusoidal movement of the crank and limb. Position transducer: during movements a vane attached to the mould moves across a window, controlling the illumination of a photo-electric cell. Force transducer: two semi-conductor strain gauges are mounted on a bracket at the end of the crank. Changes in the force on the crank distort the bracket. This distortion gives rise to resistance changes in the gauges which are used to signal force. Inset: a specimen record of limb position and force fluctuation. The smooth sinusoid is the position record, extension of the limb being shown by an upward movement. The less regular record indicates the force variation at the wrist. The mean force was 12 kg.

was set in motion by an electric motor, but the motor was then de-coupled to reduce transmitted vibration, and the fly-wheel gradually slowed down. In a single sequence of movements it was thus possible to study the forces developed in response to a whole range of frequencies. Throughout each sequence of movements the subject flexed his elbow against the crank to maintain a constant mean force; to assist him in this the mean force measured at the wrist was displayed on a meter which had a very long time constant compared with the frequencies of movement used.

The position of the limb and the force on the crank were recorded through the whole of each sequence of movements; a short section of record is included in Fig. 1. The experimental method and the method of analyzing the results will be reported in detail elsewhere.

THE FORCES RECORDED

The sinusoidally alternating forces recorded during each sequence of movements were resolved into components that were in phase with the movement and components in quadrature. The quadrature components gave more immediate information about the reflex response to movement and the description that follows will be confined to them.

Each of the histograms that make up Fig. 2 is a record of the quadrature component of this alternating force at the wrist over a whole range of frequencies; each block in the histograms indicates the average force in 10 consecutive cycles. Taking Fig. 2d as an example, one can see that at the higher frequencies the force had a positive value; the limb then presented a frictional type of resistance to the movement, the tension on the crank and couplings being greater when the limb was being pulled toward the extended position than when it was flexing back away from the fly-wheel. As the frequency of movement decreased, however, the direction of this force changed so that at 7-13 Hz the tension was greater during flexion than during extension; the limb was then doing work on the fly-wheel.

One can conclude therefore that in the sequence of movements from which Fig. 2d was obtained, there was an intermittent activation of the elbow muscles at the same frequency as the movement, which at 7-13 Hz was so timed as to have its greatest

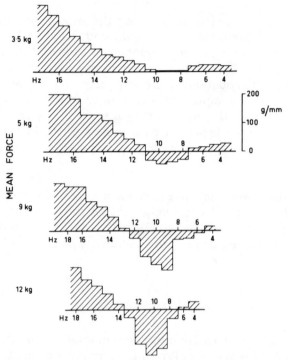

<u>Fig. 2.</u> The component of force out of phase with (in
quadrature to) the movement during a 2. 25 mm (peak to peak)
sinusoidal movement of the wrist.
Each histogram represents a whole sequence of 120-180 cycles
of movement. The quadrature component of force has been
measured for each cycle but each block in the histogram
shows the average of that force in 10 consecutive cycles expressed
as a function of the movement. A positive value indicates
resistance to the movement whereas a negative value indicates
a force that tended to maintain the movement. During each
record the movement gradually slowed down, as shown by
the frequency scales.
The four different histograms were obtained when the subject
exerted different mean flexing forces against the crank.

effect on the flexor muscles after they had actually begun to
shorten. Human subjects cannot voluntarily move their elbow
joints at frequencies greater than 6-7 Hz, and this is true even
when the limb is slung between springs that give it a natural
frequency of oscillation of more than 7 Hz. The intermittent
muscular activity that must have occurred in the present

experiments cannot therefore have been voluntary, and the fact that it remained locked to the movement over a range of frequencies from 13-7 Hz implies that it was a reflex response to the movement.

Electromyograms showed that the elbow flexor muscles were also activated intermittently when the frequency of movment was higher than 13 Hz, but the amount of force that this activity contributed could not be determined since it was obscured by the properties of the 'passive' limb.

THE EFFECT OF THE FLEXING EFFORT

In all these experiments the subject exerted a flexing force against the crank, and it is on the background of this steady flexing effort that the sinusoidal force fluctuation occurred. When this mean flexing force was changed, the response to a sinusoidal movement also changed, and in particular, the negative quadrature force attributable to reflex activity changed. The result shown in Fig. 2d was obtained while the subject flexed against the crank with a large mean force (the 12 kg measured at the wrist was about a half of this subject's absolute maximum). When he flexed with a smaller force (Fig. 2b and c), this negative quadrature component of force could still be seen at frequencies around 10 Hz, but it was smaller and it extended over a more limited frequency range. When he flexed against the crank with only a small force (Fig. 2a) the quadrature component of the force did not reverse at all, but remained positive at all frequences, indicating that work always has to be done on the limb to maintain the movement.

The reflex response to the sinusoidal movement clearly increased when the subject contracted his muscles with a larger mean force.

THE EFFECT OF AMPLITUDE OF MOVEMENT

Figure 3 was constructed in the same way as Fig. 2d, but different amplitudes of movement were used for different parts of the figure while the subject always exerted the same 12 kg mean flexing force. The force is expressed as a function of the amplitude of movement, so that the similarity of the different

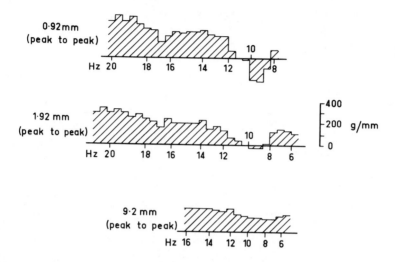

Fig. 3. The effect of amplitude of sinusoidal movement on the quadrature component of force. The histograms have been prepared in the same way as in Fig. 2, though they are from a different subject. The subject exerted a mean flexing force of 12 kg. The amplitude of movement is shown beside each histogram.

histograms for frequencies of 14 Hz or more implies that at these higher frequencies the quadrature component of the force increases in proportion to the movement amplitude.

At frequencies around 10 Hz the amplitude of movement had a different and very striking effect on the force developed. With the smaller amplitudes of movement (Fig. 3a), the quadrature component of the force was negative as it had been in Figs. 2b-d, indicating that the reflex response to the movement was then sufficiently powerful to outweigh the effect of friction within the limb. When, however, large amplitudes of movement were employed, there was no reversal of the quadrature force which remained positive at all frequencies.

With larger amplitudes of movement, therefore, either the reflex contraction was relatively less than with small movements, or the frictional resistance of the limb was greater.

THE NATURE OF THE REFLEX

The reflex response implied by this negative quadrature force was unchanged by eye closure, and it remained when cutaneous sensation in the wrist and fingers was seriously impaired by the prolonged pressure of the mould; it is likely therefore, that it arose from deep receptors within the limb. In view of the large amount of information available about the properties of muscle spindles, it is interesting to consider how far the present results can be explained in terms of their properties, and the properties of the monosynaptic stretch reflex.

Muscle spindle primary afferent fibres discharge most vigorously when the spindle is being lengthened; at the frequencies and amplitudes of movement used in these experiments the maximum afferent discharge could well have occurred when the velocity of lengthening was greatest, that is 90° in advance of the maximum length (Matthews and Stein, 1969). When the frequency of movement was 8-12 Hz the reflex muscle contraction occurred during shortening; if this were a result of the muscle spindle activity there must have been a delay of about 50 msec between the maximum spindle afferent discharge and the reflex contraction that it generated. Such a delay agrees with the timing of the biceps tendon jerk and it is the sort of delay that one might obtain from a fast, perhaps monosynaptic reflex pathway coupled to moderately fast muscle fibres; it is, however, a good deal less than the stretch reflex delay recorded at the human elbow joint by Hammond, Merton and Sutton (1956). They found a reflex increase in force which began at a much longer interval after the onset of a constant velocity extension and only reached its maximum some 100 msec or more after the onset of movement; they inferred that this reflex had a slower and perhaps longer pathway than the tendon jerk. A similar relatively slow 'functional stretch reflex' has been recorded in the human calf muscles (Melvill Jones and Watt, 1971).

The present results do not necessarily conflict with those of Hammond et al.; their subjects exerted a steady flexing force until the onset of the movement, but the forces they used were smaller than in the present experiments (about 3 kg in their plate V). When during sinusoidal movement the subjects exerted a similar small flexing force (Fig. 2a), there was less evidence of a fast reflex response to the movement and it was only when

the subject exerted larger mean forces that this response was
clearly present (Figs. 2b-d).

This result could perhaps have been expected; activity in
the motor nerve supply to a muscle group is usually accompanied
by an increase in fusimotor activity to the same muscles (Granit,
1970) and an increase in the primary afferent fibre discharge
from their muscle spindles (Vallbo, 1971). This increase in
muscle spindle sensitivity might well account for the increase
in fast reflex response to the movement.

Muscle spindles are more sensitive to small movements than
to large ones (Matthews and Stein, 1969). The afferent discharge
that accompanies movements of up to about 1% of the muscle's
range (Matthews, 1972) is a vigorous one, but an increase to a
larger amplitude of movement is not associated with a correspondingly large increase in the afferent discharge. It was hardly
surprising therefore that in the present experiments there was
more stretch reflex activity in response to a small sinusoidal
movement than to a large one; Matthews (1969) found a similar
powerful reflex response to small extensions of decerebrate cat
muscles, and this too became relatively less when the amplitude
of movement was increased.

THE ROLE OF THE STRETCH REFLEX

Sinusoidal movements have been used here as a convenient
method of examining the human stretch reflex; the limb presumably
meets other disturbances with an equally rapid reflex response
which has the same high sensitivity to small movements. The
stretch reflex may thus play a part in the early response to an
unexpected disturbance by providing sufficient resistance to limit
the displacement until such time as it takes for the nervous system
to react more completely by using more complex longer pathways.

In the present experiments the reflex was most effective when
the limb muscles were powerfully contracting. There is, however,
no reason to suppose that in mammals the fusimotor activity need
be tied to the activity of the extrafusal fibres, and one would like
to think that in normal activity the higher centres of the nervous
system can vary the fusimotor activity in whatever way is most
appropriate for the posture or movements going on at the time.

The response of a fast direct pathway can only be a fairly simple one, but it is tempting to think that the higher centres of the nervous system continuously control and alter the fusimotor activity to keep the stretch reflex 'set up' in a way that will give the most appropriate response to the sorts of disturbance that experience and foresight lead us to expect.

Acknowledgement: This work was supported by a grant from the National Fund for Research into Crippling Diseases.

REFERENCES

Granit, R., 1970. The Basis of Motor Control. Academic Press, London.

Hammond, P.N., Merton, P.A., and Sutton, G.G., 1956. Nervous gradations of muscular contraction. Brit. Med. Bul. 12, 214-218.

Matthews, P.B.C., 1969. Evidence that the secondary as well as the primary endings of the muscle spindles may be responsible for the tonic stretch reflex of the decerebrate cat. J. Physiol. 294, 365-398.

Matthews, P.B.C., 1972. Mammalian Muscle Receptors and their Central Actions. Arnold, London, 580 pp.

Matthews, P.B.C., and Stein, R.B., 1969. The sensitivity of muscle spindle afferents to small sinusoidal changes of length. J. Physiol. 200, 723-743.

Melvill Jones, G. and Watt, D.G.D., 1971. Observations on the control of stepping and hopping movement in man. J. Physiol. 219, 709-727.

Vallbo, A.B., 1971. Muscle spindle response at the onset of voluntary contraction in man. Time difference between fusimotor and skeletomotor effects. J. Physiol. 218, 405-431.

THE CONTINUITY OF MOVEMENTS

V. B. Brooks, J. D. Cooke and J. S. Thomas

Department of Physiology, University of Western
Ontario, London, Canada

A study was made of self-initiated and self-terminated elbow
movements made by Cebus monkeys during performance of a
self-paced step-tracking task. Movements were termed
"continuous" if their acceleration traces crossed the zero
line only once, and "discontinuous" if there was more than
one zero crossing. Parameters of continuous and discontinuous
movements were measured. Acceleration in continuous movements could oscillate at 7-8 Hz ("deviations"), and in discontinuous movements at 3-4 Hz ("steps"). Steps of discontinuous
movements became smaller as movements approached their
targets. Amplitudes of continuous movements and of steps
were highly correlated to their durations, and fitted the same
regression line. It is concluded that the variations of acceleration of continuous and discontinuous movements appear
locked into harmonics of the same frequency. Their relationship to physiological tremor is discussed.

INTRODUCTION

Voluntary limb movements can be made in a "continuous" or a
"discontinuous" manner. The former appear as smooth displacements and the latter as a sequence of "steps". Rhythmical human
finger, hand and arm movements have been so described by
Stetson (1905) and Stetson and Bouman (1935). The fastest
ballistic movements were assumed to have been preprogrammed

257

by the central nervous system since they were not controllable
once started (Stetson and McDill, 1923) in contrast to slower
movements that exhibited small adjustments that were thought
to have been corrections (cf. Woodworth, 1899). Similar types
have been described for monkeys' performance of a self-paced
step-tracking task (Kozlovskaya et al., 1970). Since these
self-initiated elbow movements of monkeys were however in
the mid-range of speeds between "ballistic" throws and slow
"moving fixations", they may have more in common than
appeared originally.

In this paper we have extended the study of monkeys' elbow
movements to ask the questions: how predictable and regular
are the executions of continuous and discontinuous movements?
Previous descriptions from this laboratory have been confirmed
(Kozlovskaya et al., 1970, 1973) but in addition we now show
that the detailed sequences of actions in all movements fit a
basic rhythm, whose frequency for the monkey under study was
about 7-8 Hz.

METHODS

The data included in this report were obtained primarily from
one monkey (M18L) during one experimental session (12.2.73),
with additional data for Fig. 3 from another (M12L, 21.5.73).
All illustrated relationships were also confirmed by analysis of
various samples from M12L and M20L. The motor task under
study and the apparatus have been described previously (Brooks
et al., 1973). Briefly, a Cebus monkey was trained to sit in a
primate chair and to turn a freely moving handle through a horizontal arc from one target zone to another with alternate flexions
and extensions about the elbow joint. Arrival into a target zone
was signalled by both a light and a tone. The monkey was required
to hold the handle in the target for 1 sec whereupon auditory and
visual "success" signals were given, and he then had to move the
handle to the other target within a 5 sec period as signalled by a
soft, masking timing noise. Juice reinforcement was given after
three "successes". No other restrictions were placed on the self-
paced movements from one target to the other. Control periods
of movement were alternated with four periods of about 5 min each
during which the dentate nucleus was reversibly cooled (which
constitutes a separate series of experiments to be reported elsewhere). The recording sessions lasted approximately 1 hour.

Target zones had widths of 10° of arc with their centres separated by 50° of arc. The mechanical stops on the movement of the handle were 15° of arc beyond the outer edges of the targets. A continuous record of the angular position of the handle was obtained from a precision potentiometer which was mounted with its axis at the centre of rotation of the handle.

The signal from the potentiometer was recorded on magnetic tape for later analysis with a PDP-12 computer. The position signals, that were accurate to within 0.5° of arc, were digitized (12 bit) at a sampling rate of 1 KHz and the average of consecutive sets of 10 points was written on LINC tape resulting in an effective sampling rate of 100 Hz. The velocity and acceleration records (middle and lower traces in Fig. 1) were obtained by sequential fifth point differentiation of the digitized position signal. All acceleration data, except that shown in Fig. 1, were obtained after smoothing of the acceleration by a running 5 point averaging technique. Signal frequencies above 10 Hz were severely attenuated because of the 50 msec "window" for differentiating and smoothing. The data were analyzed by programs written in machine language and FOCAL.

RESULTS

Representative "continuous" and "discontinuous" movements are shown in Fig. 1. As has been previously described, the basic pattern of a continuous movement is one in which the position (top left trace) changes smoothly from start to end point (Kozlovskaya et al., 1970). The velocity goes through one maximum (middle trace) at which time acceleration is zero (bottom trace). By contrast, a discontinuous movement contains several "steps" in the position trace (top right) and its velocity reaches several maxima (middle trace). Correspondingly there are several points at which the acceleration curve crosses zero. Steps, which may now be defined as those parts of discontinuous movements made between three consecutive occurrences of zero acceleration, occur in a cyclic manner at about 3 Hz as previously described (Kozlovskaya et al., 1970).

Contrary to previous experience, however, we now find a cyclic phenomenon also in continuous movements: the left acceleration trace of Fig. 1 shows "deviations" from smooth continuation in the form of alternating maxima and minima that

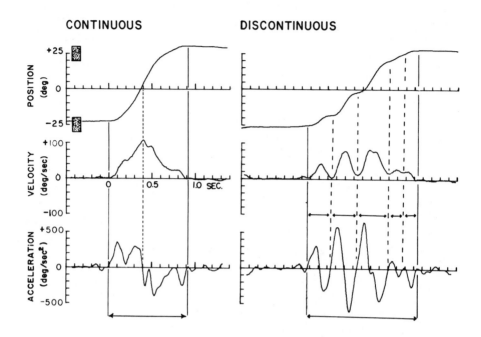

Fig. 1. "Continuous" and "discontinuous" movements are
shown in the left and right columns. Position - upper traces;
velocity - centre traces; acceleration - lower traces (plotted
by computer from position information). Solid vertical lines
bounding horizontal markers (below the traces) indicate
beginning and end of movements. Dashed vertical line for
the continuous movement (on the left) indicates maximum
velocity and the corresponding zero acceleration. Intervening
maxima and minima ("deviations") of acceleration do not
cross the zero acceleration line. Points of zero acceleration
bounding "steps" in the discontinuous movement (on the right)
are indicated by broken vertical lines separated by horizontal
markers. The monkey was performing the standard task with
targets of 10^0 width (indicated by boxes on calibration of
position trace) whose centres were separated by 50^0. Time
scale (in sec) applies to all traces, and scales of position,
velocity and acceleration apply to both continuous and discontinuous movements (M18L, 12.2.73).

appear as modulations of the acceleration sequence of the movement. Deviations in continuous movements go from one acceler-

ation maximum to the next through a minimum that does not cross zero acceleration, while steps in discontinuous movements are bounded by acceleration zero crossings. Deviations in continuous movements went unnoticed in previous work because the velocity, rather than the more revealing acceleration traces, served as prime indicators of change.

Parameters of Continuous and Discontinuous Movements

Fig. 2 presents the distributions of some parameters of all the movements made during one experimental session, classified as continuous or discontinuous by the computer program. No movements were rejected regardless of whether they went from one target completely to another, whether they terminated in a holding or a quick return, or because of any other criteria. Mean values of amplitudes cluster around inter-target distances and thus indicate that most movements of this well-trained animal fulfilled the task requirements. The present data are comparable to those published previously (cf. Fig. 3 in Kozlovskaya et al., 1973) except that durations of discontinuous movements of the current monkey were unusually brief and peak velocities of continuous movements were low.

The relationships between some of the parameters of Fig. 2 are listed in Table 1 as correlation coefficients for pairs of parameters. Strong correlations were found only for continuous movements, relating amplitude to peak, or mean, velocity or to duration. Neither peak acceleration nor deceleration were well correlated with amplitude, with the exception (for this monkey only) of peak acceleration of continuous extensions. Correlations cannot specify physiological events but they can indicate what could or could not be possible. One might therefore imagine that for task performance with continuous movements, the central nervous system could as well govern velocity as position.

Relation of "Steps" to Continuous Movements and Their Acceleration "Deviations"

As has been noted in relation to Fig. 1, acceleration in a continuous movement rises to a maximum (peak acceleration) and then decreases to a minimum (peak deceleration), reaching zero acceleration only once between these two points. A similar

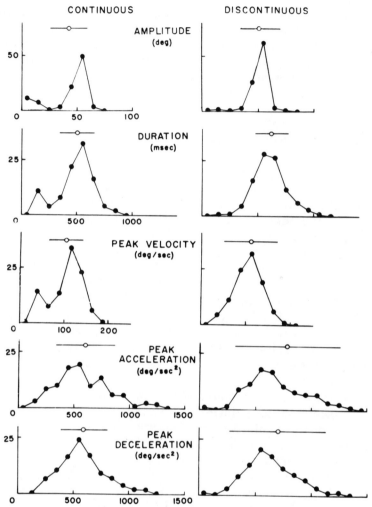

Fig. 2. Distributions of amplitudes, durations, peak velocities, peak accelerations and decelerations are shown for continuous (left) and discontinuous (right) movements. The relative frequency of occurrence, i. e. the percentages of the total number measured, are plotted on the ordinates while the abscissae plot measures of parameters defined on the drawings. Means and SDs are indicated above each curve, based on all movements made in one session: 165 continuous and 565 discontinuous movements (M18L: 12. 2. 73).

	Continuous movements		Discontinuous movements	
	Flexion	Extension	Flexion	Extension
Peak velocity vs amplitude	0.85	0.79	0.47	0.54
Mean velocity vs amplitude	0.79	0.75	0.51	0.51
Amplitude vs duration	0.79	0.63	0.16	0.19
Peak acceleration vs amplitude	0.39	0.63	0.08	0.32
Peak deceleration vs amplitude	0.02	0.38	0.05	0.30
n	109	56	256	309

Table 1. Relationships between some parameters of all continuous and discontinuous movements presented in Fig. 2 are listed
as correlation coefficients obtained from a least squares best fit
regression analysis of pairs of parameters. The number of
movements (n) upon which the calculations were based is given
in the bottom row.

pattern clearly holds for the individual steps in discontinuous movements. In a previous study steps in discontinuous movements were described as resembling very small continuous movements, and as part of a continuum in the relation between amplitude and duration (Kozlovskaya et al., 1973). This was confirmed in the present work and is illustrated in Fig. 3.

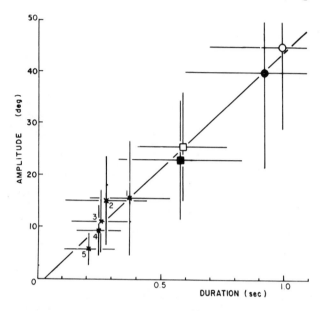

Fig. 3. Relationship between amplitudes (ordinate) and durations (abscissa) of continuous movements and steps in discontinuous movements. Mean amplitudes and durations of continuous movements (circles and squares) and of steps in discontinuous movements (crosses) are plotted. Data from two experiments; one in which the target centres were separated by 50° (circles and crosses: M18L) and one in which target centres were separated by 25° (squares: M12L). Open symbols: flexions; closed symbols: extensions. The plotted (least squares best fit regression) line has a correlation coefficient of 0.99. The numbers beside the crosses indicate the position of the step in the discontinuous movement (i.e. the first step, the second, etc.). The points are based on 109 continuous flexions and 56 continuous extensions, as well as 211 steps in 55 discontinuous movements with 50° target separation (M18L: same samples as Fig. 2 and Table 2) and 132 continuous flexions and 183 continuous extensions for 25° target separations (M12L).

Two groups of continuous movements were used, made by two monkeys working with different separations between targets. Mean amplitudes are plotted as a function of mean durations for all continuous flexions (open symbols) and extensions (closed symbols) made during the recording session. Crosses represent mean amplitudes and durations of the steps in discontinuous movements made in the experiments with the usual (50 °) target separation. The least squares best fit regression line drawn through all points follows the relation:

$$y = -1.31 + 45.06x \qquad (r = 0.99)$$

(where y is amplitude in degrees of arc and x is duration in seconds).

This relationship differs from that relating only the points for continuous movements:

$$y = -3.90 + 47.99x \qquad (r = 0.84)$$

and for steps:

$$y = -6.20 + 62.82x \qquad (r = 0.99)$$

However, in view of the large scatter of data, it seems reasonable to regard these all as one continuum. Their relation is not too different from a previous one based on size-grouped steps:

$$y = -5 + 72x \qquad \text{(Fig. 5 in Kozlovskaya et al., 1973)}.$$

The formalization of differences between successive steps is new, although it agrees with previously published tracings (Fig. 7 in Kozlovskaya et al., 1973). It is unknown how the individual steps are strung together and why the first step is of longer duration than ensuing steps. We can only conclude from our data that once it has been determined in the central nervous system that acceleration variations are to be of such amplitude as to produce what we call steps, that they then have properties which are on a continuum with continuous movements. The two types of movement may not be qualitatively different, but rather may differ only in the intensities of cyclic force application.

We may now enquire how the parts of continuous and discontinuous movements are timed to succeed one another within their

movement types. How regular is the sequential timing of acceleration deviations in continuous movements, and how are they
related to movement onset? The intervals from start of movement
to peak acceleration (Fig. 4, first dotted line) and from that peak

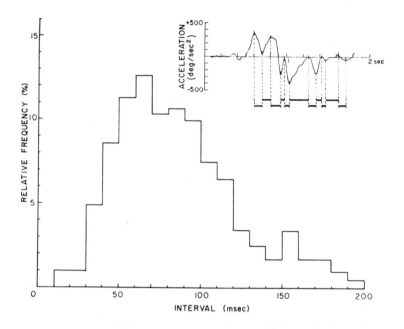

Fig. 4. Relative frequency distribution of intervals between
maxima and minima of acceleration in continuous movements.
The dashed vertical lines on the inset locate maxima and
minima of acceleration in a continuous movement. Solid lines
below the trace indicate the intervals that were measured for
the histogram to the nearest 10 msec, a minimum imposed
by the 100 Hz A/D conversion rate. The distribution is based
on a sample of 406 intervals derived from an arbitrary sample
of the initial 28 continuous movements made by M18L in that
trial.

acceleration to peak deceleration (sixth dotted line) are 0.29 +
0.18 sec and 0.40 + 0.21 sec. (The data were obtained from all
continuous movements in the 50° sample presented in Fig. 5).
These intervals are equivalent to a frequency of 0.9-1.2 Hz.
The distribution of intervals between consecutive acceleration
maxima and minima is presented in Fig. 4 as a unimodal distribution with a peak at about 65 msec, and a mean of 89 msec.

This interval could arise from a sinusoid with a period of 2 x 65 msec, i.e. 130 msec, which is equivalent to a frequency of 7-8 Hz. The skew in the curve to the right could have been produced by the selection method which required a minimum difference of $50°/sec^2$ between consecutive maxima and minima. With smaller differences, that data point was ignored and the next maximum/ minimum point found and compared, which would bias the curve towards high values of intervals. Measurement of acceleration maximum-minimum intervals yields only a crude indication of the cyclic processes involved in the production of the movements studied. Frequencies lower than 7 Hz cannot be directly measured if modulated by a strong 7 Hz component, and higher frequencies may be missed if the amplitude of their contribution is below the detection threshold. The method of analysis used in this work does not preclude the presence of frequency components other than 7 Hz, which would increase the variability of the measured intervals.

The next question was how constant the time relations were in continuous movements of the intervals from peak acceleration to peak velocity, and from peak velocity to peak deceleration. Two such intervals are indicated by the solid bars below the acceleration trace inset in Fig. 5. In contrast to Fig. 4, this distribution is periodic with peaks at 35, 140 and 255 msec. (Later peaks may occur but are not well enough defined in the present sample.) If peak acceleration, peak velocity and peak deceleration are considered to be on a sinusoid, then the first peak should represent the duration of a quarter cycle. The minimum period of the underlying sinusoid therefore would be about 140 msec, equivalent to a frequency of about 7 Hz. This is very close to the value of 8 Hz obtained when all maxima and minima of acceleration were considered, indicating that peak acceleration and deceleration occur with a relatively constant phase relation to the 8 Hz phasic activity. As was noted earlier, this more rapid oscillation of acceleration appears superimposed on a slower sinusoidal oscillation (Fig. 1).

An analysis of the steps in discontinuous movements indicates that the duration of the steps may be related to this frequency of 7-8 Hz which is present in continuous movements. Table 2 lists the means and SDs of step durations from the same sample of discontinuous movements that was used for Fig. 3. Statistical analysis showed that first step was longer than those following, that were about 250 msec. In addition, step amplitudes appeared

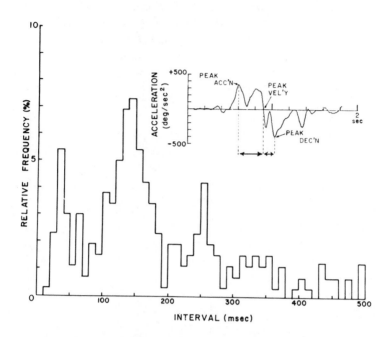

<u>Fig. 5.</u> Relative frequency distribution of intervals between
peak acceleration, deceleration and velocity of continuous
movements. The dashed vertical lines on the inset locate
the peaks of acceleration, deceleration and velocity in a
continuous movement. The horizontal arrows below the
trace indicate the intervals that were measured for the
histogram. The data were derived from all continuous movements made by M18L, same sample as in Fig. 2.

in multiples of 5 °, with the largest occurring farthest from the
target, and the smallest nearest the target.

DISCUSSION

The present work has confirmed previous descriptions of
monkeys' arm movements (Kozlovskaya et al., 1970, 1973).
The distributions of parameters (Fig. 2) were similar, except
that the continuous movements in the current sample were slower
and longer than those observed with other animals. Fig. 1 indicates a new finding, namely a basic oscillation of 1 Hz in the

Step Number	1	2	3	4	5
Mean amplitude (deg.)	15.6 (10.9)	15.1 (8.4)	10.9 (5.9)	9.2 (4.8)	5.7 (3.1)
Mean duration (msec.)	375 (162)	278 (166)	259 (118)	249 (93)	212 (103)
n	55	55	49	32	20

Table 2. Mean amplitude and duration (+ 1 SD) for the first five steps in a sample of discontinuous movements (chosen arbitrarily as the initial 55 made by M18L on 12.2.73), and presented in Fig. 3. The number of steps (n) in the sample is given in the bottom row.

acceleration of continuous movements, modulated at 7-8 Hz. Discontinuous movements exhibited steps at 3-4 Hz. Perhaps the deviations of acceleration at 7-8 Hz serve as a timing signal for steps that thus occur at the first subharmonic frequency. In fact, movements made in the step-tracking task tended to be in phase at 3 Hz, and possibly at 7-8 Hz, when the handle was vibrated at various frequencies (Thomas, Cooke and Brooks, unpublished). Similarly, the human arm resonates at 2-5 Hz to an impressed frequency spectrum (Berthoz and Metral, 1970), and the finger at 8-12 Hz to single taps (Lippold, 1970).

The properties in Results apply only to the described self-paced task. The amplitude-duration continuum (Fig. 3) does not apply, for instance, to the rapid alternating movements studied by Conrad and Brooks (1973 and unpublished) where the arm was slammed back and forth between the mechanical stops instead of coming to controlled holds in the target zones. Those movements traversed the usual distances in half the time and with 5-10 times greater peak velocities: they appeared to be the equivalents to Stetson's fastest ballistic movements.

What signs of neural control do the acceleration changes show?

Stetson and Bouman (1935) inferred that fast (ballistic) movements were centrally preprogrammed, whereas slow movements were said to be under continuous control dependent on afferent information from the limb, more recently called the "evolving movement" by Eccles (1968). Such a distinction was also made by Stark (1968) for correction of fast and slow tracking hand movements (see Brooks and Stoney, 1971, for review). The amplitudes of successive steps in discontinuous movements of monkeys seem to decrease like those in a simple proportional error control system (Table 2). This would fit the demonstrated greater dependence on sensory feedback of discontinuous movements than that of continuous movements (Kozlovskaya et al., 1973a) and the even greater independence of rapid alternations (Conrad and Brooks, unpublished). We have no proof, however, as to the degree of preprogramming in any of these movements, nor do we know whether position, or velocity, are being programmed, although the correlations in Table 1 seem to make it less likely for acceleration.

The present new observation of the cyclic tendency of acceleration changes in continuous and discontinuous movements emphasize similarities to physiological tremor, which for humans has a base frequency at about 3 Hz for the elbow (Fox and Randall, 1970) and higher rates for more distal joints (Stiles and Randall, 1967; Lippold, 1970). Tremor may have mechanical and neural origins. The former would let the limb oscillate as an underdamped system, tuning itself to a preferred frequency because of mechanical filtering. Stiles and Randall (1967) found this mechanical aspect true for the finger and hand, and Fox and Randall (1970) for the elbow: in all cases frequency was governed by moment of inertia but was unrelated to rhythms of muscular activity. Neural control was manifested by synchronous muscle action (Lippold, 1970; and dependence on afferent connections: Lippold et al., 1959) under heavy steady loads on the tremoring limb (Fox and Randall, 1970) and by demonstration of an 8-12 Hz tremor component that persisted over a range of opposing spring forces (Joyce and Rack, 1971a, b) and weights (Fox and Randall, 1970). Monkeys working against modest loads with various forcing functions (Thomas et al., 1973, and unpublished) typically also exhibited a relatively invariant tremor at 6-8 Hz whose amplitude was proportional to the forcings, suggesting that neural control outweighed mechanical resonance over the range tested.

Acknowledgement: Supported by grants from the Medical Research
Council of Canda (M-4465) and the U.S. Public Health Service
(NS-10311). We wish to thank Mr. S. Kohl for training the monkeys
and Mr. J. Pylyshyn for writing machine language computer programs.

REFERENCES

Berthoz, A. and Metral, S., 1970. Behaviour of a muscular group
  subjected to a sinusoidal and trapezoidal variation of force.
  J. Appl. Physiol. 29, 378-384.
Brooks, V.B., Kozlovskaya, I.B., Atkin, A., Horvath, F.E. and
  Uno, M., 1973. Effects of cooling the dentate nucleus on
  tracking-task performance in monkeys. J. Neurophysiol. 36,
  in press.
Brooks, V.B. and Stoney, S.D. Jr., 1971. Motor mechanisms: The
  role of the pyramidal system in motor control. Ann. Rev.
  Physiol. 33, 337-392.
Conrad, B. and Brooks, V.B., 1973. Effects of cooling the dentate
  nucleus on rapid alternating arm movements. Can. Physiol. 4, 29.
Eccles, J.C., 1969. The dynamic loop hypothesis of movement control.
  In Information Processing in the Nervous System. Springer-Verlag,
  N.Y. pp. 245-269.
Fox, J.R. and Randall, J.E., 1970. Relationship between forearm
  tremor and the biceps electromyogram. J. Appl. Physiol. 29,
  103-108.
Joyce, G.C. and Rack, P.M.H., 1971a. The effect of force on elbow
  tremor. J. Physiol. 216, 29-30P.
Joyce, G.C. and Rack, P.M.H., 1971b. The effect of load on elbow
  tremor. J. Physiol. 217, 36-37P.
Kozlovskaya, I., Uno, M. and Brooks, V.B., 1970. Performance of
  a step-tracking task by monkeys. Comm. Behav. Biol. 5, 153-156.
Kozlovskaya, I.B., Atkin, A., Horvath, F.E., Uno, M. and Brooks,
  V.B., 1973. Mechanisms of motor control of two types of tracking
  movements in monkeys. Proc. 2nd Int. Symp. on Motor Control,
  Varna, Bulgaria. Agressologie 14A, 49-57.
Lippold, O.C.J., 1970. Oscillation in the stretch reflex arc and
  the origin of the rhythmical 8-12 c/s component of the physiological tremor. J. Physiol. 206, 359-382.
Lippold, O.C.J., Redfearn, J.W.T. and Vuco, J., 1959. The influence
  of afferent and descending pathways on the rhythmical and
  arhythmical components of muscular activity in man and anaesthetized cat. J. Physiol. 146, 1-9.
Stark, L., 1968. Neurological Control Systems. Plenum Press, N.Y.
  428 pp.
Stetson, R.H., 1905. A motor theory of rhythm and discrete succession. I. Psychol. Rev. 12, 250-270.
Stetson, R.H. and McGill, J.A., 1923. Mechanisms of the different
  types of movements. Psychol. Monographs 32, 18-40.

Stetson, R.H. and Bouman, H.D., 1935. The coordination of simple
    skilled movements. Arch. Neerland. Physiol. 20, 179-254.
Stiles, R.N. and Randall, J.E., 1967. Mechanical factors in hand
    tremor frequency. J. Appl. Physiol. 23, 324-330.
Thomas, J.S., Cooke, J.D. and Brooks, V.B., 1973. Movement re-
    organization during reversible dentate dysfunction and feed-
    back forcings. Fed. Proc. 32, 419.
Woodworth, R.S., 1899. The accuracy of voluntary movement.
    Psychol. Monographs 3, 1-114.

POSTURAL CONTROL: A QUANTITATIVE STUDY

OF NERVOUS SYSTEM FUNCTIONS IN THE DOG

R. E. Talbott

Department of Physiology, University of Oregon
Medical School, Portland, Oregon

External manifestations of postural control in the dog have
been measured under static and dynamic conditions. During
quiet standing, trained dogs were found to exhibit laterally
symmetric weight distribution and to carry approximately 60%
of their weight on their front legs. Lateral symmetry of weight
distribution was also the rule during the postural reaction to
momentary (ramp) or continuous (sinusoidal) displacement of
the support platform on which the dogs stood. A Fourier
analysis of data obtained during sinusoidal oscillation of the
table provided an indication of the amount of harmonic distortion generated by the dog. It was found that records of body
position were relatively free from distortion, thus implying a
relatively linear transformation of the input signal. However,
the motions of the various hindlimb joints and the changes in
vertical forces which were engendered by the table oscillation
all showed considerable distortion. Hence, the components of
the postural control system might be seen to behave in essentially non-linear fashion (or to be governed by time varying
parameters) while the basic system output- body position in
space - apparently exhibits low pass filter characteristics and
hence resembles certain characteristics usually associated
with linear systems. Irrespective of the mechanism responsible
for the observed distortions, the set of coefficients for any
particular output measure provides a statistically reliable
indicator of system performance, and the set of coefficients
in essence becomes a defining characteristic of the dog's

postural behaviour under these experimental conditions. On this latter fact is founded the basis for comparing normal and abnormal performance of this behaviour.

For the past several years our experiments on animal posture have been oriented toward solving a very broad problem in neurophysiology. Briefly stated, that problem is this: given an animal which is as free from constraints of an artificial nature as possible, how does that animal use his nervous system, in toto, to produce an integrated behaviour? Such a question is obviously much too vague to be tested experimentally; nevertheless, our goal has been to define some class of behaviour with which we, as experimenters, could interact and for which we could provide a quantitative description. The extension of that goal would be to delve into the intricacies of the nervous system and to tease out those aspects of supposed function which bear important or determinant relation to the behaviour studied.

A conceptual orientation to our experiments can be obtained from the block diagram for the dog postural control system which is shown in Fig. 1. Certain terms used in this diagram are purposefully vague. Thus, the Volitional Reference incorporates many concepts and points of view about how a nervous system in a higher mammal might formulate a construct of the behaviour which we wish to study. The box containing Decoding, Integration, etc., represents a gross lumping of what are most certainly multiple neural pathways which are intermingled and interactive. The diagram does serve, however, to focus attention on a whole nervous system which is utilized to generate some well defined output - in this case, the control of body position in response to a disturbance. No attempt has been made to incorporate the types of hierarchies advocated by Allweis (1971; cf. also Jones, 1973) nor has adequate representation been provided for some of the important subsystems which make up the complete postural control system (e.g. Rosenthal et al., 1970; Roberts et al., 1971; Nashner, 1971, 1972; Fernandez and Goldberg, 1971; Melvill Jones and Watt, 1971; Melvill Jones and Milsum, 1971; Mannard and Stein, 1973; Houk, 1972). What is emphasized here is the view of a unified nervous system whose parts we wish to understand in relation to a unified output rather than summing together a set of independently studied parts of the system and subsequently trying to reconstitute both the nervous system and its output. These two approaches can, of course, interact symbiotically to

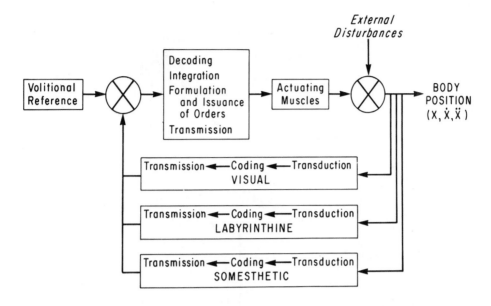

Fig. 1. Model system for the control of posture in the dog. The volitional reference implies those features of the dog's mental function which serve to identify the experimental postural control problem. By combining the problem identification, as an abstraction, with various feedback (visual, labyrinthine, somaesthetic) signals the stage is set to decode and to integrate the information into a coherent set of neural orders which will be transmitted to the relevant muscles of the body and thereby yield a change in the net balance between the tensions exerted by these muscles. This shift in relative tension will combine with the external disturbance in such a manner that the output of the postural control system, body position (and its derivatives), will be brought into good juxtaposition with respect to the volitional reference.

provide more fruitful results than would be achieved by either in isolation.

Our experimental paradigm is illustrated in Fig. 2. The dog is trained, by means of positive reinforcement (McIntire, 1968), to adopt an upright posture when placed upon the shake table or support platform. The dog's task is to maintain this posture even during periods in which the table is moved. During periods of

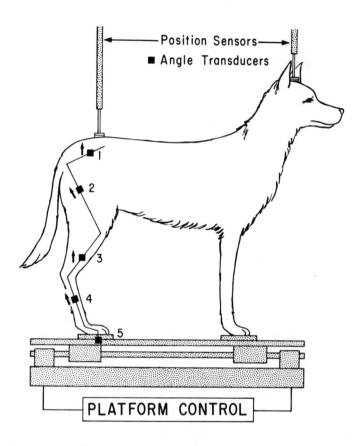

Fig. 2.   Position of the dog on the shake table and the location of the sensors used to monitor postural reactions. The shake table or moveable support platform is confined to a single direction of travel - headward and tailward. Changes in the joint angles are measured by the pairs of transducers affixed to both sides of the hip, knee, ankle and phalangeal (toe) joints of the right hind leg. The longitudinal position of the head and pelvis is determined from the voltage drops across potentiometers connected to the levers which are attached to the animal. The animal stands on a set of four blocks: these blocks might be vertical force transducers, horizontal force transducers, or just wood, depending upon the experimental objective.

quiet stance and relative motion (i.e. motion of the dog induced by table motion) several output variables are measured to provide a quantitative description of the dog's postural control. Among these output variables are the positions of the head and pelvis (Brookhart et al., 1970), the changes in the angles (Reed and Reynolds, 1969), formed at the hip, knee and ankle, and phalangeal (toe) joints of the right hind leg, and the vertical (Petersen et al., 1965) and horizontal (Cross, 1972) forces exerted by the dog's four paws. The table position is also monitored in order to have a quantitative record of the input or forcing function. The details of our data collection and reduction procedures are fully described elsewhere (Petersen, 1968; Talbott and Brookhart, in preparation).

These experiments on postural control require that the dog be capable of stable or replicable behaviour when he is positioned on the moveable platform. Fig. 3 shows the results of a test of postural stability in which the dogs were standing quietly for a period of time and the centre of gravity was calculated from the records of vertical force from the four paws (Brookhart et al., 1965). Based on these data, it is reasonable to infer that dogs are indeed capable of stable quiet standing and that such stance patterns are replicable. Though some dog to dog differences were apparent, as revealed in Fig. 3, all dogs in this experimental situation appear to bear about 60% of their weight on their front legs and to divide the weight distribution equally to the two sides.

The response to dynamic conditions must also be stable and replicable and in addition must show the same degree of lateral symmetry which exists in the quiet standing situation. Previous studies (Mori and Brookhart, 1968; Brookhart et al., 1970) demonstrated fulfillment of these requirements for dogs making a postural correction in response to brief ramp displacements of the support platform. The constancy of response was not confined to vertical force outputs but was also found in the position records, and, more importantly, in the sudden shifts in the level of muscle activity (revealed by the electromyograms from several thigh muscles). These changes in muscle activity occurred in two preferred time zones (20-25 msec and 55-60 msec) following the onset of the displacement in either headward or tailward direction. The uniformity of EMG timing, despite differences in the overall qualities of the disturbance and despite elimination of somaesthetic input from the paws (Mori et al., 1970), suggested that the temporal characteristics of the reaction are determined by attributes of the central control mechanism rather than by the pattern of

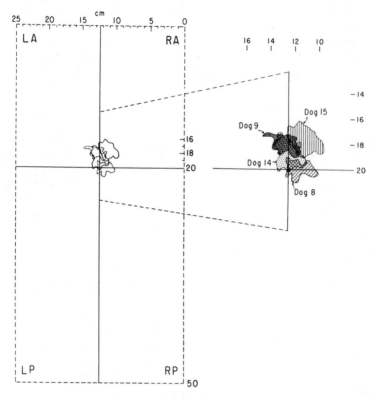

Fig. 3. Summary of centre of gravity recordings from 10
trials for each of 4 dogs. The centre of gravity was derived
from vertical force records from the four paws during
periods of quiet standing. The left side of the figure depicts
the entire horizontal plane of the support platform which was
bounded by the positions of the paws on the force transducers.
Lateral symmetry in the stance is apparent and a headward
displacement of the centre of gravity (about 60% of the weight
on the anterior feet) was also common to all of the dogs. The
right side of the figure provides an enlarged view of the areas
(extremes of deviation) covered by the centres of gravity.
From this data it can be surmised that dogs are capable of
assuming the command posture in a stable and replicable
fashion (Brookhart et al., 1965).

afferent activity associated with the ramp displacement. The
corrective changes in body position which followed a brief displacement of the table had latencies around 100-150 msec. This

long latency reflected the fact that time is required to alter the
tension exerted by a muscle following a change in its level of
neural drive. By calculating the torques generated at the various
fore-and hind leg joints, Cross (1972) predicted the probable
time course for the tension changes which would accompany the
compensatory changes in body position following a brief displacement. The character and timing of both the torque and position
changes suggest similarities to the 'functional stretch reflex'
described by Melvill Jones and Watt (1971), but such similarity
in external manifestation cannot be taken to imply similarity in
mechanism.

The response to a ramp or step displacement is complicated
by the fact that the motion of the table cannot occur rapidly
enough to really appear as a step function without causing foot
slippage. There will always be positive and negative accelerations
sufficiently separated in time to be discerned as two distinct
stimuli. Thus, the use of Fourier transform methods on data
derived from ramp displacements, in the manner suggested by
Milner-Brown et al. (1973), may not be appropriate since the output of the postural control system under these conditions probably
does not represent a true impulse response. What frequency response characteristics would be derived by performing a Fourier
transform on the ramp displacement data has not yet been determined. Rather, we elected to study the dog postural response to
steady state sinusoidal oscillation of the table and to assess the
frequency response directly.

Fig. 4 provides an example of the first 256 data points from a
single trial of sinusoidal forcing. The analog signal for the hip
angle changes was sampled at about 160/sec, interpolated to 128
samples/cycle of the forcing frequency, and calibrated (Talbott
and Brookhart, in preparation; Petersen, 1968). A total of 1,024
data points (8 cycles/table motion) per channel for both the input
and the outputs were subjected to Fourier analysis to yield 512
sine and 512 cosine coefficients; by further calculation, the
associated magnitude and phase coefficients were obtained. There
are obvious harmonic distortions in this and all other measures
of postural response to sinusoidal forcing. Drift, or change in
the output signal which occurs at lower frequency than the input
frequency, is also found. But this sample record does not give
sufficient information to evaluate the relative contribution of drift
to the overall harmonic distortion found in the response measures.

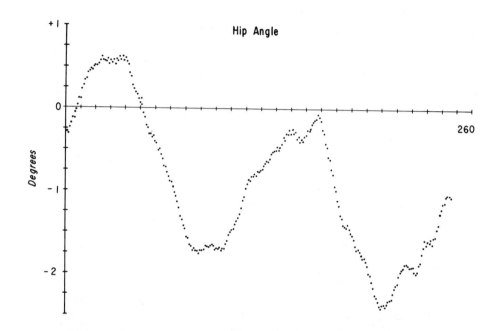

Fig. 4. First 256 data points (2 cycles) for hip angle change
during a single trial of one dog. The data points are derived
from digitized analog voltages by calibrating and interpolating
the raw data to yield 128 points/cycle of the driving frequency
(separation of $2.8125°$). The presence of both harmonic distortion and of drift is apparent in this sample record. Of these
two contaminating features of the dog's response to sinusoidal
motion, drift (i. e. changes in output which occur slower than
the forcing frequency) proved to be a random event bearing no
systematic relation to the presence of the driving disturbance.
Harmonic distortion, especially at multiples of the input
frequency, appears to be an inherent aspect of the mode of
response adopted by the dog. Table motion was 8 cm, peak to
peak, at a frequency of 1 Hz.

Such slow changes in output were essentially random occurrences
bearing no particular phase or magnitude relation to the driving
function: over many trials the effects due to drift could clearly
be differentiated from effects more directly related to the presence
of the driving function. Some question might be raised that, in the
presence of drift, the criterion of steady state is not met. On an

individual trial basis (e.g. a continuous train of 10 cycles of input)
this may be true; however, the statistical properties of these
responses to sinusoidal displacement seem to allow the conclusion
that a quasi steady state was achieved such that residual harmonic
distortion (that part remaining after removing the drift contribution)
was a characteristic of the postural control systems mode of
operation). This problem of interpreting the existence of distortion
in the output records will be discussed further later.

The Fourier coefficients which are related to the input frequency
clearly would characterize data of the type shown in Fig. 4. In
Fig. 5, the sine and cosine coefficients for the input frequency
have been used to trace the response properties of the vertical
forces exerted by the paws. Three input frequencies were used
(0.5, 1.0, 2.0 Hz all at 8 cm, peak to peak). The responses
from the left and right vertical force transducers can be seen to
superimpose thus providing further evidence that the dog behaves
in a laterally symmetric manner in both the static and dynamic
conditions. The phase plane representation of the response data
in Fig. 5 also shows that changes in the mean amplitude (magnitude of the vector from the origin to the mean sine-cosine
coefficients) and the mean phase (zero degrees for the input lies
along the positive sine axis) are functions of the input frequency.
The trajectories for these changes are similar in the anterior
and posterior vertical forces.

In Fig. 6 the mean values of amplitude and phase coefficients
for 7 dogs are plotted. Since lateral symmetry was established
for the response to sinusoidal oscillation, only data for angle
changes of the right hind leg have been collected on a routine
basis, and similar changes for the left hind leg are assumed to
be present. The frequency response characteristic for position
resembles that expected from a second order linear system
(Mannard and Stein, 1973; Milsum, 1966). The response
parameters describing joint angle changes have characteristics
more like pulse integrators. In both cases, however, the linear
systems analogies may not be appropriate.

The presence of harmonic distortion of higher frequency than
the driving frequency was obvious in the sample record in Fig. 4.
The question now becomes, does this distortion represent an
inherent characteristic of the dog postural control system or is
it just an incidental outcome due to the way the experiment was
performed? Fig. 7 shows data from two different dogs: one set

VERTICAL FORCE - FOURIER COEFFICIENT

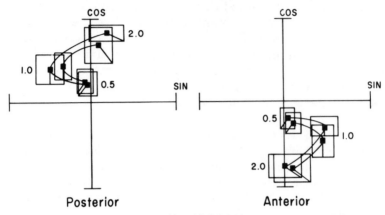

Fig. 5. Trajectories for the vertical forces exerted by the left and right anterior and the left and right posterior paws during sinusoidal motion of the support platform. The mean and standard deviation is plotted (N = 30) for the sine and cosine Fourier coefficients which represent the frequency of the input (forcing function). Data are from a single dog; table motion was 8 cm, peak to peak amplitude, and 0.5, 1.0 and 2.0 Hz. These trajectories indicate that the dog was laterally symmetric during response to dynamic input. The trajectories of the anterior and posterior paws are roughly 180° out of phase with each other, which indicates that the dog was essentially rocking back and forth from his hind to fore legs as the table oscillated. The amplitude of this rocking increased as the frequency of the input increased. The input, being essentially a pure sine function, would appear as a point on the positive sine axis. Calibration for vertical force: 1 kg = 1,000 mv (Petersen, unpublished).

of data (A and B) is represented as the sine and cosine coefficients while the other set of data (C) is in the form of amplitude and phase coefficients. The eighth harmonic represents the input

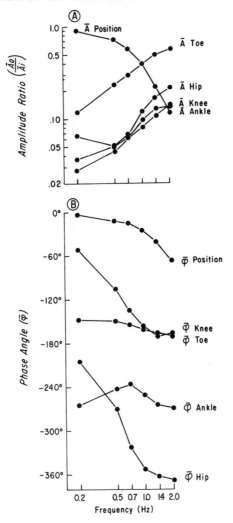

Fig. 6. Describing function for several frequencies of oscillation at fixed amplitude (8 cm, peak to peak). The mean values
of the driving frequency amplitude and phase coefficients are
plotted for data from 7 dogs (177-180 trials, 20 or 30 trials
per dog). The frequency response characteristic for position
resembles that found with a second order linear system having
a damping ratio around 0.9; however, given the existence of
probable non-linear behaviour it is also possible to view the
position response curve as representing the sinusoidal describing function for velocity limiting. The frequency response
curves for the joint angle changes exhibit high pass filter

Fig. 6, contd. characteristics and are similar to the kind of
behaviour found with pulse frequency integrators; these
curves also resemble amplitude limiting or saturation
characteristics.

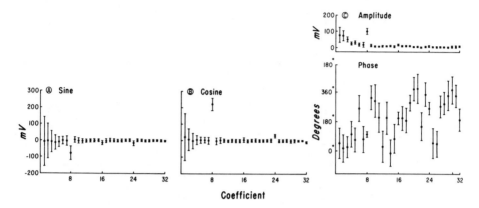

Fig. 7. First 32 Fourier coefficients for changes in ankle
angle of two dogs. A and B. The sine and cosine coefficients
for one dog are plotted as the mean and standard deviation
over 30 trials in which the forcing function had a peak to
peak amplitude of 8 cm and a frequency of 1 Hz. The eighth
harmonic represents the input frequency. Hence it can be
seen that only the harmonics which are integral multiples
of the input harmonic are characterized by non-zero mean
values and standard deviations which do not incorporate zero.
C. The mean and standard deviations of the amplitude and
phase coefficients from another dog (N = 10). Since the
amplitude coefficient is never negative, the first 7 averaged
amplitude coefficients appear large compared to the eighth
or input harmonic. However, the phase coefficients for
these same first 7 harmonics exhibit large variances, and,
in agreement with the data in A and B, this would argue for
these drift components in the response being random
fluctuations. The conversion factor for the sine, cosine and
magnitude coefficients is 200 mv per degree of angle change.

frequency (1 Hz). Drift accounts for the energy found in the first
7 coefficients. The zero mean values of the sine and cosine
coefficients and the large deviations for these first several
coefficients in A, B and C indicate the random nature of drift.
The integral multiples of the input frequency (i. e. f_8, f_{16}, etc.)

are non-zero. Since the drift associated coefficients above the eighth harmonic are essentially zero, the existence of non-zero harmonics at multiples of the input frequency tends to reinforce the notion that the various response parameters represent the behaviour of an underlying non-linear control system.

The degree of this underlying non-linear control is different for the various output measures as shown in Fig. 8. These graphs of the describing function and of the non-linear remnant were made on the expectation that the data might resemble similar graphs for various classes of simple non-linearities, such as a power function relation between the input and the output (Graham and McKuer, 1961, Chap. 4). The data in Fig. 8 does not resemble the straight lines expected for a power function relation, nor does it resemble any of the other varieties of simple amplitude dependent non-linearities. The graphs in Fig. 8 demonstrate, however, that the toe angle change exhibits less distortion (harmonic content) than the knee angle change (13% distortion versus 18% distortion, respectively, at 8 cm using the first 8 multiples of the input frequency coefficient).

The above description of the postural behaviour of the dog suggests that this mode of nervous system operation represents a system whose behaviour is inherently non-linear. How badly non-linear is the system and can one model the system response by utilizing transfer functions derived by the usual linear systems analysis approach? This question will not be answered because insufficient data exist at present to determine which output variables are the relevant ones that the nervous system of the dog considers essential for solution of the postural control problem and which are related but non-essential. The output variable most sensitive to changes in sensory feedback (Talbott and Brookhart, in preparation; Reynolds, Talbott and Brookhart, unpublished) seems to be body position (cf. Houk, 1972), and that output variable is also the one which behaves most nearly like a linear system parameter. The angle changes, or by extrapolation, the torque changes at the joint (Cross, 1972), however, seem to represent either non-linear or time varying parameters (Gelb and Vander Velde, 1968) systems. This is surprising since, in isolation, the subsystems for these joint motions appear to behave quite linearly (Rosenthal et al., 1970; Mannard and Stein, 1973; Berthoz et al., 1971; Roberts et al., 1971; but cf. Houk et al., 1970). It is all the more surprising since the degree of angle change induced in our animals during

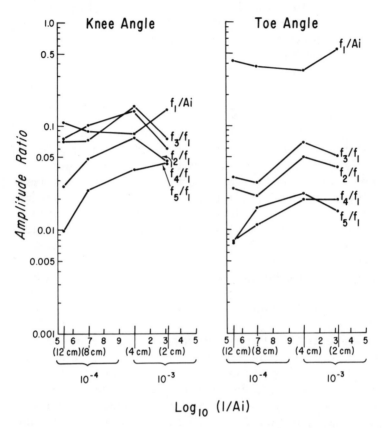

Fig. 8. Describing function and remnant for knee and toe
angle changes in response to 1 Hz disturbance at different
amplitudes. All ratios and reciprocals were calculated from
the mean amplitude Fourier coefficients (N = 20) expressed
in terms of millivolts so that dimensionless ratios were
obtained. The corresponding peak to peak amplitudes in
centimeters are indicated for the table motion. Straight lines
on these log-log plots would indicate a power function relation
between the input and the output. In these graphs, f_1 is the
coefficient for the input frequency and the other coefficients
represent integral multiples of that frequency. Based on the
relative amplitude of the f_1 coefficients, it is clear that
there is more movement at the toe joint than at the knee joint.
From the ratios of the higher harmonics to the driving
frequency harmonic, it can be inferred that there is a greater
degree of distortion in the motion of the knee joint.

response to sinusoidal oscillation is quite small, perhaps mimicing small signal analysis, relative to the large changes found during locomotion (Engberg and Lundberg, 1969). Hence, we expect even greater non-linearities in certain output variables as the displacements become larger and faster in order to approximate other types of motions which occur naturally.

At this stage of development of our experimental exploration of postural control in the dog, at least two avenues are open. The first is to pursue a quantitative mathematical model for the overall postural control system. The approach of Spekreijse and Oosting (1970) might be used to sort out the linear and non-linear aspects of the system. Alternatively, the white-noise approach of Marmarelis and McCann (1973) might be used by deriving the number and order of the kernels needed to describe the system response. However, as indicated above, the level of knowledge about the dog postural control system has not yet been attained at which such a pursuit of an overall mathematical model would be very useful. We need first to obtain measures of a sufficient number of forces and torques to completely specify the system and then to extend the static analysis done by Cross (1972) to the dynamic condition.

The second avenue is of more immediate appeal. That entails viewing the results of a harmonic analysis of the dog's response to sinusoidal input as an end in itself. Viewed in this way, the data analysis provides a set of parameters (coefficients) which fully characterize the behaviour (insofar as the variables chosen for measurement can characterize the behaviour). The logical utility of this set of derived parameters is a basis of comparison by which modifications of response can be determined (Talbott and Brookhart, in preparation; Reynolds, Talbott and Brookhart, unpublished; Albers et al., 1973; Contini et al., 1965, pp. 427). By this approach we would effectively substitute one form of pattern recognition (the set of coefficients) for another (the raw data). Our short term goal is thus to collect and compare the normal and abnormal dog postural behaviour in terms of a Fourier analysis of their response data. From this latter approach will come a quantitative assessment of the relative role of the many neural components which collectively make up the postural control system of the dog.

Acknowledgements: This research was supported by NIH Grant NS-04744, NIH Research Career development Award 5-K04-NS-70021, and NSF grant GB-35416. The research described in this report involved animals maintained in animal care facilities fully accredited by AALAC and the research was conducted according to the 'Guiding Principles in the Care and Use of Animals' of the American Physiological Society.

REFERENCES

Albers, J.W., Potvin, A.R., Tourtellotte, W.W., Pew, R.W. and Stribley, R.F., 1973. Quantification of hand tremor in the clinical neurological examination. I.E.E.E. Trans. Biomed. Eng. BME-20, 27-37.

Allweis, C., 1971. Control system diagrams in physiology, biology and medicine. Israel J. Med. Sci. 7 (Suppl.), 84 pp.

Berthoz, A., Roberts, W.J. and Rosenthal, N.P., 1971. Dynamic characteristics of stretch reflex using force inputs. J. Neurophysiol. 34, 612-619.

Brookhart, J.M., Mori, S. and Reynolds, P.J., 1970. Postural reactions to two directions of displacement in dogs. Amer. J. Physiol. 218, 719-725.

Brookhart, J.M., Parmeggiani, P.L., Petersen, W.A. and Stone, S.A., 1965. Postural stability in the dog. Amer. J. Physiol. 208, 1047-1057.

Contini, R., Gage, H. and Drillis, R., 1965. Human gait characteristics. In Biomechanics and Related Bioengineering Topics. (Ed. Kenedi, R.M.) Pergamon Press, Oxford, Chapter 34.

Cross, C.E., 1972. Analysis of Postural Dynamics in the Dog. Ph.D. Thesis, Dept. Elec. Eng., Oregon State Univ., Corvallis, Oregon.

Engberg, I. and Lundberg, A., 1969. An electromyographic analysis of muscular activity in the hindlimb of the cat during unrestrained locomotion. Acta Physiol. Scand. 75, 614-630.

Fernandez, C. and Goldberg, J.M., 1971. Physiology of peripheral neurons innervating semicircular canals of the squirrel monkey. II. Response to sinusoidal stimulation and dynamics of peripheral vestibular system. J. Neurophysiol. 34, 661-675.

Gelb, A. and Vander Velde, W.E., 1968. Multiple-Input Describing Functions and Nonlinear System Design. McGraw-Hill Book Co., N.Y. 665 pp.

Graham, D. and McRuer, D., 1961. Analysis of Nonlinear Control Systems. John Wiley and Sons, N.Y. 482 pp.

Houk, J., 1972. On the significance of various command signals during voluntary control. Brain Res. 40, 49-53.

Houk, J.C., Singer, J.J. and Goldman, M.R., 1970. An evaluation of length and force feedback to soleus muscles of decerebrate cats. J. Neurophysiol. 33, 784-811.

Jones, R.W., 1973. Principles of Biological Regulation. Academic Press, N.Y. 359 pp.

Mannard, A. and Stein, R.B., 1973. Determination of the frequency response of isometric soleus muscle in the cat using random nerve stimulation. J. Physiol. 229, 275-296.

Marmarelis, P.Z. and McCann, G.D., 1973. Development and application of white-noise modeling techniques for studies of insect visual nervous system. Kybernetik 12, 74-89.

McIntire, R.W., 1968. Dog training, reinforcement and behavior in unrestricted environments. Amer. Psychol. 23, 830-831.

Melvill Jones, G. and Milsum, J.H., 1971. Frequency-response analysis of central vestibular unit activity resulting from rotational stimulation of the semicircular canals. J. Physiol. 219, 191-216.

Melvill Jones, G. and Watt, D.G.D., 1971. Observations on the control of stepping and hopping movements in man. J. Physiol. 219, 709-728.

Milner-Brown, H.S., Stein, R.B. and Yemm, R., 1973. The contractile properties of human motor units during voluntary isometric contractions. J. Physiol. 228, 285-306.

Milsum, J.H., 1966. Biological Control Systems Analysis. McGraw-Hill Book Co., New York, 466 pp.

Mori, S. and Brookhart, J.M., 1968. Characteristics of the postural reactions of the dog to a controlled disturbance. Amer. J. Physiol. 215, 339-348.

Mori, S., Reynolds, P.J. and Brookhart, J.M., 1970. Contribution of pedal afferents to postural control in the dog. Amer. J. Physiol. 218, 726-734.

Nashner, L.M., 1971. A model describing vestibular detection of body sway motion. Acta Otolaryng. 72, 429-436.

Nashner, L.M., 1972. Vestibular postural control model. Kybernetik 10, 106-110.

Petersen, W.A., 1968. A flexible data acquisition and formatting system for input to digital computers. I.E.E.E. Region IV Conference Report, paper 2-C-2, 7 pp.

Petersen, W.A., Brookhart, J.M. and Stone, S.A., 1965. A strain-gage platform for force measurements. J. Appl. Physiol. 20, 1095-1097.

Reed, D.J. and Reynolds, P.J., 1969. A joint angle detector. J. Appl. Physiol. 27, 745-748.

Roberts, W.J., Rosenthal, N.P. and Terzuolo, C.A., 1971. A control model of stretch reflex. J. Neurophysiol. 34, 620-634.

Rosenthal, N.P., McKean, T.A., Roberts, W.J. and Terzuolo, C.A., 1970. Frequency analysis of stretch reflex and its main subsystems in triceps surae muscles of the cat. J. Neurophysiol. 33, 713-749.

Spekreijse, J. and Oosting, H., 1970. Linearizing: a method for analysing and synthesizing nonlinear systems. Kybernetik 7, 22-31.

VESTIBULAR AND REFLEX CONTROL OF NORMAL STANDING

L. M. Nashner

Laboratory of Neurophysiology, Good Samaritan
Hospital and Medical Centre, Portland, Oregon

The regulation of antero-posterior body sway about the ankle joints has been the object of this study of human posture control. The stabilizing influences of two of the relevant sensory systems have been studied: (1) postural responses initiated by the vestibular system as a consequence of body sway motion and (2) muscle proprioceptive reflexes and sensory systems of the ankle joints responding to ankle joint rotation during body sway.

A servo-controlled platform was used to open the feedback loop between body sway motion and associated ankle joint rotation, thus removing proprioceptive, joint and cutaneous sensation related to body sway. The vestibular senses, not normally important for control of standing, were thus forced to become the initiators of the stabilizing torque responses at the ankle joints. The response parameters observed under these conditions formed the basis for constructing a model of vestibular control of standing while on the platform. The model predicted a clear functional separation between the stabilizing influences of the angular acceleration sensors (semicircular canals) and the linear acceleration sensors (utricular otoliths).

Electrical stimulation of the vestibular system while a subject's head was turned to face over a shoulder (75-250 μ amp; 150-500 msec duration) evoked a brief change in background level of EMG activity in the gastrocnemius muscle with a

latency of 100 msec and duration of approximately 350 msec.
Corresponding to the evoked changes in EMG level, small
changes in torque exerted about the ankle joints were seen
after approximately 200 msec. The response could be either
an increase or a decrease in the firing rate. The direction of
change could be affected in the following two ways: (1) by
reversing the direction of the stimulating currents, or (2) by
rotating the head 180° from facing over one shoulder to facing
over the other. With the head in the forward position, no
changes in EMG level or torque were observed. Electrical
stimuli which were sustained for 5 sec evoked a change in the
orientation of the body in addition to the brief change in EMG
level.

Electrical stimulation was used in conjunction with the servoplatform technique to study the adaptive interaction of vestibular evoked responses with sensory feedback from the ankle
joints. The brief changes in EMG level in the first 600 msec
following electrical stimulation were not affected by the presence or absence of ankle joint rotation associated with body
sway. Rotation of the ankle joints provided a strong modifying
influence on compensatory responses and sway orientation
following the 600 msec period. Removing all ankle joint rotation increased the effect of current on sway orientation by a
factor of 3-5 times normal. Reinforcing the ankle rotations
associated with sway a factor of 2 times by counter-rotating
the platform reduced the effect on orientation by a corresponding
factor of 2 times. Based on the results, a possible mechanism
for the interaction of vestibular and reflex control of posture is
proposed.

The function of proprioceptive stretch reflexes in humans is
not well understood. Are they of lesser consequence (e.g. Melvill-
Jones and Watt, 1971a), or do they play a significant role in controlling muscle length or tension during movement (e.g. Marsden
et al., 1972)? Recent experiments on posture control in humans
indicated that resistance of the ankle joints to rotation may play
a significant role in regulation of body sway, depending on the
conditions of the task. This finding did not resolve the question,
but rather served to illustrate that a conclusion concerning reflex
function is influenced by the characteristics of the task under
study. Pre-programmed, central control is an alternate explanation for the origin of rapid compensatory responses during posture

control and gait. A systems model was developed from experimental results which described how the vestibular system controlled posture centrally under a different set of task conditions. Finally, a hypothesis was presented to describe how information from rotation of the ankle joints and from the vestibular system may be combined to control orientation of body sway. Experiments placed a strong emphasis on describing changes in posture control strategy depending on the conditions of the task. Roles of reflexes and central programs were not seen as fixed but rather depended on the parameters of the task.

Tasks chosen for study were simple but sufficient to demonstrate adaptation of stimulus-response relationships. Regulation of antero-posterior sway about the ankle joints was observed during a variety of test conditions altering relationships between body movements and rotation of the ankle joints. Conditions were limited to those requiring only regulation of ankle torque; no complex stepping or relative movements of upper body parts were required. Measuring responses evoked by a particular sensory feedback system is difficult in actively performing human subjects. A technique was developed to study vestibular control of posture by removing information relating to sway orientation from rotation of the ankle joints and by concurrently removing visual cues (Nashner, 1971). The role of the ankle joints in control of sway was determined by comparing vestibular performance with controlled amounts of information from ankle joint rotation. After a brief review of the experiments on human posture control, the results are discussed as they relate to central and peripheral control of postural sway.

VESTIBULAR CONTROL OF POSTURE

Forcing a subject to rely on vestibular information to control antero-posterior sway required opening the sensory feedback loops dependent on rotation of the ankle joints and on vision. Rotation of the ankle joints correlated with antero-posterior sway was removed by servodriving the rotational axis of a platform to track body sway motion, thus maintaining fixed ankle joint angles during sway (Fig. 1). The servodriven platform was used to create a special situation in which to study the properties of compensatory responses to sway induced by the experimenter (Nashner, 1971). The functional dependence of a compensatory response latency on the rate of free-fall sway was determined, translating the platform

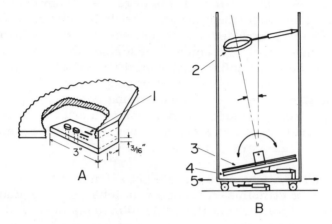

Fig. 1. The two degree-of-freedom platform. A. A force
measuring flexure showing 1 the mounting of the four strain
gauges. B. A view of the rotating and translating members of
the platform with 2 the belt and the potentiometer which measure the antero-posterior body sway angle, 3 the force plate
measuring ankle torque, 4 the rotating member, and 5 the
translating member.

either forward or backward to induce anterior or posterior sway.
Latency of compensatory torque responses was found to decrease
with increasing rates of induced sway, reaching an asymptotic
minimum at 185 msec. The angle of sway subtended at the time of
the response was minimum at slow rates, then increased as the
response times approached a minimum (Fig. 2). Visual information had no significant effect on the latency time, but did have
a strong effect on subsequent portions of the compensatory responses. However, the use of visual information is yet to be
studied. All experiments here were conducted with eyes closed.

There have been a number of studies relating postural responses
(Bizzo and Baron, 1972; Coats, 1972, 1973; Dzendolet, 1963;
Njiokiktjien and Folkerts, 1971) to electrical stimulation of the
vestibular system. The method was introduced in this study as a
way of providing an "internal" vestibular stimulus, one not disturbing body position directly. Because in past studies the
properties of responses to electrical vestibular stimulation were
uncertain, initial experiments defined the parameters of postural

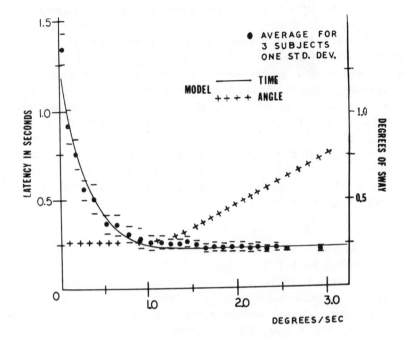

Fig. 2. Average latency times for three subjects to detect antero-posterior sway as a function of the rate of induced sway. Subjects stood on the servodriven platform with eyes closed. Data are compared to responses predicted by the vestibular posture control model.

responses (Nashner and Wolfson, 1973) in a more quantitative way. Controlled pulses of current were introduced between the mastoid bones and the responses in gastrocnemius-soleus (GS) muscles were determined as a measure of the resulting disturbances to posture. Results of the experiments can be summarized as follows: (1) depending on orientation of the head and polarity of the stimulus, a 250 μa current lasting at least 75 msec evoked a reflex response in GS muscles with a 100 msec latency and a duration of approximately 350 msec. (2) GS responses to electrical vestibular stimulation were modulated by position of the head. With head facing forward no responses were evoked, while a 180°

change in head position from facing over one shoulder to facing over the other reversed the effect of the stimulus. (3) Reversing the direction of current also reversed the response evoked for a given orientation of the head. (4) The brief response in GS muscles caused a measurable disturbance to posture. The properties of the GS response during the first 600 msec were not affected by motion of the servoplatform or by duration of the stimulus beyond the 75 msec minimum. However, servodriving the platform to remove ankle joint rotation correlated with sway or maintaining the current for longer periods of time both had strong effects on later components of the postural response to the electrical stimulation. The properties of the initial portions of the postural responses to electrical vestibular stimulation are summarized in Fig. 3.

The above experiments can be considered in terms of a vestibular posture control model (Nashner, 1972), combining the experimental results with models of the vestibular sensors and a model of the dynamics of antero-posterior body sway. The model (Fig. 4) described the function of the posture control system in the following categories: (1) effects of body sway motion on the semicircular canals and on the utricular otoliths, (2) dynamic characteristics of the canals and the otoliths, and (3) characteristics of the relationships between vestibular responses and postural responses. The model was developed in two stages. First, models of the semicircular canals (Meiry, 1966; Young, 1968) and utricular otoliths (Young and Meiry, 1968) were analyzed to determine the response characteristics of these sensors to postural sway. A model for detection of postural sway by the semicircular canals resulted. Second, the detection model was one component within a more extensive model of the posture control system. Properties of the interface between vestibular output and postural responses were determined by matching characteristics of the complete posture control model with postural response sequences measured experimentally.

Several hypotheses about vestibular control of posture were drawn from the model. There was a dynamic separation of function between the semicircular canals and the utricular otoliths. The utricular otoliths, responding only to specific force, could not resolve conflicting gravitational and tangential acceleration forces during the free-fall and the compensatory response phases of control. As a result, the sign of the otolith response with respect to the direction of swaying was reversed during the free-fall

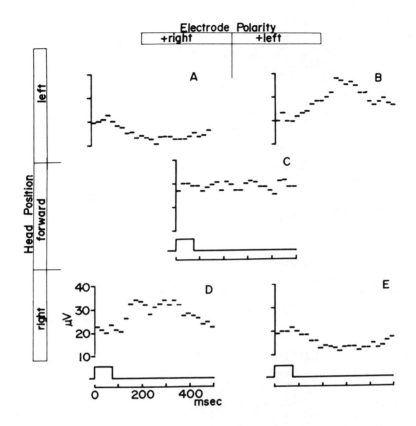

Fig. 3. Transient EMG responses in GS muscles elicited by
250 μa, 150 msec galvanic current pulses. A, B, D and E are
grouped according to the position of the head and the polarity
of the stimulus. Positive electrode was on the right mastoid in
C. Lower traces show time scale in msec and a representation
of the stimulus. Each EMG response record in μV is the result
of averaging the summed electrical activity of both GS muscles
during 256 trials, 64 performed on each of the 4 subjects.
Averaging was performed digitally using a PDP-12 computer.

phase as compared to the response evoked by static orientation or
by a slow movement. Sensing angular acceleration, the semicircular
canals did not suffer from this ambiguity but had no static sensi-

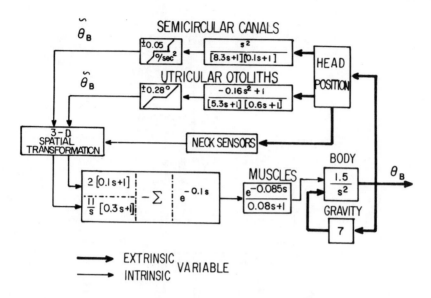

Fig. 4. The vestibular posture control model.

tivity to orientation with respect to gravity. The model predicted
that these conflicts are resolved; the canals provided dynamic sway
information during transient sway sequences; and the otoliths, a
low frequency vertical reference.

A neural integration of the semicircular canal response was
necessary to determine sway orientation during the free-fall and
initial compensatory phases of the postural response. During
these phases, interactions between gravitational and tangential
acceleration was greatest, so that indication of orientation from
the otoliths was dynamically incorrect. A simple linear summation
of canal and otolith responses was assumed in the model. This
assumption required a continuous integration of the canal output.
The combination of canal and otolith information is most likely
more complex than a linear summation, so that a more general
interpretation of the model would have been that the integration
was required during the brief periods in which large tangential
accelerations were encountered. Then the integrator need only
be a slowly responding first order system, a more likely physiological process. A neural integration of canal output in the control of
horizontal eye movements of this type was observed by Carpenter
(1972). Using artificial stimulation of the VIIIth nerve in decerebrate cats, reflex changes in the limbs were related to position

even though the receptor output signal indicated velocity (Partridge and Kim, 1969).

The effect of head position on the relationship between vestibular stimulation and postural responses corresponded to a spatial transformation of a vector from one frame of reference, the head, to another, the body. Body sway motion in a given direction requires a compensatory postural response appropriate to that direction. However, motion in a given direction will stimulate the vestibular sensors in quite different ways, depending on orientation of the head. A transformation, depending on orientation of the head with respect to the body is required if the vestibular system is to have a stabilizing influence on posture independent of head orientation. The experiments showed that such a transformation operated both on the short latency and long term postural responses evoked by electrical vestibular stimulation.

STABILIZING ROLE OF THE ANKLE JOINTS

While standing on a fixed base, resistance to sway is provided by rotating the ankle joints. Both the inherent properties of muscle and active reflex responses tend to resist rotation. The stabilizing role of feedback from rotation of the ankle joints was studied by measuring the modifying influence of feedback from the ankles on postural responses evoked by electrical vestibular stimulation. GS responses and postural sway were evoked using 250 μa, 8 sec current pulses, while the equivalent gain of information from the ankle joints was varied. An equivalent ankle feedback gain of 1 corresponded to standing on a fixed platform, allowing normal rotation of the ankle joints in relation to sway. Gains less than 1 were achieved by servodriving the platform to remove ankle joint rotation relative to postural sway. The platform servo was counterrotated to enhance the effects of body sway on ankle rotation to achieve equivalent ankle feedback gains greater than 1. Four subjects have thus far been tested in a preliminary study. Two are shown to illustrate the range of differences among the subjects. Subjects a and b responded very similarly when equivalent gains were 1 or greater. For gains less than 1 responses of a were well damped, while those of b were oscillatory (Fig. 5A). If feedback from the ankle joints was allowed at frequencies above 1 rad/sec by slowing the frequency response of the platform servo, responses of b were no longer oscillatory (Fig. 5B). Fig. 6 shows the average steady state bias for a and b as a function of the equivalent ankle

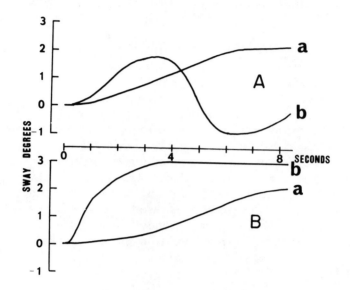

Fig. 5. A. Average body sway responses (64 trials) of two
subjects evoked by 250 μa, 8 sec current pulses to the vestibular system. Subjects stood on the servodriven platform with
eyes closed. B. Average body sway responses (64 trials) with
the same subjects and stimulus parameters. The gain of the
platform servo was the same but its response time was lengthened to 1 sec.

feedback gain. For equivalent gains greater than 1 the effect of
electrical stimulation decreased in direct proportion to the increase in gain, suggesting that the compensatory response was directly dependent   to the amount of ankle joint rotation. The steady
state effect of the stimulus was about 4 times greater with an
equivalent ankle joint gain of 0 than with an equivalent gain of 1.

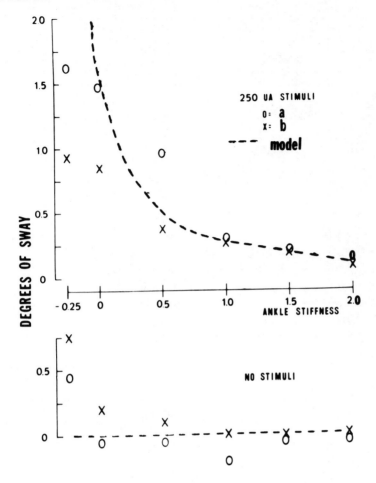

Fig. 6. The average steady state bias in body sway evoked by 250 μa, 8 sec current pulses to the vestibular system, 0 for subject a and X for subject b. Dotted line shows the bias angle predicted by the static vestibular ankle feedback model presented in Fig. 9.

There were significant differences in the time sequence of compensatory responses depending on the equivalent ankle joint gain (Fig. 7). The EMG and torque responses were unaffected by the equivalent ankle joint gain during the first 600 msec after the onset of the stimulus. Significant differences were noted after 600 msec, the earliest time for the onset of a compensatory response. When the equivalent gain was 1 or greater, the compensatory response began at about 600 msec, reaching a peak at 1 sec and then

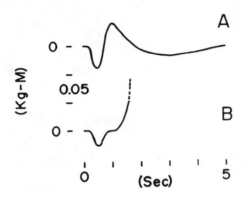

Fig. 7. Average ankle torque responses in one subject
(250 μa; 5 sec) with head turned right and positive electrode
on the right mastoid. A shows response to 64 trials on the
rigid platform. B shows response to 64 trials on the servodriven platform.

decaying. Without feedback from the ankles the compensatory
response was delayed until 1.1 sec, then was much larger because
the body was allowed to fall further before its onset.

Results of the vestibular posture control study (Nashner, 1971,
1972) are reviewed to explain the changes in postural responses
with changes in the feedback from the ankle joints. The vestibular
study concluded that compensatory responses to induced sway
motion were initiated by the vestibular system when there was no
feedback from the ankle joints. The average latency of compensatory responses at the slowest rates of induced sway was 1300
± 150 msec (mean ± S. D.). This latency is similar to that of a
compensatory response following an electrical stimulus when
there was no feedback from the ankle joints (1100 ± 125 msec).
This similarity suggests that in the absence of ankle joint feedback
the compensatory responses to sway evoked by electrical stimulation were also initiated by the vestibular system. The signifi-

cantly shorter latencies seen on the fixed or counter-rotated platform were probably due to more sensitive, shorter latency responses evoked by ankle joint rotations.

Two hypotheses about the stabilizing role of the ankle joint feedback could account for the above results: (1) There was a summation of information about body orientation from the vestibular system and from the ankle joints. Increasing the gain of the ankle feedback loop increased the total gain of the system, thus reducing sensitivity of the system to internal disturbances. (2) The posture control system used information from the ankle joint preferentially, such that increasing the amount of ankle feedback reduced the influence of vestibular control on postural responses. The first hypothesis is favoured because the initial phases of GS response to vestibular stimuli were unaffected by information from the ankle joints.

The stabilizing influence of ankle angle feedback covers the full dynamic range of body movements. Both the dynamic and static components of body sway could be significantly reduced depending on the task under study. Fig. 8 illustrates the additional dynamic stability provided by the ankle feedback, comparing Fourier coefficients of body motion during quiet standing on the fixed versus the servo-controlled platform. For random movement, ankle joint feedback reduced motion primarily at the higher frequencies. Fig. 5 shows that higher frequency information from the ankle joints could damp the oscillation of postural responses to electrical vestibular stimulation. The steady state bias of body sway was reduced by feedback information from the ankle joints (Fig. 6). A simple static feedback model was formulated to illustrate the proposed mechanism for the combined vestibular ankle feedback control of postural sway (Fig. 9). The model established relative magnitudes for ankle and vestibular feedback gains. Assumptions were that: (1) vestibular and ankle joint information about sway orientation summed linearly, (2) electrical vestibular stimulation evoked an internal disturbance within the vestibular feedback loop, and (3) gain of the vestibular feedback loop remained fixed, independent of changes in equivalent ankle feedback gain. An ankle feedback gain 2.7 times that of the vestibular gain was required to predict the strong modifying influence of ankle feedback on static orientation. The model indicated that under normal conditions the ankle joints provide the major contribution to stabilize sway.

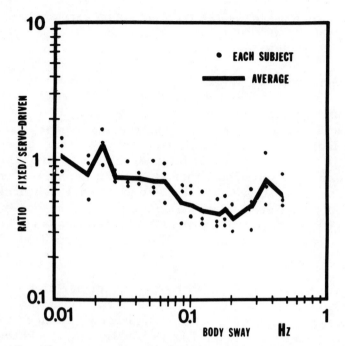

Fig. 8. The amplitude ratio comparing Fourier coefficients of body sway standing on the fixed platform versus the servo-driven platform. Subjects' eyes were closed in both cases.

DISCUSSION

The experiments on control of postural sway in human subjects have thus far directed attention on two types of sensory feedback control, from the vestibular system and from senses effected by rotation of the ankle joints. Conclusions drawn from the experiments and models assumed that the servoplatform can isolate vestibular control of posture. Proof of this technique can be made only be inference provided by the following statements. Standing on the fixed platform did not require vestibular or visual information (Nashner, 1970). Clinical studies showed that performance without these senses was limited if the supporting

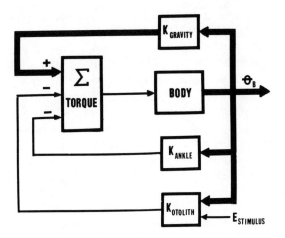

Fig. 9. A static feedback model for the control of body sway (Θ_B) jointly by the vestibular system and the ankle joints. $T_G(\Theta)$ is the relationship of gravitational torque to sway angle. $T_A(\Theta)$ and $T_O(\Theta)$ are respectively the stabilizing torque components from ankle joint and otolithic feedback depending on sway angle. E represents the disturbance of an electrical stimulus. Static stability is defined as the angle at which the three torques sum to zero for a given magnitude of E and values for T_A and T_O.

base is irregular or non-rigid (e.g. Fregly and Graybiel, 1968; Fregly et al., 1972). A subject without vestibular function was unable to remain stable on the servodriven platform, with or without vision (Nashner, 1970). Experiments on normal subjects using electrical vestibular stimulation showed that sensitivity to an internal vestibular disturbance increased 4 times when standing on the servodriven platform.

There has been considerable debate regarding the role of stretch reflexes in humans. Herman (1970) stated that the commonly held view that reflex activity is not present in normal muscle is open to serious question. Marsden et al. (1971, 1972) demonstrated properties of a proprioceptive length servo in human subjects performing voluntary tracking tasks. However, from a study of stepping, hopping and responses to falling in humans, Melvill-Jones and Watt (1971a, b) concluded that control was exercised primarily by central programs with reflexes playing a less signi-

ficant role. This study has shown that primary control of postural
sway can be effected either by muscle and reflex responses at the
ankle joints or centrally by the vestibular system. The principle
mechanism of control depended upon the conditions of the task.
Resistance of the ankle joints to rotation played a significant role
in stabilizing sway when subjects stood on a fixed platform. If
information from the ankle joints was removed, control was executed centrally by the vestibular system. Both types of control,
reflexive and central programs, were used in motor control, with
the conditions of the task determining the relative roles played by
each. The tasks studied here involved regulation of body sway to
small disturbances about a fixed operating point. The task used
by Marsden et al. (1971) could also be described as simple regulation, during a tracking task, while those of Melvill-Jones and
Watt (1971a) involved larger, more complex movements. Reflexive control may be more useful during regulation, and central
pre-programming, during active control of movements.

A number of details must be considered before attempting to
attribute ankle joint regulation of postural sway to some form of
reflex servo. The limited range of movements during postural
sway were possibly within a region in which muscle exhibits a
high resistance to stretch. Sway movements of $\pm 1.0°$ corresponded
to approximately ± 0.9 mm changes in GS length, $\pm 0.5\%$ of total
GS length. With normal ankle rotation allowed, postural sway
responses to electrical vestibular stimulation were at most half
this amount, approximately $\pm 0.25\%$ of GS length. Hill (1968) reported a short-range elastic resistance to stretch for 0.2% length
changes in frog sartorius muscle. Nichols and Houk (1973) observed a resistance to stretch which was much greater during
the first 0.4 mm (approximately 0.45%) than during the remainder
of a 3.5 mm stretch of cat soleus muscle. Within this region of
high resistance, active reflexes had little modifying influence.
Active reflexes had significant effects on later portions of the
response to stretch. The high resistance region of GS muscle
possibly accounted for stability of small disturbances to posture.
Regulation of sway within this limited range possibly did not
require significant contributions from proprioceptive reflexes
or central commands.

The earliest active compensatory responses to body sway attributable to ankle rotation were seen beginning 600 msec after
onset of an electrical stimulus to the vestibular system. Subtrac-
ting the latency of the GS response to the stimulus and the delays

between EMG and muscle responses, there was still about a 300 msec latency for the compensatory response. Marsden et al. (1971) showed servo action of the arm during compensatory responses commencing 50 msec after a change in controller dynamics. EMG responses resembling those of a length servo acted for 200 msec thereafter. Because of their long latency, compensatory responses to sway could have been initiated either at a spinal or at a central level. Clearly, more study is required to determine the role of feedback from ankle joint rotation in stabilizing posture. Currently, the properties of muscle and the exact timing of active reflex responses to stretch are being measured as a function of the parameters of the task. The vestibular posture control model provides a means for accurately predicting the first onset of responses initiated centrally by the vestibular system. Within this predictable latency period, a minimum of 100 msec, a window is provided during which compensatory responses initiated by spinal mechanisms will be observed.

REFERENCES

Bizzo, G., and Baron, J.B., 1972. Aspect cybernetique dés deplacements du centre de gravité du corps induits par des stimulations labyrinthiques électriques rectangulaires ou sinusoidales, Agressologie 13 B, 41-50.

Carpenter, R.H.S., 1972. Cerebellectomy and the transfer function of the vestibulo-ocular reflex in the decerebrate cat. Proc. Roy. Soc. Lond. 181, 353-372.

Coats, A.C., 1972. The sinusoidal galvanic body-sway response. Acta Otolaryngol. 74, 155-162.

Coats, A.C., 1973. Effect of varying stimulus parameters on the galvanic body-sway response. Ann. Otolaryngol. Rhinol. Laryngol. 82, 96-102.

Dzendolet, E., 1963. Sinusoidal electrical stimulation of human vestibular apparatus. Percept. Mot. Skills 17, 171-185.

Fregly, A.R., and Graybiel, A., 1968. An ataxia test battery not requiring rails. Aerosp. Med. 39, 277-282.

Fregly, A.R., Graybiel, A., and Smith, M.J., 1972. Walk on floor eyes closed (WOFEC): a new addition to an ataxia test battery. Aerosp. Med. 43, 395-399.

Herman, R., 1970. The myotatic reflex. Brain 93, 273-312.

Hill, D.K., 1968. Tension due to interaction between sliding filaments in resting muscle. The effect of stimulation. J. Physiol. 199, 637-684.

Marsden, C.D., Merton, P.A., and Morton, H.B., 1971. Changes in loop gain with force in the human muscle servo. J. Physiol. 222, 32-34.

Marsden, C.D., Merton, P.A., and Morton, H.B., 1972. Servo action
    in human voluntary movement. Nature 238, 140–143.
Meiry, J.L., 1966. The vestibular system and human dynamic space
    orientation. NASA-CR-628.
Melvill-Jones, G., and Watt, D.G.D., 1971a. Observations on the
    control of stepping and hopping movements in man. J. Physiol.
    219, 709–727.
Melvill-Jones, G., and Watt, D.G.D., 1971b. Muscular control of
    landing from unexpected falls in man. J. Physiol. 219, 729–737.
Nashner, L.M., 1970. Sensory feedback in human posture control.
    M.I.T. Rep. MVT-70-3.
Nashner, L.M., 1971. A model describing vestibular detection of
    body sway motion. Acta Otolaryngol. 72, 429–436.
Nashner, L.M., 1972. Vestibular posture control model. Kybernetik
    10, 106–110.
Nashner, L.M., and Wolfson, P., 1973. Influence of head position
    and proprioceptive cue on short latency postural reflexes evoked
    by galvanic stimulation of the human labyrinth. Brain Res.
    In press.
Nichols, T.R., and Houk, J.C., 1973. Reflex compensation for
    variations in the mechanical properties of a muscle. Science
    181, 182–184.
Njiokiktjien, Ch., and Folkerts, J.F., 1971. Displacement of the
    body's centre of gravity at galvanic stimulation of the labyrinth.
    Confin. Neurol. 33, 46–54.
Partridge, L.D., and Kim, J.H., 1969. Dynamic characteristics of
    response in a vestibulomotor reflex. J. Neurophysiol. 32,
    485–495.
Young, L.R., 1968. The current status of vestibular system models.
    Automat. 5, 369–374.
Young, L.R., and Meiry, J.L., 1968. A revised dynamic otolith model.
    Aerosp. Med. 39, 606–609.

A CEREBELLO-THALAMO-CORTICAL PATHWAY CONTROLLING FUSIMOTOR ACTIVITY

S. Gilman

Department of Neurology, College of Physicians and Surgeons of Columbia University, New York

The mechanisms underlying the beneficial effects of lesions in ventrolateral nucleus of thalamus (VLN) in humans with disorders of posture and movement have not been clarified with certainty. In experimental animals, lesions in VLN produced with a cooling probe decrease significantly the responses of medial gastrocnemius (MG) spindle primary afferents to extension of the gastrocnemius muscle. Lesions in a nearby thalamic nucleus, pulvinar, do not depress the responses of MG spindle primary afferents. Earlier studies have shown that the technique of sampling spindle afferent responses used in these experiments provides a reliable indication of the level of tonic activity of fusimotor neurones innervating the MG muscle spindle primaries. It is concluded that (1) the VLN has a net excitatory effect on fusimotor neurones projecting to hindlimb extensor muscles; (2) the VLN is part of a specific pathway for facilitation of fusimotor neurone activity; (3) lesions of VLN have a beneficial effect on limb rigidity in humans through a decrease of spindle afferent responses resulting from the depression of fusimotor activity.

Complete ablation of the cerebellum, including the deep nuclei, results in a marked depression of the responses of MG muscle spindle afferents to extension of the gastrocnemius muscle. Bilateral section of the superior cerebellar peduncles (SCP) to interrupt the major outflow of the lateral nuclei of the cerebellum to the VLN also decreases the responses of spindle

309

primaries. The degree of depression of the responses following
SCP section is less than that resulting from total cerebellectomy
and strikingly similar to that resulting from lesions of VLN.

Ablation of precentral areas 4 and 6 in the monkey results in
a marked depression of spindle afferent responses to extension
during the first week postoperatively. Subsequently there is a
return to control levels, complete at about 2 months after ablation. Bilateral pyramidotomy in the monkey also depresses the
responses of spindle primaries in the first week after operation.
There is a gradual recovery of responses during the subsequent
2 months, but the responses do not recover to control levels.
In monkeys with lesions of cerebellum, precentral cortex and
pyramidal tracts, there is a correlation between the degree of
hypotonia (decreased resistance to passive manipulation) of the
limbs and the level of activity of the spindle primaries. These
experiments indicate that a central circuit important to postural
mechanisms involving the fusimotor system consists of the cerebellar nuclei, the VLN, the precentral cortex and the medullary
pyramidal tracts.

INTRODUCTION

Compelling anatomical, physiological and clinical evidence indicates that the ventrolateral nucleus of the thalamus (VLN) is a
structure vital to the control of posture and locomotion in higher
animals and man. It is particularly important in the pathophysiology
of disorders of posture and movement in humans. Anatomically, the
VLN receives the output of the lentiform nucleus by way of the ansa
lenticularis and of the rostral projections of the cerebellum by way
of the brachium conjunctivum (Nauta and Mehler, 1966, 1969;
Mettler, 1972). Physiologically, stimulation of either the ansa
lenticularis or the brachium conjunctivum evokes monosynaptic
EPSPs in a majority of VLN cells, as demonstrated by intracellular
recordings (Desiraju and Purpura, 1969; Purpura, 1972a, b). The
EPSPs generated by stimulation of brachium conjunctivum are often
followed by IPSPs whereas the EPSPs activated from the ansa lenticularis are only rarely followed by IPSPs (Purpura et al., 1965;
Purpura, 1972b). Neurones in the VLN show spontaneous rhythmic
bursting when recorded in cats anaesthetized with barbiturate
(Andersen et al., 1969) or chloralose (Massion et al., 1965) and
in monkeys anaesthetized with chloralose (Albe-Fessard et al.,
1966). In paralyzed, unanaesthetized cats, high frequency bursts

occur only during slow wave sleep with EEG synchronization (Dormont, 1968; Lamarre et al., 1971; Steriade et al., 1971). Correspondingly, in chronic monkeys, VLN units discharge in bursts when the animal is immobile and drowsy (Lamarre and Joffroy, 1970, 1971). Monkeys with lesions in the tegmentum of the brain stem at about the level of the substantia nigra show spontaneous limb tremor movements (Ward et al., 1948; Cordeau et al., 1960; Poirier, Lamarre et al., 1966; Poirier, Sourkes et al., 1966). In these animals, neurones in the VLN discharge in bursts, some of which show precise temporal relationships with the limb tremor (Lamarre and Cordeau, 1967; Lamarre and Joffroy, 1970; Jasper et al., 1972). The discharge of these units does not result passively from the movements of the limbs since the discharge patterns persist following complete cessation of the tremor movements by administration of Flaxedil (Lamarre and Joffroy, 1970). The function of the cerebral motor cortex is important in the production of the tremor and burst activity, since focal cooling in the cortex results in complete cessation of tremor, and alteration of the frequency of the burst (Jasper et al., 1972). Lesions of the VLN in the monkey arrest the tremor produced in animals with tegmental lesions (Battista et al., 1970). Corresponding to these studies in animals, recordings of thalamic unit discharge in humans during stereotaxic surgery for Parkinson's disease have revealed cells in the VLN which fire in bursts at the frequency of the limb tremor (Albe-Fessard et al., 1966; Jasper and Bertrand, 1966). Lesions in the VLN have a striking effect upon tremor and abnormalities of posture in humans. A lesion of the posterior two-thirds of the VLN consistently reduces or abolishes the rigidity and tremor associated with Parkinson's disease (Cooper, 1971).

The mechanismsunderlying the beneficial effects of VLN lesions in humans with disorders of posture and movement have not been clarified with certainty. The physiological data concerning rhythmical activity in VLN neurones suggest that VLN lesions may interrupt the activity of neurones important in the initiation or maintenance of tremor of various origins. Conflicting theories have been advanced to explain the beneficial effects of VLN lesions on limb rigidity. Hassler (1956, 1966) proposes that a depression of fusimotor activity underlies the rigidity of Parkinson's disease and suggests that thalamic lesions restore the decreased fusimotor discharge to normal levels by reducing thalamic inhibition of fusimotor activity. An opposing theory (Asai et al., 1960; Rushworth, 1961, 1962) proposes that fusimotor activity is enhanced in

Parkinson's disease and that lesions of the VLN relieve rigidity
through a reduction of tonic fusimotor activity. The latter theory
is supported by the finding that the activity of muscle spindle
primary afferents is enhanced in Parkinsonian patients at rest
(Hagbarth et al., 1970).

LESIONS IN VENTROLATERAL NUCLEUS

One method of exploring the relationship between VLN and fusimotor neurones is to determine in experimental animals whether
lesions in VLN result in a depression or an enhancement of fusimotor activity. A study of this nature has been carried out using
freezing lesions of VLN in lightly anaesthetized cats and examining
the responses of muscle spindle primary afferents to extension of
the muscle of origin of the afferent (Gilman, Lieberman et al.,
1971; Lieberman et al., 1972, 1973). This procedure provides an
index of the level of tonic activity of fusimotor neurones innervating
the spindles studied (Gilman and Ebel, 1970). The details of the
experimental procedure, including the characteristics of the cryogenic probe and the resulting lesions, are described elsewhere
(Gilman, Lieberman et al., 1971; Lieberman et al., 1973). The
lesions produced by the probe are approximately spherical and
vary in diameter as a function of tip temperature. Histological
examination of the lesions, including both cell and fibre stains,
reveals necrosis occurring consistently from temperatures of
-30° to -60°C. A temperature of -20° consistently produces
tissue necrosis but inconsistently produces hemorrhage detectable
on gross and microscopic examination.

The cooling probe was inserted into the VLN of 6 cats. The
afferent responses to extension of the gastrocnemius muscle of 45
medial gastrocnemius spindle primaries were recorded to obtain
control values, then these responses were re-recorded serially
after cooling in 10°-20° steps. In the data analysis, the values
observed during the control recordings were compared with those
obtained at -20° since this temperature consistently produced
lesions confined to the VLN. The responses of 28 units were used
in the final analysis; the remaining 17 units were eliminated from
the analysis because of inaccurate placement of the lesion or inade-
quate administration of anaesthesia. The data obtained under control and -20° cooling conditions were compared with the data
following ventral root (VR) section to eliminate all fusimotor
innervation. Fig. 1 contains the responses of a representative unit

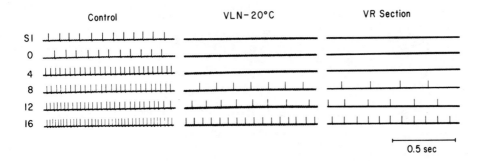

Fig. 1. Responses of a single medial gastrocnemius (MG) muscle spindle primary afferent recorded from a small filament of S_1 dorsal root in a cat. The gastrocnemius muscle is extended statically to various lengths as indicated: SL indicates the muscle is slack, free of external tension; 0 indicates extension of the muscle until 1-2 g of tension have been applied; subsequent numbers 4-16 indicate further extension in mm beyond 0 length. Note rise of threshold to firing and decrease of discharge rate after cooling in contralateral VLN and further decrease after section of ipsilateral ventral roots innervating gastrocnemius muscle.

and Fig. 2 a graph of mean frequencies at each muscle length for all units recorded in the control condition, the 28 units obtained during VLN cooling to -20°, and following VR section. Statistical analysis of the data, presented in detail elsewhere (Lieberman et al., 1973) revealed that spindle afferent discharge is depressed significantly by cooling to -20° and further depressed significantly by subsequent VR section.

In 5 other animals, the cooling probe was inserted into the pulvinar and the afferent responses to extension of the gastrocnemius muscle of 31 MG spindle primaries were recorded to obtain control values. The purpose of this experiment was to determine whether the effects observed during VLN cooling result specifically from a lesion placed in that location or whether similar effects may result from cooling another nearby thalamic nucleus. The responses were recorded serially after cooling in 10°-20° steps. We selected

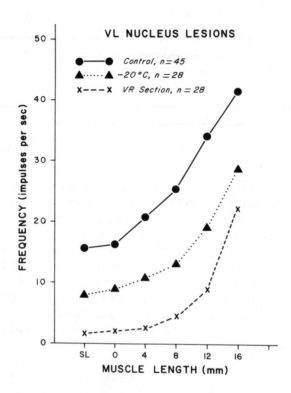

Fig. 2. Mean discharge frequencies of spindle primary afferents
of MG muscle as a function of gastrocnemius muscle length in
lightly anaesthetized cats, showing responses from 45 units
prior to cooling, 28 units after cooling in VLN, and the same 28
units after section of ventral roots innervating gastrocnemius
muscle.

for analysis the data obtained at -20° for comparison with the
effects of cooling VLN to this temperature and also the data from
cooling to -40°, which produced large lesions extending into nearby
structures. Finally, the effects of VR section were studied. Fig. 3
contains a graph of mean frequencies at each muscle length for all
units in the control condition, during cooling to -20°, -40°, and
after VR section. The analysis of these data revealed a significant
increase of discharge rate from cooling to -20°, no significant
change in rate from subsequent cooling to -40°, but a significant
decrease in rate from final VR section. The details of the statistical

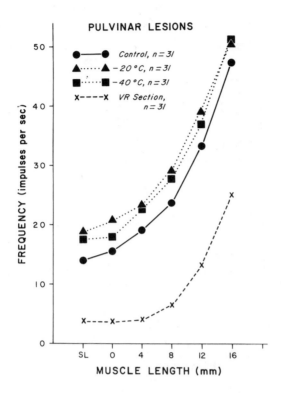

Fig. 3. Mean discharge frequencies of spindle primary after-ents of MG muscle as a function of gastrocnemius muscle length in lightly anaesthetized cats, showing responses from the same units prior to and after cooling pulvinar to -20° and -40 °C, and after sectioning ventral roots innervating gastrocnemius muscle.

analysis are presented elsewhere (Lieberman et al., 1973).

The finding of an increase of discharge rate after cooling in pulvinar introduces the possibility that the change of rate results from the physiological effects of the cooling procedure or from some experimental artifact, such as a progressive decrease in the level of anaesthesia. To study the latter possibility, a "sham" experiment was performed; the responses of 8 units were recorded serially during a simulated control determination, 4 simulated cooling determinations, and after actual VR section. The data obtained from this experiment are graphed in Fig. 4. Statistical analysis of differences in discharge rate between the control level and that

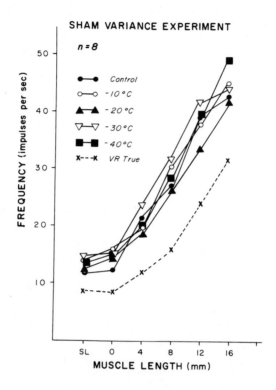

Fig. 4. Mean discharge frequencies of spindle primary afferents of MG muscle as a function of gastrocnemius muscle length
in a single lightly anaesthetized cat. Individual curves represent
data recorded seriatim from the same 8 units over a time
interval equivalent to that required for serial cooling to the
temperatures shown. Lowest curve shows effects of sectioning
ventral roots innervating the gastrocnemius muscle.

obtained during the simulated -20° cooling condition revealed no
significant change of the response levels (Lieberman et al., 1973).
However, subsequent VR section depressed the responses significantly, from both the control levels and those obtained during
"sham" -20° cooling. Thus, it appears likely that the increase
of spindle afferent responses during pulvinar cooling did not result
from some artifact of the experimental procedure, and may represent a physiological phenomenon.

These experimental findings demonstrate that lesions in the

VLN decrease significantly the responses to extension of spindle primary afferents in the MG muscle. Earlier studies have shown that the present technique of sampling spindle afferent responses provides a reliable indication of the level of tonic activity of fusimotor neurones innervating the muscle spindles studied (Gilman and McDonald, 1967; Gilman and Ebel, 1970). Consequently, the present data indicate that VLN lesions decrease the tonic activity of fusimotor neurones innervating MG muscle spindle primaries. Furthermore, the fact that pulvinar lesions do not depress the responses of MG spindle primary afferents suggests that VLN lesions interrupt a specific pathway facilitating fusimotor responses which is not disturbed by destruction of a large nearby thalamic nucleus. These findings support the concept that the VLN mediates a tonic neocerebellar facilitation of cerebral cortical activity influencing segmental postural reflex responses through fusimotor neurones (Dow and Moruzzi, 1958; Gilman, 1969, 1970).

EFFECTS OF CEREBELLAR LESIONS

Complete ablation of the cerebellum in cats, including the deep nuclei, results in a severe depression of the responses of MG muscle spindle afferents to extension of the gastrocnemius muscle (Fig. 5). Since the output of the cerebellar cortex is thought to be exclusively inhibitory (Eccles et al., 1967; Ito, 1970), it is presumed that this tonic facilitatory influence must be derived from the deep cerebellar nuclei, which produce predominantly excitatory influences upon thalamic neurones (Purpura, 1972b; Sakata et al., 1966; Saski et al., 1972). Bilateral section of the superior cerebellar peduncles (SCP) to interrupt the major outflow of the lateral nuclei of the cerebellum to the VLN results in a depression of the responses of muscle spindle primaries to muscle extension (Fig. 5). The degree of depression is less than that produced by total cerebellectomy, but the spindle responses are significantly less than those of the controls. It is of interest to compare the curve relating impulse frequency to muscle length from the animals with SCP section with the curve from the animals with lesions of VLN. The resemblance is most remarkable, particularly in light of the fact that the experiments on VLN were performed on a separate series of animals several years after the experiments on superior cerebellar peduncle were performed. These data provide strong evidence indicating that the lesions of SCP and VLN interrupt to a similar extent a strong tonic facilitatory mechanism influencing the activity of spinal fusimotor neurones.

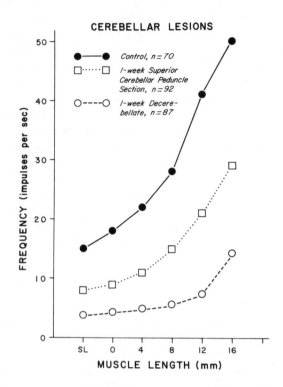

Fig. 5. Mean discharge frequencies of spindle primary afferents of MG muscle as a function of gastrocnemius muscle length in three groups of cats: control, completely decerebellate; and after bilateral section of superior cerebellar peduncles.

It appears likely that the neurones arising in VLN which affect fusimotor activity utilize a circuit involving the cerebral cortex, since the major projection site of the VLN is the precentral cortex (Walker, 1934, 1936, 1938; Chow and Pribram, 1956). However, certain experiments have suggested that other pathways may also be involved. For example, Yanagisawa et al. (1963) found that stimulation of VLN resulted in alteration of the activity of muscle spindle afferents in hindlimb muscles, and that these effects were not influenced by ablation of sensorimotor cortex or section of the medullary pyramids. However, bilateral lesions in the midbrain tegmentum reduced or abolished the effects. They proposed that the effects are mediated by a pathway between the VLN and the midbrain tegmentum involving the medial and intralaminar thalamic nuclei, corpus striatum, and globus pallidus. Spuler et al. (1962) suggested that a pathway involving the hypothalamus and other dien-cephalic structures mediates the spinal effects of VLN stimulation. Thus, VLN effects on fusimotor neurones at the spinal level may occur by means of several different pathways. Nevertheless, there is reason to believe that one of the major important pathways in primates and man is through the precentral cortex. The recent experiments of Jasper et al. (1972) indicate that cooling restricted to a focal point on the motor cortex reduces the tremor produced by brainstem tegmental lesions and also alters the rhythmic dis-charges of neurones located in VLN. In addition, recent experi-ments have demonstrated that ablation of portions of precentral cortex have a strong influence upon the activity of fusimotor neurones at spinal levels, with consequent profound alteration of the activity of spindle afferent responses (Gilman, Marco and Lieberman, 1971; Gilman et al., 1973).

EFFECTS OF CEREBRAL CORTICAL AND PYRAMIDAL TRACT LESIONS

Studies of the effects of precentral cortex lesions upon fusi-motor neurone activity were carried out in monkeys utilizing the format of some of the experiments described above. Ablation of cortical areas 4 and 6 in pre-Rolandic cortex was selected because of the dense projection of VLN neurones to area 4. In addition, ablations in this region result in a hypotonic hemiplegia initially which later evolves into a hypertonic hemiplegia (Denny-Brown, 1966). The details of the operative procedure, the findings on electromyographic examination of the limbs over time, and a detailed description of the histological findings are provided else-where (Gilman, Marco and Lieberman, 1971; Gilman et al., 1973). For the first 4-6 weeks after unilateral cortical ablation, the opposite limbs developed a hypotonic hemiparesis. During the third week the resistance to passive manipulation of the limbs increased until it became equal to that of the limbs opposite the intact cortex. During the fourth to sixth weeks, a definite heightening of resistance to dorsiflexion of the ankle and wrist emerged. At that time the deep tendon reflexes of the limbs became hyperactive and abnormally spreading. During the subsequent month, a further increase of plastic resistance to manipulation appeared in the shoulder, wrist, and ankle opposite the ablation. However, little or no increase of resistance appeared at the knee, and the resistance at the elbow was variable, usually slightly greater in the hemiparetic limbs than the others.

The afferent responses of 39 MG muscle spindle primaries
were recorded from 2 monkeys during the seventh day after ablation
of areas 4 and 6 in the hemisphere contralateral to the side of
recording. In Fig. 6, the mean values of these responses at each

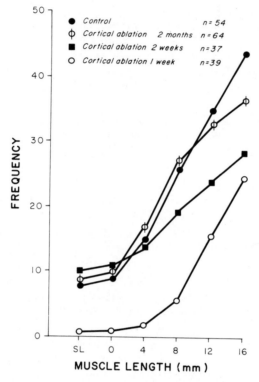

Fig. 6. Mean discharge frequencies of muscle spindle primary
afferents of MG muscle as a function of gastrocnemius muscle
length in monkeys lightly anaesthetized. Data taken from previously unoperated controls and animals 1 week, 2 weeks and 2
months after ablation of areas 4 and 6 in contralateral cerebral
cortex.

muscle length are compared with those recorded from previously
unoperated controls. Statistical analysis of these data (Gilman et
al., 1973), indicates that the frequencies from the group with
cortical ablations are significantly less than those of the control
animals. To determine whether a heightening of spindle afferent
response accompanied the limb hypertonia occurring in the monkey

with chronic ablations of areas 4 and 6, the afferent responses of 64 MG muscle spindle primaries were recorded from 6 monkeys during the phase of hypertonic hemiparesis resulting from the ablations. Recordings were taken from these animals when they were clinically stable and maximum hypertonia had been observed for 1 week. In most cases maximum hypertonia occurred 2 months after operation. Fig. 6 shows graphs of the mean values of these responses at each muscle length in comparison with those obtained from previously unoperated controls. Statistical comparison of mean discharge frequencies of these two groups, averaged across all muscle lengths, revealed no significant differences (Gilman et al., 1973). Thus, the responses of spindle primary afferents in MG muscle to extension of the muscle become depressed during the phase of hypotonic hemiplegia following ablation of areas 4 and 6, then recover to control levels during the phase of hypertonia. The time sequence of recovery was examined further with recordings taken from two animals 2 weeks after ablation, during the hypotonic hemiparetic phase. The results are illustrated in Fig. 6, which presents the mean values of these responses at each muscle length in comparison with those obtained from control animals and animals 1 week and 2 months after ablation of areas 4 and 6. The responses from the animals 2 weeks after ablation are significantly different from those of the controls and also different from those of the 1 week and of the 2 months animals (Gilman et al., 1973).

These experiments demonstrate that the animals with ablation of cortical areas 4 and 6 during the first postoperative week show a hypotonic hemiplegia in association with a significant depression of the responses of spindle primaries to muscle extension. However, 2 weeks after the ablation, when the animals still show a hypotonic hemiplegia, considerable restoration of spindle activity has occurred, suggesting that compensatory processes, whatever their nature, begin to function long in advance of increased deep tendon reflexes or heightened resistance to passive manipulation of the limbs. Recordings during the phase of hypertonia show clearcut findings; the spindle responses return to control levels but do not exceed them. Thus, these studies provide no evidence that tonic over-action of the fusimotor efferent spindle afferent system constitutes a fundamental "release" mechanism in the pathogenesis of hypertonia following cortical ablations of the type used in the present study. However, this finding does not rule out the possibility that fusimotor hyperexcitability underlies other types of limb hypertonia, particularly that of naturally occurring Parkinson's disease (Hagbarth et al., 1970).

The agranular frontal cortex is the site of origin of a large
number of fibres projecting to the spinal cord by way of the
medullary pyramids (Lassek, 1954). Section of the medullary
pyramids bilaterally in the monkey results in a depression of
the myotatic reflexes of the limbs, loss of contactual orienting
responses of the hands and feet, and loss of discrete use of
individual digits (Tower, 1940; Goldberger, 1969; Lawrence
and Kuypers, 1968; Gilman and Marco, 1971). The depressed
myotatic reflexes are manifested by hypotonia (diminished
resistance to passive manipulation) of the limbs, abnormalities
of posture, and alterations of the deep tendon reflexes. In the
animal with chronic pyramid section, hypotonia diminishes
but does not disappear, even 6 months after operation (Gilman
and Marco, 1971). To determine whether the clinical hypotonia
was associated with an alteration of spindle afferent responses
to muscle extension, monkeys with pyramidotomy were studied
under light anaesthesia, and the results compared with those
obtained from unoperated controls and from monkeys with complete cerebellar ablation (Gilman, Marco and Ebel, 1971).
The afferent responses of 38 MG muscle spindle primaries were
recorded from 3 monkeys during the first week after bilateral
section of the medullary pyramids. These responses were significantly depressed in comparison with the responses obtained
from 54 MG primaries recorded in control animals (Fig. 7).
However, the responses recorded in animals with pyramidotomy
were not different from those obtained in monkeys with complete
cerebellectomy of equal duration, approximately 1 week (Gilman,
1969). These observations indicated that the depression of
spindle afferent responses in pyramid-sectioned and in decerebellate animals may result from interruption of a common pathway which is facilitatory to the fusimotor neurones in the lumbosacral spinal cord. To test this possibility, the responses to
extension of MG muscle spindle primary afferents were recorded
in an animal with bilateral pyramid section of 7 days duration.
Then the cerebellar hemispheres and dentate nuclei were ablated
bilaterally by suction and the responses of the same units were
recorded again. As shown in Fig. 8, the ablation did not alter
substantially the responses of these units. It is possible that the
pyramid lesions had depressed the spindle afferent responses so
severely that further depression from a cerebellar lesion would
be undetected. However, complete interruption of all fusimotor
innervation of MG muscle spindles by section of the ipsilateral
ventral roots L_2-S_2 decreased these responses further (Fig. 8).
Consequently, fusimotor activity derived from other sources

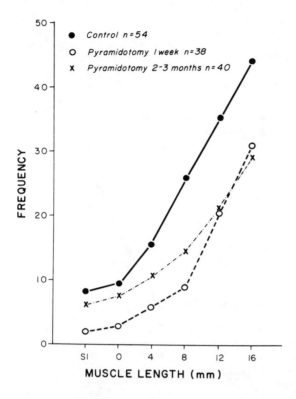

Fig. 7. Mean discharge frequencies of muscle spindle primary afferents of MG muscle as a function of gastrocnemius muscle length in monkeys lightly anaesthetized. Data taken from previously unoperated controls and animals 1 week and 2 months after bilateral section of medullary pyramidal tracts.

persisted in the pyramid-sectioned decerebellate animals.

Clinical examination of animals with chronic pyramidotomy revealed evidence of partial recovery of myotatic responses (Gilman and Marco, 1971). To determine whether muscle spindle afferent responses show similar recovery of responses, recordings were made of the responses of 40 spindle primaries in 4 monkeys with pyramidotomy of 2 to 3 months duration. As shown in Fig. 7, at most muscle lengths the afferent responses of the chronic-pyramid animals were greater than those of the acute-pyramid animals, but remained less than those of the controls. A statistical

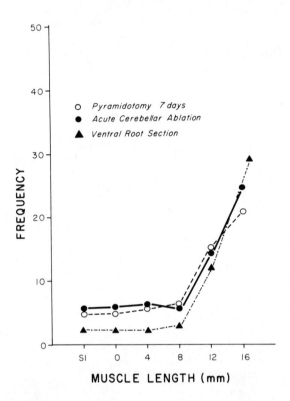

Fig. 8. Mean discharge frequencies of 8 muscle spindle primary afferents of MG muscle as a function of gastrocnmeius muscle length in a single monkey lightly anaesthetized. Open circles indicate responses 7 days after bilateral pyramidotomy. Filled circles show responses of the same units recorded again after acute ablation of cerebellar hemispheres and dentate nuclei bilaterally. Triangles show responses of the same units recorded again after section of ventral roots innervating gastrocnemius muscle.

analysis of these differences has been presented (Gilman, Marco and Ebel, 1971).

These studies have demonstrated that hypotonia, a decrease of the resistance to passive manipulation of the limbs, results from recent lesions in the cerebellum, precentral cortex, or medullary pyramids in the monkey. In each of these preparations, direct recordings from spindle primary afferents reveal a marked depression of the responses to muscle extension, indicating that the lesions have produced a decrease of tonic fusimotor activity innervating the spindles under study. The similarity of the resulting frequency-length curves along with experiments in which serial ablations have been performed indicate that the hypotonia from these various lesions results from the interruption of a central circuit important to postural mechanisms involving the fusimotor system. The circuit involves the cerebellar nuclei, the VLN, precentral cortex, and the medullary pyramidal tracts. However, it should be emphasized that in each of the experimental preparations tested, elimination of fusimotor activity by ventral root section usually decreases further the level of spindle activity, demonstrating that other systems are important in the control of fusimotor activity. In particular, it seems likely that reticulo-spinal and vestibulo-spinal pathways are important in the modulation of spindle afferent activity through effects on fusimotor neurones (Gernandt and Gilman, 1961; Cook et al., 1969a, b).

Acknowledgements: Some of the figures in this paper are reproduced through the courtesy of the editors of Brain and J. Neurophysiol. This work has been supported in part by USPHS Grants NS 05184, NS 02682, and NS 02356.

REFERENCES

Albe-Fessard, D., Guiot, G., Lamarre, Y., and Arfel, G., 1966. Activation of thalamo-cortical projections related to tremorogenic processes. In The Thalamus. (Eds. Purpura, D.P. and Yahr, M.D.) Columbia Univ. Press, N.Y., pp. 237-253.

Andersen, P., Olsen, L., Skede, K., and Sveen, O., 1969. Mechanisms of thalamo-cortical rhythmic activity with special reference to the motor system. In 3rd Symposium on Parkinson's Disease. (Eds. Gillingham, F.J., and Donaldson, I.M.L.) Livingston, Edinb. pp. 112-118.

Asai, K., Hufschmidt, H.J., and Schaltenbrand, G., 1960. The passive muscle relaxation in Parkinsonism: Myographic studies of the pathophysiology of the rigor. J. Nerv. Ment. Dis. 130, 449-455.

Battista, A.F., Nakatani, S., Goldstein, M., and Anagnoste, B., 1970. Effect of harmaline in monkeys with central nervous system lesions. Exp. Neurol. 28, 513-524.

Chow, K.L., and Pribram, K.H., 1956. Cortical projection of the thalamic ventrolateral nuclear group in monkeys. J. Comp. Neurol. 104, 57-76.

Cook, W.A. Jr., Cangiano, A., and Pompeiano, O., 1969a. Dorsal root potentials in the lumbar cord evoked from the vestibular system. Arch. Ital. Biol. 107, 275-295.

Cook, W.A. Jr., Cangiano, A., and Pompeiano, O., 1969b. Vestibular control of transmission in primary afferents to the lumbar spinal cord. Arch. Ital Biol. 107, 296-320.

Cooper, I.S., 1971. Motor functions of the thalamus with recent observations concerning the role of the pulvinar. Int. J. Neurol. 8, 238-259.

Cordeau, J.P., Gybels, J., Jasper, H., and Poirier, L.J., 1960. Microelectrode studies of unit discharges in the sensorimotor cortex. Investigations in monkeys with experimental tremor. Neurol. 10, 591-600.

Denny-Brown, D., 1966. The Cerebral Control of Movement. Liverpool Univ. Press, Liverpool.

Desiraju, T., and Purpura, D.P., 1969. Synaptic convergence of cerebellar and lenticular projections to thalamus. Brain Res. 15, 544-547.

Dormont, J.F., 1968. Activité unitaire dans le noyau ventral latéral chez le chat éveillé. J. Physiol. (Paris) Suppl. 1, 60, 242.

Dow, R.S., and Moruzzi, G., 1958. The Physiology and Pathology of the Cerebellum. The Univ. of Minn. Press, Minneapolis.

Eccles, J.C., Ito, M., and Szentágothai, J., 1967. The Cerebellum as a Neuronal Machine. Springer, N.Y.

Gernandt, B.E., and Gilman, S., 1961. Differential supraspinal control of spinal centers. Exp. Neurol. 3, 307-324.

Gilman, S., 1969. The mechanism of cerebellar hypotonia: An experimental study in the monkey. Brain 92, 621-638.

Gilman, S., 1970. The nature of cerebellar dyssynergia. In Modern Trends in Neurology (Ed., Williams, D.) Butterworths, Lond. pp. 60-79.

Gilman, S., and Ebel, H.C., 1970. Fusimotor neuron responses to natural stimuli as a function of prestimulus fusimotor activity in decerebellate cats. Brain Res. 21, 367-384.

Gilman, S., Lieberman, J.S., and Copack, P., 1971. A thalamic mechanism of postural control. Int. J. Neurol. 8, 260-275.

Gilman, S., Lieberman, J.S., and Marco, L.A., 1973. Spinal mechanisms underlying the effects of unilateral ablation of areas 4 and 6 in monkeys. Brain. In press.

Gilman, S., and Marco, L.A., 1971. Effects of medullary pyramidotomy in the monkey. I. Clinical and electromyographic abnormalities. Brain 94, 495-514.

Gilman, S., Marco, L.A., and Ebel, H.C., 1971. Effects of medullary pyramidotomy in the monkey. II. Abnormalities of spindle afferent responses. Brain 94, 515-530.

Gilman, S., Marco, L.A., and Lieberman, J.S., 1971. Experimental hypertonia in the monkey: Interruption of pyramidal or pyramidal-extrapyramidal cortical projections. Tr. Amer. Neurol. Ass. 96, 162-168.

Gilman, S., and McDonald, W.I., 1967. Cerebellar facilitation of muscle spindle activity. J. Neurophysiol. 30, 1494-1512.

Goldberger, M.E., 1969. The extrapyramidal systems of the spinal cord. II. Results of combined pyramidal and extrapyramidal lesions in the Macaque. J. Comp. Neurol. 135, 1-26.

Hagbarth, K.-E., Hongell, A., and Wallin, G., 1970. Parkinson's Disease: Afferent muscle nerve activity in rigid patients. A preliminary report. Acta Med. Upsal. 75, 70-76.

Hassler, R., 1956. Die extrapyramidalen Rindensysteme und die zentrale Regelung der Motorik. Deut. Z. Nervenheilk. 175, 233-258.

Hassler, R., 1966. Thalamic regulation of muscle tone and the speed of movements. In The Thalamus. (Eds. Purpura, D.P. and Yahr, M.D.) Columbia Univ. Press, N.Y., pp. 419-438.

Ito, M., 1970. Neurophysiological aspects of the cerebellar motor control system. Int. J. Neurol. 7, 162-176.

Jasper, H.H., and Bertrand, G., 1966. Thalamic units involved in somatic sensation and voluntary and involuntary movements in man. In The Thalamus. (Eds. Purpura, D.P. and Yahr, M.D.) Columbia Univ. Press, N.Y., pp. 365-390.

Jasper, H., Lamarre, Y., and Joffroy, A., 1972. The effect of local cooling of the motor cortex upon experimental Parkinson-like tremor, shivering, voluntary movements, and thalamic unit activity in the monkey. In Corticothalamic Projections and Sensorimotor Activities. (Eds. Frigyesi, T.L., Rinvik, E., and Yahr, M.D.). Raven Press, N.Y., pp. 461-473.

Lamarre, Y., and Cordeau, J.P., 1967. Étude du mécanisme physio-pathologique responsable, chez le singe, d'un tremblement experimental de type Parkinsonien. Actual. Neurophysiol. 7, 141-166.

Lamarre, Y., Filion, M., and Cordeau, J.P., 1971. Neuronal dis-charges of the ventrolateral nucleus of the thalamus during sleep and wakefulness in the cat. I. Spontaneous activity. Exp. Brain Res. 12, 480-498.

Lamarre, Y., and Joffroy, A.J., 1970. Thalamic unit activity in monkey with experimental tremor. In L-DOPA and Parkinsonism. (Eds. Barbeau, A., and McDowell, F.H.). F.A. Davis, Phila., pp. 163-170.

Lamarre, Y., and Joffroy, A.J., 1971. Spontaneous unit activity in the ventrolateral thalamus of the chronic monkey. Int. J. Neurol. 8, 190-197.

Lassek, A.M., 1954. The pyramidal tract: Its status in medicine. Charles C. Thomas, Springfield.

Lawrence, D.G., and Kuypers, H.G.J.M., 1968. The functional organization of the motor system in the monkey. I. The effects of bilateral pyramidal lesions. Brain 91, 1-14.

Lieberman, J.S., Copack, P., and Gilman, S., 1972. Effects of focal freezing in ventrolateral nucleus and pulvinar on muscle spindle afferent responses. Neurol. 22, 438.

Lieberman, J.S., Copack, P.B., and Gilman, S., 1973. Fusimotor effects of cryogenic lesions in ventrolateral nucleus and pulvinar. In preparation.

Massion, J., Angaut, P., and Albe-Fessard, D., 1965. Activités evoquees chez le chat dans la région du nucleus ventralis lateralis par diverses stimulations sensorielles. II. Étude microphysiologique. EEG Clin. Neurophysiol. 19, 452-469.

Mettler, F.A., 1972. The corticothalamic projection: the structural substrate for the control of the thalamus by the cerebral cortex. In Corticothalamic Projections and Sensorimotor Activities. (Eds. Frigyesi, T.L., Rinvik, E., and Yahr, M.D.). Raven Press, N.Y., pp. 1-19.

Nauta, W.J.H., and Mehler, W.R., 1966. Projections of the lentiform nucleus in the monkey. Brain Res. 1, 3-42.

Nauta, W.J.H., and Mehler, W.R., 1969. Fiber connections of the basal ganglia. In Psychotropic Drugs and Dysfunction of the Basal Ganglia. (Eds. Crane, G., and Gardner, R. Jr.). Public Health Service Publ. No. 1938, U.S. Government Printing Office, Wash., D.C., pp. 68-72.

Poirier, L.J., Lamarre, Y., and Cordeau, J.P., 1966. Neuroanatomical study of an experimental postural tremor in monkeys. Second symposium of Parkinson's disease. J. Neurosurg. Suppl. 24, 191-193.

Poirier, L.J., Sourkes, T.L., Bouvier, G., Boucher, R., and Carabin, S., 1966. Striatal amines, experimental tremor and the effect of harmaline in the monkey. Brain 89, 37-52.

Purpura, D.P., 1972a. Intracellular studies of synaptic organizations in the mammalian brain. In Structure and Function of Synapses. (Eds. Pappas, G.D., and Purpura, D.P.). Raven Press, N.Y., pp. 257-302.

Purpura, D.P., 1972b. Synaptic mechanisms in coordination of activity in thalamic internuncial common paths. In Corticothalamic Projections and Sensorimotor Activities. (Eds. Frigyesi, T.L., Rinvek, E., and Yahr, M.D.). Raven Press, N.Y., pp. 21-56.

Purpura, D.P., Scarff, T., and McMurtry, J.G., 1965. Intracellular study of internuclear inhibition in ventrolateral thalamic neurons. J. Neurophysiol. 28, 487-496.

Rushworth, G., 1961. The gamma system in Parkinsonism. Int. J. Neurol. 2, 34-50.

Rushworth, G., 1962. Muscle tone and the muscle spindle in clinical neurology. In Modern Trends in Neurology, Vol. 3. (Ed. Williams, D.). Butterworths, Inc., Wash., D.C., pp. 36-56.

Sakata, H., Ishijima, T., and Toyoda, Y., 1966. Single unit studies on ventrolateral nucleus of the thalamus in cat: its relation to the cerebellum, motor cortex and basal ganglia. Jap. J. Physiol. 16, 42-60.

Sasaki, K., Matsuda, Y., Kawaguchi, S., and Mizuno, N., 1972. On the cerebello-thalamo-cerebral pathway for the parietal cortex. Exp. Brain Res. 16, 89-103.

Spuler, H., Szekely, E.G., and Spiegel, E.A., 1962. Stimulation
of the ventrolateral regions of the thalamus. Its effect upon
tremor induced by midbrain stimulation in cats. Arch. Neurol.
6, 208-219.
Steriade, M., Apostol, V., and Oakson, G., 1971. Control of
unitary activities in cerebellothalamic pathway during wakefulness and synchronized sleep. J. Neurophysiol. 34, 389-413.
Tower, S.S., 1940. Pyramidal lesion in the monkey. Brain 63,
36-90.
Walker, A.E., 1934. The thalamic projection to the central gyri
in macacus rhesus. J. Comp. Neurol. 60, 161-184.
Walker, A.E., 1936. An experimental study of the thalamo-cortical
projection in the macaque monkey. J. Comp. Neurol. 64, 1-39.
Walker, A.E., 1938. The Primate Thalamus. Univ. Chicago Press,
Chicago.
Ward, A.A. Jr., McCulloch, W.S., and Magoun, H.W., 1948. Pro-
duction of an alternating tremor at rest in monkeys. J.
Neurophysiol. 11, 317-330.
Yanagisawa, N., Narabayashi, H., and Shimazu, H., 1963. Thalamic
influences on the gamma motor system. Arch. Neurol. 9, 348-357.

THE SUPPLEMENTARY MOTOR AREA -- A CONTROL SYSTEM FOR POSTURE?

M. Wiesendanger, J.J. Séguin and H. Künzle

Department of Physiology, University of Western
Ontario, London, Canada, and the Institut für
Hirnforschung, Universität Zürich, Switzerland

The supplementary motor area (SMA) is interconnected
with the precentral motor cortex and receives its main
afferents from the somatosensory areas I, II and 5; it is
therefore most likely concerned with somatosensori-motor
integration. In primates, there is no anatomical evidence
of a thalamic relay to the SMA or of a direct projection to
the spinal cord. Stimulation of corticospinal fibres evoked
antidromic discharges in the precentral tail and hindleg
areas (as defined by intracortical stimulation), but not in
the SMA. Indirect influences on the motor apparatus may
be exerted through the red nucleus, the pontine nuclei, and
bilaterally via the precentral motor cortices and the
striatum. Experiments in monkeys in which conventional
serial surface (-) stimulation was used were complemented
by experiments using also single pulse (+) and intracortical
train (-) stimulation. Prolonged repetitive stimulation of
the SMA at high intensities (1.5-2.5 ma) readily evoked
movements of the contralateral upper limb. However, EMG
bursts followed each pulse and occurred with the same
latencies as those obtained with weak stimuli from the precentral forelimb area. The thresholds also showed a steady
increase as the stimulating electrode was moved from the
best precentral point towards the SMA. Thus, spread of
current to the precentral cortex was probably the dominant
factor producing the arm responses upon SMA stimulation.
This was supported by experiments in monkeys with large

331

lesions of the precentral forelimb area. Strong repetitive
stimulation evoked, apart from tail or hindleg movements,
a slow contraction chiefly of shoulder girdle muscles out-
lasting stimulation for several seconds. The firing of motor
units was not related to stimulus frequency. These "genuine"
motor effects from the SMA were complex synergies, and a
somatotopic organization was not established. Strong single
pulses (up to 7 ma) and short trains of intracortical stimuli
(up to 2 ma) failed to evoke twitches in the presence of precentral cortical lesions. The results are compatible with
the view that the SMA exerts a control on postural mechanisms
involving mainly the proximal muscles.

Electrical stimulation of fore- and hindlimb nerves elicited
field potentials in the SMA and also single unit discharges
(latencies 10-30 msec) with considerable spatial convergence.
The behavioural deficit of forced grasping following SMA
lesions might have its neuronal counterpart in a tonic inhibition
exerted by the SMA on the transcortical grasp reflex sub-
served by the somatic afferent pathway and the pyramidal
tract. In preliminary experiments, a moderate inhibition
from the SMA on precentral cells was observed. It is concluded
that there is a marked difference between the characteristics
of the SMA and the primary motor cortex, and it is conceivable
that the SMA has a higher position in the motor control
hierarchy than the motor cortex. This is also indicated by
observations of a neglect in the use of the nonparetic arm in
monkeys and patients with SMA lesions.

The supplementary motor area (SMA), buried within the medial
longitudinal fissure anterior to the hindleg and tail areas, has been
explored with stimulating electrodes in patients (Penfield and
Jasper, 1954), and this led to the mapping experiments in monkeys
and various other species (for recent review see Jameson et al.,
1968). The simiusculi (diagrammatic maps in the shape of a dis-
torted monkey) of the precentral motor cortex and of the SMA,
described by Woolsey et al. (1950) have been published in numerous
textbooks. As yet, it appears to us that the functional significance
of the SMA is far from being understood and that several problems
remain controversial. From results of ablation experiments in
monkeys, Travis (1955) concluded that the SMA is mainly concerned
with somatotopically organized control of muscle tone. The inference is sometimes made (Bowsher, 1970) that hemiplegic spasticity

in man results from a combined lesion of capsular fibres from
the precentral cortex (leading to paresis) and from the SMA
(leading to spasticity). Travis' (1955) results have, however,
been contested by Coxe and Landau (1965), who did not find
'... any significant lasting changes in muscle tonus, tendon
reflex activity or posture'. Whether the SMA exerts a direct
influence on the spinal cord (Bertrand, 1956; Nyberg-Hansen,
1969) has also been questioned (Smith et al., 1958; DeVito and
Smith, 1959). Remarkable progress has been made in recent
years in elucidating with degeneration techniques the hodology
of the various cortical areas. We will first summarize the
afferent and efferent connections to the SMA; this information
will then be related to our own experimental findings.

STRUCTURAL RELATIONS OF THE SMA

The SMA has no clearcut cytoarchitectonic boundaries and
cannot be considered as a primary cortical area since it has no
specific input from a well defined thalamic relay (Akert and
Woolsey, 1954; see also Fig. 18.4 in Akert, 1964). In Fig. 1
an attempt has been made to summarize the present knowledge
of the afferent and efferent connections of the SMA. Most
importantly, it has been shown that the SMA has a direct input
from the somatosensory areas I, II and 5 and that these relations
are not reciprocal; this is in contrast to the reciprocal relationship of the SMA with the precentral motor cortex (Jones and
Powell, 1969, 1970). Since a spinal projection from the SMA
has not been found anatomically in monkeys (DeVito and Smith,
1959), it appears that the SMA exerts its influence on the motor
system via the precentral motor cortex and via subcortical
structures (Kemp and Powell, 1970; Kuypers and Lawrence,
1967) believed to be parts of motor feedback loops (Kemp and
Powell, 1971). The results described in this paragraph have
been obtained with silver degeneration methods. For comparison
one monkey (Macacus irus) has been investigated with the auto-
radiographic tracing method. H3-proline was injected into the
SMA, and the brain was investigated after a survival period of
51 hours. In agreement with previous results, an ipsilateral
projection to the pontine nuclei (including n. teg. pontis) and
an ipsilateral projection to the red nucleus were found. No
labelled material was detected at levels caudal to the pontine
nuclei. Surprisingly little labelling was seen in the precentral
motor cortex, bilaterally in area 6 and unilaterally in area 4

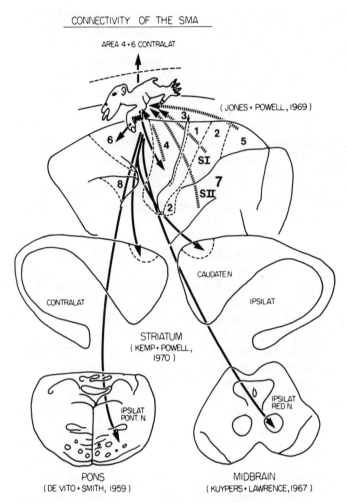

CONNECTIVITY OF THE SMA

Fig. 1. Afferent and efferent connections of the SMA as revealed by anterograde degeneration techniques.

(sparing the face area). The bilateral projection to the striatum was not confined to the head of the caudate nucleus, but extended further back in both, the caudate nucleus (corpus) and the putamen. A clear unilateral labelling was also present in cells of various thalamic nuclei (VA, VLo, VLc, VPLo, VPI. CM and Pcn).

MOTOR EFFECTS PRODUCED BY ELECTRICAL
STIMULATION OF THE SMA

The motor effects elicited by prolonged serial stimulation of what is now called the SMA caught the attention of neurologists because they resembled the seizure patterns occurring in the presence of foci within the mesial cortex of area 6; mass movements on the contralateral side (especially lifting of the arm); adversive movements of the head, eyes and trunk; vocalization and arrest of speech (Penfield and Jasper, 1954). Intracortical stimulation with an array of electrodes allowed Talairach and Bancaud (1966) to stimulate altogether 766 different points within the human SMA. This stereo-encephalographic technique has been used in patients in order to localize epileptogenic foci. Typical responses obtained by these authors are in good agreement with older reports: speech arrest, vocalization, deviation of eyes and head, and tonic raising of the arm. Thus, stimulation of the SMA in patients revealed a characteristic pattern of complex synergies with no apparent somatotopic organization comparable to that in the precentral motor cortex. In contrast to these results from humans are those obtained by Woolsey et al. (1950) in monkeys with 'late pentobarbital anaesthesia'. A simiusculus similar to that of the precentral cortex was used to depict the somatotopic organization of the SMA. It was noted that the area was smaller and more difficult to explore than the precentral cortex, and that motor responses required higher stimulus intensities.

Since it is not clear whether or not this area is an output system with fairly direct access to the spinal motor apparatus and whether it is endowed with somatotopic characteristics we have reinvestigated the motor effects produced by electrical stimulation of the SMA. The results discussed above were obtained with repetitive cathodal stimulation. In the present experiments, two additional techniques were used: 1. Single surface anodal pulses of 5 msec duration (Liddell and Phillips, 1950) which elicits twitches in distal muscles when applied to the precentral cortex. It was previously shown that these motor effects in primates are dependent on an intact pyramidal tract (Felix and Wiesendanger, 1971). 2. Trains of cathodal pulses applied intracortically through microelectrodes which allowed an extremely localized excitation of motor cortical neurones in cebus monkeys (Asanuma and Rosén, 1972). It was shown earlier in cats (Asanuma and Sakata, 1967) that minimal motor responses to intracortical microstimulation are mediated by the pyramidal tract. In the

present series of experiments, stimulation of the SMA was
performed in 10 macaques and 3 cebus monkeys under N_2O
anaesthesia supplemented by additional small doses of short
acting barbiturates (Thiopental[R], Surital[R]). The sagittal
sinus was reflected to the opposite side and access to the mesial
wall was obtained by inserting small cotton balls, soaked in
warm paraffin oil, into the medial longitudinal fissure in order
to separate the mesial surface of the cortex from the falx. The
cortex was also widely exposed in the peri-Rolandic region for
comparison of thresholds in the SMA with those of the precentral
motor cortex. Electromyographic responses were recorded with
pairs of fine needle electrodes, insulated except at the tips. The
stimulation points of the cortex were marked on a photograph of
the exposed cortex taken during surgery. One macaque had a
large chronic lesion of the precentral forelimb area on one side
and bilateral chronic lesions of the bulbar pyramids. Two cebus
monkeys had large chronic lesions of the precentral forelimb
areas.

Movements could be elicited upon repetitive stimulation of
the mesial cortex in the region of the SMA, and the patterns of
movements, indicated in the figurine chart of Fig. 2 (intact right
cortex), are roughly comparable to those obtained by Woolsey et
al. (1950). In particular, it was confirmed that movements of
the forelimb occurred upon stimulation of sites rostral to the
precentral leg and tail areas (the latter being rather large in
cebus monkeys). Analysis of the electromyographic response of
the hand and forearm muscles revealed that each pulse of
repetitive stimulation at 30-50 Hz, after a summation time of
several seconds, elicited a synchronized burst of activity. The
latencies of the EMG bursts recorded in intrinsic hand muscles
(9-14 msec) and of the flexors and extensors of the wrist and
fingers (5.5-8 msec) were, however, in the same range as
those for similar responses elicited by stimulation of the precentral hand area. The same was true for the responses evoked
by single anodal pulses. This finding makes it likely that the
forelimb responses to SMA stimulation were caused by current
spread to the precentral forelimb region. This is also supported
by the results of 3 experiments in which the cortex was systematically mapped from the precentral forelimb area towards the
SMA with repetitive and single pulses. Stimulation thresholds
for EMG responses in arm muscles increased steadily as the
electrode was moved nearer to the SMA. Essentially the same
result was seen upon intracortical stimulation with a micro-

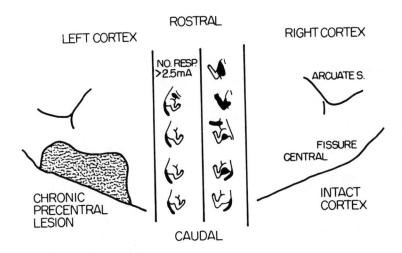

Fig. 2. Patterns of movements elicited by repetitive
cathodal stimulation (50 Hz, 1 msec pulses) at various
points of the marginal gyrus of the mesial surface. Left
cortex had a large, chronic precentral lesion (sparing some
of the motor cortex at the depth of the central fissure).
Note the scarcity of forelimb movements upon stimulation
of left SMA as compared to the effects elicited from the
intact cortex. Cebus monkey, N_2O/Surital anaesthesia.

electrode. As illustrated in Fig. 3, in which the penetrations
and thresholds for minimal EMG responses in the hand muscles
at the 'best' cortical depth are marked. A very high intensity
was needed to elicit EMG responses as soon as the electrode
tracks were outside the precentral hand area. These results
strongly indicate that spread of current to the precentral motor
cortex (with perhaps additional background facilitation mediated
by fibres from the SMA to the precentral cortex) was the
dominant factor in causing the movements elicited by stimulation
of the SMA.

In order to detect some concealed 'genuine' effects of the
SMA stimulation, experiments were also done on animals with
chronic precentral lesions (forelimb area). It could be assumed
that movements produced by electrical stimulation of the SMA
in these animals were little, if at all, contaminated by effects

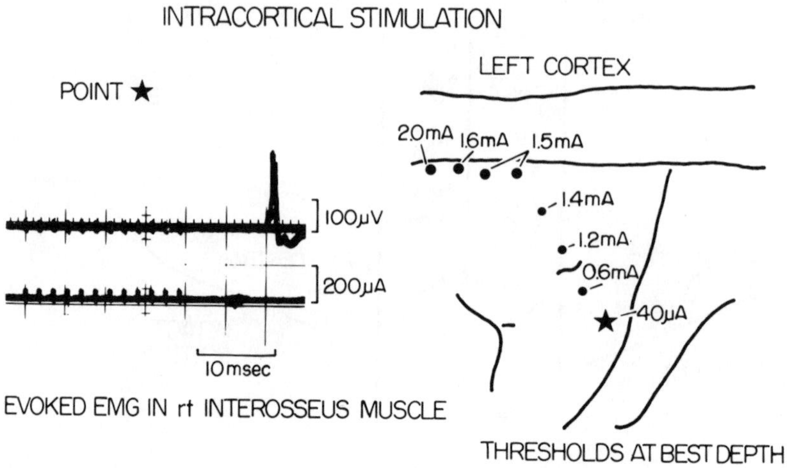

INTRACORTICAL STIMULATION

POINT ★

LEFT CORTEX

EVOKED EMG IN rt INTEROSSEUS MUSCLE

THRESHOLDS AT BEST DEPTH

Fig. 3. Thresholds for EMG response elicited by intracortical train stimuli (-) applied with a tungsten low
resistance microelectrode at "best" depth. On the left,
threshold response of the interosseus muscle; stimulation
at the "best" precentral penetration. Note increase of
threshold intensity (ma) as penetrations were made nearer
to the SMA. Cebus monkey, N_2O/Surital anaesthesia.

originating from the precentral motor cortex. In the macaque
(which had also a bilateral pyramidal lesion) repetitive stimulation of the SMA elicited, after a summation period of several
seconds, a slow, tonic raising of the arm which persisted for
up to half a minute after cessation of stimulation. This pattern
was strikingly different from the much more localized contractions
observed in intact animals upon precentral stimulation. Sometimes
SMA stimulation caused arm movements which were seen in
isolation; sometimes the hindleg and tail were involved as well.
Motor units were firing asynchronously, i.e. the discharge rate
was not related to the frequency of stimulation and the tonic activation again outlasted the period of stimulation. In the two cebus
monkeys with precentral lesions, stimulation of the most rostral
parts of the SMA elicited a tonic retraction of the shoulder, but
tail movements occurred at lower thresholds and over a wide
field of the mesial cortex (Fig. 2, left cortex). In all three
animals we failed to discern a somatotopy. Stimulation of most
points, especially of the more caudal ones in the SMA, involved

also the tail and hindlegs, but this might readily be explained
by the proximity of the precentral hindlimb and tail areas which
were left intact in these animals. Single anodal pulses at intensities of up to 7 ma evoked no responses in forelimb muscles.
With intracortical train stimulation, the highest current passing
through the microelectrode (about 2 ma) likewise failed to activate
motor units of the upper limbs (only a few such trials were made
at the end of an exploration with surface stimulation because such
high currents were likely to produce electrolytic lesions).

The present results are in keeping with those recorded by
Penfield and Welch (1951), who found that when "...the primary
motor arm area is excised, hand movements are no longer
elicitable from the mesial cortex, but at higher threshold more
proximal movements can be produced from this region". In
summary, our stimulation experiments on animals without precentral forelimb area, indicate that some tonic contractions,
predominantly of the proximal muscles of the upper limb, can be
elicited by prolonged and strong stimulation but not by single
pulse anodal or discrete intracortical stimulation. These movements were strikingly different from the discrete patterns evoked
from the precentral motor cortex. The results can be taken to
indicate that the SMA exerts an influence, via indirect routes,
on the spinal motor apparatus, especially on motor units of
proximal muscles. Although the present findings make it
unlikely that the pyramidal tract is involved in the direct
mediation of motor effects from the SMA to the spinal cord, the
problem was further investigated in two experiments. Cortical
cells were identified as corticospinal by antidromic invasion
from stimulation of the dorsolateral funiculus. In Fig. 4, an
area posterior to the co-ordinate A 22 is shown in which several
penetrations with a microelectrode were done. In each track,
pyramidal tract neurones were encountered. Stimulation through
the same microelectrode resulted in twitch movements of the tail.
Rostral to A 22, however, no pyramidal tract cells were found.
Thus, there seemed to be a rather sharp division between the
'pyramidal cortex' (tail area of the cebus monkey) and the 'non-
pyramidal' cortex which would lie in Woolsey's forelimb area
of the SMA. The finding of Bertrand (1956) of a typical pyramidal
tract response to SMA stimulation seemed at the time to support
the view of a corticospinal projection from the SMA. However,
it was shown by Smith et al. (1958) that the pyramidal response
was probably due to spread of current to the precentral cortex.
This is in agreement with our failure to record antidromic responses

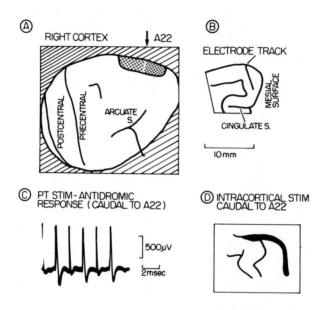

Fig. 4. A. Area of exposed cortex. Microelectrode penetrations as indicated in B. In penetrations made caudal to
A 22, many cells were encountered which were fired anti-
dromically upon pyramidal tract stimulation (cervical 2) as
shown in C. Intracortical stimulation in this area elicited
tail twitches (D). No pyramidal tract cells were found in
tracks rostral to A 22 and intracortical stimulation elicited
no tail twitches. Cebus monkey, N_2O/Surital anaesthesia.

from pyramidal tract cells in the region of the SMA.

SOMATOSENSORY INFLUENCE ON THE SMA

As already mentioned, the SMA receives its main input from
somatosensory areas. In 4 experiments (2 macaques, and 2 cebus
monkeys) we have investigated the afferent input organization by
recording the field and unitary responses to electrical stimulation
of peripheral nerves. The following are the main results of these
preliminary experiments: 1. Averaged field potentials evoked by
stimulation of forelimb nerves (median, radial) and hindlimb nerves
(sciatic, femoral) were recorded over Woolsey's forelimb area

in the SMA. The latencies ranged from 10-30 msec for the forelimb nerves and from 15-30 msec for the hindlimb nerves. 2. The
amplitudes of all field potentials increased as the penetrating
electrode was placed nearer to the hindlimb area of the precentral
gyrus. 3. Stimulation of hindlimb and forelimb nerves were
equally effective in Woolsey's forelimb area of the SMA. 4. Many
cells were found which were not excited by strong repetitive
nerve stimuli. However, those neurones (n=23) which were
excited had a pronounced convergence from two or more nerves
of the upper and lower extremities (Fig. 5). The relative contribution of the various somatosensory submodalities and of natural

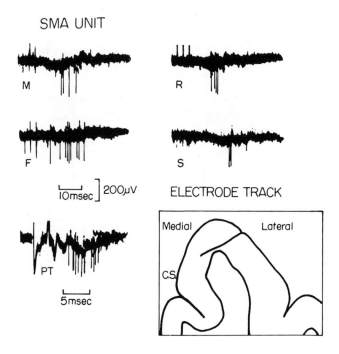

Fig. 5. Recording from a single neurone of the SMA.
Microelectrode penetration from lateral surface through
marginal gyrus. c. s. = cingulate sulcus. Note absence
of antidromic response to strong pyramidal tract (PT)
stimulation and pronounced convergence upon train
stimulation of the median (M), radial (R), sciatic (S),
and femoral (F) nerves. Macaque, N$_2$O/Surital
anaesthesia.

stimulation has not yet been tested. Results obtained by Libet
et al. (1973) in patients indicate that the SMA is a zone of convergence also for visual and acoustic signals. Thus, a considerable amount of integration is taking place in this area. Forced
grasping is a prominent though reversible sign of an SMA lesion
(Penfield and Welch, 1951; Travis, 1955). It is also known that
the grasp reflex requires an intact precentral-pyramidal system
(Denny-Brown, 1966). The neural basis of the grasp reflex was
described in terms of tight input-output columns of the precentral
cortex (Brooks, 1971). It is therefore conceivable that the SMA
exerts a tonic inhibitory action on this precentral cortical reflex.
We studied the effect of SMA stimulation on precentral units in
order to detect possible modulations exerted on precentral units
which could account, at the behavioural level, for forced grasping.
The results, so far, have been inconsistent in that in a few cells
only, a moderate suppression of spontaneous or peripherally evoked
activity of precentral units has been observed. Excitation of precentral units (PT and non-PT neurones) occurred with strong
(about 1 ma) train stimuli applied to the SMA at latencies of
3. 0 to 9. 0 msec.

DISCUSSION AND CONCLUSION

Relationship of the SMA to Other Cortical Areas

The anatomical relationship of the SMA strongly suggests
that this area is concerned with somatosensori-motor integration.
Although the SMA has sometimes been viewed as a smaller version
of the precentral motor cortex, forming together with sensori-
motor area II (buried in the Sylvian fissure) a "trilogy" of motor
cortical representation (Woolsey et al., 1950), there is a sharp
anatomical distinction between the primary cortical areas and
the SMA. The primary motor area, but not the SMA, has a specific
(point-to-point) cortico-thalamic relationship (Akert and Woolsey,
1954). Also, as pointed out by Jones and Powell (1970), the SMA
has a higher level of complexity (similar to the somato-sensory
area 5 of the parietal cortex) since it represents a first stage
of convergence from primary areas.

The Problem of Somatotopic Organization

A degree of somatotopic organization, which one would
assume from Woolsey's figurine representation, has not been
found upon electrical stimulation of the SMA in patients nor in
monkeys with acute (Penfield and Welch, 1951) or chronic
(present experiments) ablations of the precentral motor cortex.
The reason for the discrepancy between these and Woolsey's
experiments lies, in our opinion, more in the interpretation
than in the actual results as discussed previously. On anatomical
grounds alone, one would assume that a certain degree of somatotopy would be preserved since both the somatosensory areas as
well as the precentral motor area were found to project somatotopically to the SMA (Jones and Powell, 1969; Pandya and Vignolo,
1971). However, in our recordings within the SMA we found no
clear evidence of a somatotopically organized input. In fact,
single unit recordings revealed a rather pronounced degree of
convergence from hind- and forelimbs.

Is the SMA Involved in the Control of Posture?

A definite answer to this question cannot yet be given. As
mentioned in the Introduction, the view that monkeys with SMA
lesions display a pronounced spasticity (Travis, 1955) could not
be confirmed in a more recent study by Coxe and Landau (1965).
That the SMA is involved in postural adjustments might be inferred
from its bilateral projection to the basal ganglia, and by the
observation that "pure" motor effects obtained by SMA stimulation
mainly concern proximal muscles in the form of complex synergies.
The persistence of a posture induced by electrical stimulation and
the long lasting firing of motor units after cessation of stimulation
could indicate that the SMA has a predominant effect on the gamma
loop; direct evidence on this point is, however, lacking. Forced
grasping, i.e. the release of this reflex following SMA lesions
(Penfield and Welch, 1951; Travis, 1955) further indicates that
this area is involved in a tonic modulation of a transcortical-
pyramidal reflex underlying the grasp reflex (Denny-Brown, 1966;
Rosén and Asanuma, 1972). Some inhibitory effects from the SMA
on precentral units, although not conspicuous in our experiments,
would point in this direction.

Is the SMA Involved at a Higher Level of Sensori-Motor Integration?

Apart from its possible role in modulation of postural reflexes, one might consider another hypothesis derived from observation on animals (Penfield and Welch, 1951) and patients (Waltrégny, 1972) with SMA lesions; it was noted that the arm contralateral to the lesion, although not paretic, seemed to be somewhat neglected. Could it be that certain motor tasks requiring learning from proprioceptive or cutaneous feedback are controlled from the SMA? There is some evidence that the cortex on the lateral surface around the arcuate sulcus is necessary for motor tasks which seem to depend largely on 'proprioceptive, i.e. response-produced, cues' (Goldman and Rosvold, 1970). Both this area and the SMA belong to cortical area 6, and stimulation of them in humans produces similar effects (Foester, 1936). Thus, the 'programming' of certain motor habits may rely on 'modality specific memory' (Goldman and Rosvold, 1970). Electrical stimulation experiments and gross observations of motor deficits produced by SMA lesions are unlikely to produce essentially new information about the role of the SMA in motor control. The combined use of refined motor tasks requiring somatosensory cues and of simultaneous recordings of unitary activity in the SMA might be a rewarding approach for a better understanding of the functional significance of this area.

Acknowledgement: The research was performed at the Institute für Hirnforschung der Universität Zürich, Switzerland, and at the Department of Physiology, University of Western Ontario, London, Canada. Financial support received from the following institutions is gratefully acknowledged: Swiss National Foundation for Scientific Research (Grants 3.415.70, 3.133.69); the 'Dr. E. Slack-Gyr-Foundation', Zürich (Switzerland); Medical Research Council (Canada). The technical help of Mrs. S. Stauch (Zürich) and Mrs. P. Dhanarjan (London, Ontario) is much appreciated. The authors wish to thank Dr. P.G. Dellow for his helpful comments and criticism.

REFERENCES

Akert, K., 1964. Comparative anatomy of frontal cortex and thalamofrontal connections. In The frontal granular cortex and behavior. (Eds. Warren, J.M., and Akert, K.). McGraw-Hill, N.Y., p. 381.

Akert, K., and Woolsey, C.N., 1954. Ventrolateral nuclear group of
     the thalamus and its projection upon the precentral motor cortex
     of the monkey (Macaca mulatta). Fed. Proc. 13, 1-2.
Asanuma, H., and Rosén, I., 1972. Topographical organization of
     cortical efferent zones projecting to distal forelimb muscles in
     monkey. Exp. Brain Res. 14, 243-256.
Asanuma, H., and Sakata, H., 1967. Functional organization of a
     cortical efferent system examined with focal depth stimulation
     in cats. J. Neurophysiol. 30, 35-54.
Bertrand, G., 1956. Spinal efferent pathways from the supplementary
     motor area. Brain 79, 461-473.
Bowsher, D., 1970. Introduction to the anatomy and physiology of the
     nervous system. 2nd edition. Blackwell Sci. Publ. Oxford and
     Edinburgh, 133 pp.
Brooks, V.B., 1971. Tight cortical input-output coupling. Neurosci.
     Res. Prog. Bull. 9 (No. 1), 51-56.
Coxe, W.S., and Landau, W.M., 1965. Observations upon the effect of
     supplementary motor cortex ablation in the monkey. Brain 88,
     763-772.
Denny-Brown, D., 1966. The Cerebral Control of Movement. Liverpool
     Univ. Press, 130 pp.
DeVito, J.L., and Smith, O.A., 1959. Projections from the mesial
     frontal cortex (supplementary motor area) to the cerebral hemi-
     spheres and brain stem of the Macaca mulatta. J. Comp. Neurol.
     111, 261-278.
Felix, D., and Wiesendanger, M., 1971. Pyramidal and non-pyramidal
     motor cortical effects on distal forelimb. muscles of monkeys.
     Exp. Brain Res. 12, 81-91.
Foerster, O., 1936. Motor cortex in man in the light of Hughling
     Jackson's doctrines. Brain 59, 135-159.
Goldman, P.S., and Rosvold, H.E., 1970. Localization of function
     within the dorsolateral prefrontal cortex of the Rhesus monkey.
     Exp. Neurol. 27, 291-304.
Jameson, H.D., Arumugasamy, N., and Hardin, W.B., 1968. The
     supplementary motor area of the racoon. Brain Res. 11, 628-637.
Jones, E.G., and Powell, T.P.S., 1969. Connexions of the somatic
     sensory cortex of the Rhesus monkey. I. Ipsilateral cortical
     connexions. Brain 92, 477-502.
Jones, E.G., and Powell, T.P.S., 1970. An anatomical study of
     converging sensory pathways within the cerebral cortex of the
     monkey. Brain 93, 793-820.
Kemp, J.M., and Powell, T.P.S., 1970. The cortico-striate projection
     in the monkey. Brain 93, 525-546.
Kemp, J.M., and Powell, T.P.S., 1971. The connexions of the striatum
     and globus pallidus: synthesis and speculation. Phil. Trans. Roy.
     Soc. Lond. B 262, 441-457.
Kuypers, H.G.J.M., and Lawrence, D.G., 1967. Cortical projections to
     the red nucleus and the brain stem in the Rhesus monkey. Brain
     Res. 4, 151-188.

Libet, B., Alberts, W.W., Wright, E.W., Jr., Lewis, M., and Feinstein, B., 1973. Some cortical mechanisms mediating conscious sensory responses and the somatosensory qualities in man. In Somatosensory System. (Ed. Kornhuber, H.H.). Georg Thieme, Stuttgart, In Press.

Liddell, E.G.T., and Phillips, C.G., 1950. Overlapping areas in the motor cortex of the baboon. J. Physiol. 112, 392-399.

Nyberg-Hansen, R., 1969. Corticospinal fibres from the medial aspect of the cerebral hemisphere in the cat. An experimental study with the Nauta method. Exp. Brain Res. 7, 120-132.

Pandya, D.N., and Vignolo, L.A., 1971. Intra- and interhemispheric projections of the precentral and arcuate areas in the Rhesus monkey. Brain Res. 26, 217-233.

Penfield, W., and Jasper, H., 1954. Epilepsy and the functional anatomy of the human brain. Little, Brown Co., Boston. pp. 88-106.

Penfield, W., and Welch, K., 1951. The supplementary motor area of the cerebral cortex. A clinical and experimental study. Arch. Neurol. Psychiat. 66, 289-317.

Rosén, J., and Asanuma, H., 1972. Peripheral afferent inputs to the forelimb area of the monkey motor cortex: Input-output relations. Exp. Brain Res. 14, 257-273.

Smith, O.A., DeVito, J.L., and Patton, H.D., 1958. Electro-physiological analysis of supplementary motor area. Fed. Proc. 17, 151.

Talairach, J., and Bancaud, J., 1966. The supplementary motor area in man. (Anatomo-functional findings by stereo-electroencephalo-graphy in epilepsy). Int. J. Neurol. 5, 330-347.

Travis, A.M., 1955. Neurological deficiencies following supplementary motor area lesions in Macaca mulatta. Brain 78, 155-173.

Waltrégny, A., 1972. L'épilepsie de l'aire motrice supplémentaire (AMS). Méd. Hyg. 815-816.

Woolsey, C.N., Settlage, P.H., Meyer, D.R., Sencer, W., Hamuy, T.P., and Travis, A.M., 1950. Patterns of localization in precentral and "supplementary" motor areas and their relation to the concept of a premotor area. In Patterns of Organization in the Central Nervous System. Res. Publ. Ass. Nerv. Ment. Dis. 30, 238-264.

LOADING REFLEXES DURING TWO TYPES OF VOLUNTARY MUSCLE CONTRACTIONS

A. W. Monster

Department of Rehabilitation Medicine, Temple
University, Philadelphia, Pennsylvania

Small step load changes were superimposed on a constant
load applied to the extensor muscles of the human ankle
joint. Comparison of the induced loading reflex during:
(1) steady muscle contraction supporting a constant load,
and (2) a voluntary movement under this same load, shows
in both bases two peaks in the reflex electromyogram.
The first peak is much reduced during voluntary movement
and is also most affected by the rate of stretch. The size
and latency of the second peak is strongly dependent on the
contractile state of the muscle at the time of load application. Both peaks are separated by inhibition; this
depression in motoneurone firing sometimes dominates
the loading response, minimizing the effectiveness of the
load compensation reflex.

There is substantial evidence that muscle afferents are able
to play an important role in the feedback control of movement and
posture (Matthews, 1972). Functional studies have, however, not
been overly comprehensive and have not necessarily provided adequate explanations of the functional significance of the fusimotor-
muscle afferent system in voluntary muscle contraction. Neither
has there been sufficient reason to minimize the role of other
groups of muscle afferents and pressure and tactile receptors in
the feedback control and integration of voluntary motor activity.

The servo hypothesis of voluntary muscle contraction (Merton,
1953) has now been abandoned in favour of the more general alpha-

gamma co-activation hypothesis (Granit, 1955, 1968). It has, however, become increasingly clear that normal voluntary inner-vation patterns are likely to be complex and also to involve central control of the excitability of a variety of spinal inter-neurones (e.g. Lundberg, 1970; Hultborn et al., 1968), including those mediating muscle afferent activity within spinal reflex loops and others of which the primary function may be to provide supraspinal mechanisms with a temporal-spatial representation of the state of the spinal reflex system.

Whether or not the consequences of the evoked afferent dis-charges are mostly at the spinal cord level remains to be seen. Indications to the contrary arise from the close integration of ascending and descending information at different levels of the sensori-motor hierarchy (Oscarsson, 1970), including the possible observation of a short latency transcortical reflex (Evarts, 1968; Phillips, 1969). Studies of normal motor function are necessary to provide natural modulation of the excitability of identified pathways, and to resolve the historical dichotomy between the notions of reflex control and central patterning control (Evarts et al., 1970).

It therefore seemed relevant to examine differences in the state of the reflex system during two types of voluntary motor acts: the first a postural type, supporting a constant load iso-tonically; the other a voluntary isotonic movement. Specifically, we have addressed ourselves to the questions: (1) Is the earliest component of the loading reflex (i.e. spinal monosynaptic stretch reflex) different for voluntary movement, as compared to postural type activity, and (2) What are the sizes, latencies and possible origins of any later components of the loading response during these two types of voluntary motor acts?

METHODS

Small load pulses of controlled size and shape were super-imposed on a constant load (preload) isotonically supported by the calf muscles either during a voluntarily maintained constant muscle length (postural activity) or during movement. The subject was supine, with the back slightly elevated so as to monitor a visual display. One foot was attached to a motor driven mechanical transducer assembly that could rotate the ankle joint. Rotation speed of the ankle joint, muscle length at which stimuli were applied, size of the preload and size and duration of the super-imposed load pulses were carefully controlled. Load pulses

were applied at random time intervals during the steady contraction and were randomly applied during successive movements. Movements were executed at a natural speed (once
every 5-10 sec) and were self-paced. Electrical activity was
recorded differentially with surface electrodes from the ankle
flexors and extensors, and from the tibial nerve (in the popliteal fossa). Since stretch reflex responses elicited by loading
are non-synchronous, the electromyographic (EMG) activity
was rectified, low-pass filtered ($\tau \approx .01$ or $.001$ sec) and
averaged by summation. The EMG-time integral as well as
the peak values of the rectified EMG wave were used to assess
the magnitude of the reflex induced modulation of alpha motoneurone pool excitability. Averaging was required in order to
keep the size of the load disturbance (pulse) small and to
operate the stretch reflex in a reasonably linear range. The
number of samples varied from 8 to 32. Loading responses
were recorded also from the forearm flexors and from the
masseter, which elevates the lower part of the jaw. Selective
nerve blocks (Matthews and Rushworth, 1957a, b) were performed using a local anaesthetic (Xylocaine 0.5%), which was
slowly infiltrated around the tibial nerve. This was followed
by an examination below the level of the block to assess temperature, touch, phasic stretch reflex and motor response; the
examination was repeated every 10 min.

RESULTS

A sudden increase in load on a voluntary contracting muscle
evoked a reflex response. This loading response was dependent
on the size and duration of the load, the rate of load application,
muscle length, motoneurone pool excitability and on the contractile
state of the muscle at the time the load was applied. In this study,
all load pulses were applied in the relaxed position, which was
usually 5-10° into plantar flexion. Movement was initiated in a
slightly dorsiflexed position. There was then sufficient range for
the subject to settle into a smooth movement trajectory before
the load pulse was applied again at 5-10° into plantar flexion.
Preloads and load pulses were less than 10% of maximum voluntary
strength. Muscle length at load pulse application and preload were
also selected so as to provide a sufficient amount of background
electromyographic activity on which the reflex induced temporal-
spatial sequence of excitatory and inhibitory effects could be

superimposed.

LOADING RESPONSE DURING A STEADY
VOLUNTARY CONTRACTION

A typical loading response modulating EMG output during a sustained voluntary extensor contraction is shown in Fig. 1A. It is characterized by an excitatory phasic discharge (1) a period of depression immediately following the phasic discharge, (2) and a gradual recovery which includes an excitatory phase at a variable latency (3). The shape of both excitatory phases may be complex (bi- or trimodal) depending on the properties of the load pulse, the size of the voluntary contraction (i. e. preload) and muscle length. When the rate of loading is high the initial phasic discharge often shows two peaks at 20-30 msec apart, with the first occurring 25-30 msec following application of the load pulse. A very early depression, preceding the phasic component of the loading reflex is sometimes seen if rate of loading is high and the muscle prestretched. The recovery curve, i. e. the duration of the depression and the size of the later period of increased alpha motoneurone discharge, is similar to that of an H-reflex evoked by an electrical stimulus applied directly to the mixed peripheral muscle nerve; this similarity is most pronounced if the loading pulse is of short duration and stretch is synchronous (Fig. 1, compare A and B). The depression (2 in Fig. 1A) is sometimes seen in the absence of a phasic response and the latency of the late excitatory phase (3) may be quite short, such as shown in the jaw jerk of Fig. 1C.

The exact shape of the recovery curve is similar in flexors and extensors and is dependent on a number of parameters. Different preloads elicit different size phasic discharges as well as recovery curves, with increasing preloads causing an earlier recovery and even sustained periodic discharges (Fig. 2A). A short loading pulse applied towards dorsiflexion (extensor stretch) in the dorsiflexed position causes stretch of the antagonist during the rebound and the response clearly shows the interaction within the myotatic unit (Fig. 2B), i. e. flexors and extensors firing in reciprocal fashion.

The size of the initial electromyographic potential (1 in Fig. 1A) is probably a fair representation of the size of the stretch evoked afferent input and a measure of spindle sensitivity to the

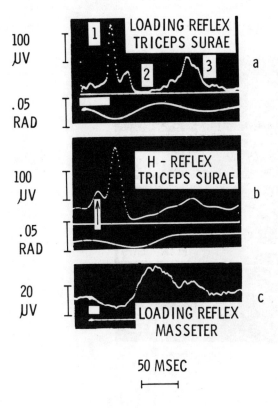

Fig. 1. Comparison of reflex response of triceps surae (A and B) and masseter (C). Size of load pulse in (A) and of the electrical stimulus in (B) were selected so as to cause the same size phasic reflex response in both cases. Loading pulse to masseter muscle was applied by dropping a small weight attached to a bite plate on the lower jaw; markers show duration of load pulse and arrow marks occurrence of electrical stimulus: load was applied so as to stretch the contracting muscle and (for the triceps surae) to cause ankle rotation towards dorsiflexion.

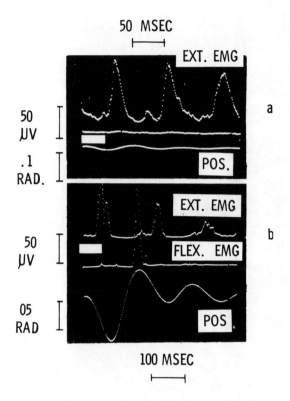

Fig. 2. Loading responses of triceps surae muscle when:
(a) supporting a large preload (20% of maximum voluntary
contraction) and (b) with the extensor muscle tightly stretched
by rotating the ankle 15° into dorsiflexion; markers show
duration of load pulse; joint rotation is indicated by label
"pos".

dynamic component of stretch. The more direct approach of
recording the afferent discharge from the tibial nerve in the
poplital fossae was found to be technically feasible, but much
more cumbersome and probably not more accurate. The

relationship between the initial rate of extensor stretch and the size of the phasic reflex response is shown in Fig. 3 (solid line).

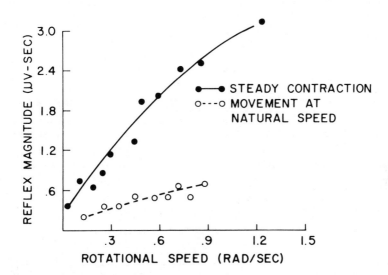

Fig. 3. Comparison of dynamic sensitivity of loading reflex during the two types of motor act. Reflex magnitude was determined from the change in the integral of the rectified and smoothed electromyographic potential measured from the initial diversion of the integral base line till its first peak. Rotational speed was derived from the derivative of the ankle position. Load pulses were in both cases applied in the normally relaxed position. Each point is average of 16 measurements on one subject at 3 different days.

Because of the asynchronous discharge especially at slow loading speed, it was necessary to base the size of the stretch reflex on the change in the time-integral of the EMG (IEMG) measured from its initial baseline to the peak reached within the first 60-70 msec following diversion from the baseline. Dynamic sensitivity during this type of postural activity is exemplified by the gradient of the curve in Fig. 3. Notice the

linear relationship between rate of stretch and reflex size up to
. 6 rad/sec ($\approx$ 50 mm/sec). The sizes of the stretches were usually
less than 5° ankle rotation and the initial dynamic response was
elicited early in the stretch cycle. The duration of the load
pulse was chosen long enough so as to evoke a maximal phasic
reflex. There was little difference between flexor and extensor
loading reflexes; afferent effects that are symmetrical appear to
dominate the postural loading response.

LOADING RESPONSE DURING VOLUNTARY EXTENSION MOVEMENTS

Simple voluntary movements such as flexion and extension
can be reproduced quite accurately. Natural speed of movement
depends on the subject's intention (effort) which is affected by the
(pre) load against which the movement is performed. The amount
of EMG activity elicited during an isotonic voluntary movement is
large compared to the condition in which a similar preload is iso-
tonically supported at a constant muscle length. EMG activity
declines when the extensor shortens, going into plantar flexion.
Both the increased EMG discharge during movement and the gradual decline, reflect the force-velocity relationship of the contracting
muscle. Typical loading responses for increasing size preload
are shown in Figs. 4A and B. Notice that a stretch reflex is
evoked in Fig. 4A, although the movement continues in the
intended direction and the muscle undergoes no external stretch.
The main characteristics of the reflex responses shown in Fig. 4
are the small, less phasic and later initial response as compared
to Figs. 1 and 2, and again the occurrence of two excitatory phases.
These two phases may be separated by a period of inhibition and
this depression is least pronounced if the load is small (compare
the two examples in Fig. 4). Notice from the integral of the EMG
that at the large preload (Fig. 4B), the reflex is not very effective
in compensating for the sudden load disturbance; to the contrary,
the inhibitory phase dominates the response.

The size and nature of the reflex response is quite dependent
on the subject's intension, e.g. forcefulness and speed of movement. The initial phasic response becomes more pronounced as
the movement is executed slower, and it follows from the
increasing similarity of postural and slow movement responses
that we are dealing with a continuous spectrum. Pronounced
difference   between a postural and a fairly forceful movement
response to loading is shown in Fig. 5 (left half); notice that the

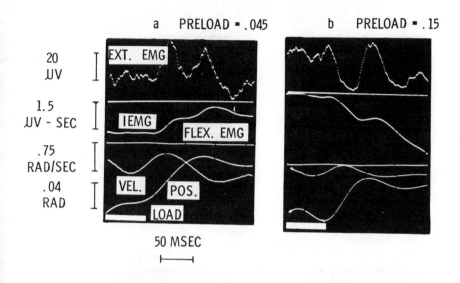

20
JV

1.5
JV - SEC

.75
RAD/SEC

.04
RAD

a   PRELOAD ▪ .045   b   PRELOAD ▪ .15

EXT. EMG

IEMG

FLEX. EMG

VEL.   POS.

LOAD

50 MSEC

Fig. 4. Effect of size of opposing load (preload + load pulse) on the loading reflex during an extensor movement. Baseline for ext. EMG-time integral (IEMG) was set at start of load pulse (relaxed position) to show effectiveness of loading reflex, i. e. change in integral; markers show duration of load pulse; "vel" is angular velocity.

rate of loading by the load pulse, was varied. The relationship between the rate of muscle stretch (ankle rotation) and the size of the initial stretch reflex evoked during movement was derived in a typical subject as described earlier. This is summarized in Fig. 3 for comparison (broken line).

A selective nerve block greatly affected the postural response (Fig. 5, top). Notice the complete absence of any reflex effect postblock except, in this case, a very gradual increase in EMG with increasing stretch. EMG patterns of the loading reflex during movement were much less affected; the amount of stretch induced by the load pulse increased somewhat postblock. The subject also executed the movement less forcefully and fatigued more quickly.

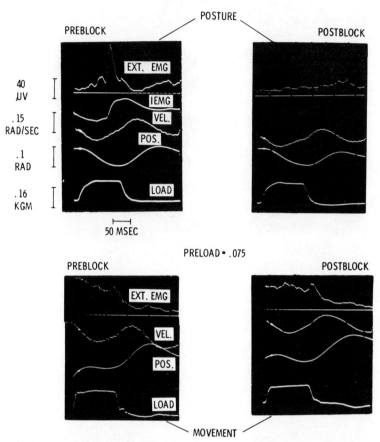

Fig. 5. Comparison of changes in loading reflex for both
types of voluntary extensor contraction and pre- and post-
block condition; tibial nerve was selectively blocked with
8 cc of .5% Xylocaine and the loading reflex was tested in
the absence of fusimotor innervation.

Because of the observed limited load compensation effects
of the spinal stretch reflex during forceful movement, it was of
interest to compare this reflex response to an electrically evoked
monosynaptic reflex superimposed on both types of voluntary
muscle contraction. An afferent volley, strong enough to elicit
a near maximal H-reflex in the triceps surae, was compared for
both experimental conditions. While the normal H-reflex recovery
curve (Fig. 1B) is observed during postural activity, recovery is
faster during voluntary movement and the effects of the synchronous
input on the movement trajectory are negligible when the move-

ment is executed more forcefully.

DISCUSSION

These experiments attempt to establish whether there are significant differences in the load compensation response of the reflex apparatus during two types of voluntary motor acts.

With respect to the initial phasic response, it was found that dynamic sensitivity is reduced during extension movements of the foot executed at a natural speed (Fig. 3). It was also shown that many parameters (e.g. speed of movement, load, muscle length, subject's intention) affect the precise temporal-spatial pattern of the loading reflex, and therefore emphasis should not be placed on the magnitude of the relative differences in dynamic sensitivity (i.e. the slopes of the curves) with one exception: the size of the initial phasic reflex component is always smaller during movement than during posture, for a comparable amount of stretch. Since the latency of the reflex was hardly affected, changes in fusimotor bias affecting the sensitivity of primary endings may well be responsible. Static fusimotor effects are necessary to compensate for muscle shortening and to prevent spindle unloading during voluntary movement (Koeze et al., 1968; Lennerstrand and Thoden, 1968). That spindle stretch is maintained during (relatively slow) voluntary muscle shortening has been substantiated by direct recordings of afferent fiber discharges from human peripheral nerve (Vallbo, 1970) and from similar observations during muscle contraction in other experimental situations (Matthews, 1972, Ch. 10).

Calculation of the rate of stretch resulting from the sudden increase in load was based on the amount of ankle joint rotation and this may be a source of several inaccuracies: (1) Although the load pulse was applied to the muscle at the same external muscle length under both experimental conditions inaccuracies in muscle length measurement may be introduced by differences in the contractile state, and (2) the rheologic properties of muscle, specifically its extensibility, are also dependent on the contractile state and the mechanical transduction of the load pulse into effective muscle (and spindle) stretch may therefore not always be the same (see for instance Nichols and Houk, 1973). The fact that the initial phasic stretch response often shows a double peak may be due to the muscle's mechanical response to stretch.

However, alternative hypotheses involving reflex effects, for example from inhibitory afferents such as Golgi tendon organs, cannot be ruled out without further experiments. No inhibitory phase was present when a stretch reflex was absent in the post-block condition (Fig. 5).

The presence of a significant inhibitory effect independent from the occurrence of a phasic stretch response in the jaw jerk from Fig. 1C was surprising since then no contraction induced spindle unloading can occur. This inhibition may be due to an overlap of excitatory and inhibitory effects in view of the short central latency, to the tightness of this muscle as well as to inputs from cutaneous afferents.

Interaction within the myotatic unit dominates the later phases of the loading responses in Fig. 1 and 2. The initial phasic response leads to muscle shortening, spindle unloading and increased recurrent inhibition due to motor unit synchronization. The amount of muscle shortening depends on the contractile state of the myotatic unit, preload and muscle length. It was shown that if the muscle is prestretched, short load pulses cause a synchronized reflex discharge which induces a recovery curve that is nearly identical to that following an H-reflex (Figs. 1A vs B). Both the peak latency of the late excitatory phase (3) in Fig. 1A and the rate of decay of reflex oscillation are affected by mechanical factors, i.e. spindle stretch in the extrafusal relaxation cycle and by the contractile properties of muscle (Monster, 1973b). The response was changed by the amount of preload and the isotonic measuring condition clearly shows the close correlation with ankle rotation (Fig. 2).

The short latency of the late excitatory phase in the masseter muscle is of interest for two reasons: (1) because it is likely to reflect the faster firing rates, higher contractile speed and shorter period of after-hyperpolarization (Kernell, 1965) associated with muscles of which the cortical representation is more extensive (Tokizane and Shimazu, 1964), and (2) because the shorter duration of the inhibitory period may be related to its functional necessity to participate in short latency transcortical effects (Marsden et al., 1973). The origin of the relatively large late excitatory phase in Fig. 1C can, at least partially, be attributed to increased motor unit synchronization following widespread motoneurone pool depression.

Reflex patterns were qualitatively similar during posture and voluntary movement but quantitative differences were substantial. A stretch reflex is evoked even if the movement continues to progress in the intended direction (Fig. 4A) and this represents a reflex response induced by misalignment between planned and actual movement trajectory. The inhibitory period separating the two excitatory phases was attained more gradually and was of shorter duration during movement. This may be the result of a strong continuing excitatory supraspinal drive on the motoneuronal pool. Inhibition may occur in the absence of a phasic stretch reflex, especially if the load pulse is applied gradually. Comparison of the responses to increasing loads (going in Fig. 4 from A to B) indicates that the threshold of the inhibitory effect is higher than that of the (excitatory) spindle stretch reflex. Autogenetic inhibitory effects may be exhibited during movement (Sears, 1973). Inhibitory responses dominate most in the presence of an already substantial preload or an unexpectedly large load pulse. In other words, servo action during movement is observed only within the pre- scribed loading limits and may include an essential predictive element (sensori-motor expectation).

The spinal loading reflex during voluntary movement (Figs. 4 and 5) may not be as significant as has often been assumed. The muscular component provides most of the resis- tance to stretch during loading especially when loads are changing quickly. The increased muscle stretch in the post-block loading response during movement (Fig. 5, bottom) is at least partially due to a less forceful initiation of the movement and not so much to the absence of an active spinal reflex. Utilization of afferent information and proper adjustment of effort to demand may be first of all at supraspinal levels. A high degree of spatial specificity in ascending stretch receptor afferent information (Rosén and Sjölund, 1972) may become relevant for a proper adjustment of effort to demand during voluntary muscle contraction (Granit, 1972), for precise calibration of movement (Monster, 1973c), for the execution of movements more complex than the flexion-extension patterns studied here and for learning new motor skills. It has been proposed on the basis of single unit pyramidal tract recordings that a relatively simple representation of the final motor output descends (Evarts, 1968). There is also some evidence from electrospinogram recordings in humans (Monster, 1973a) that a short latency descending discharge is evoked by a

strong Ia volley (latency of loop ~35 msec to lower thoracic cord).
The concept of a reflex may, however, be too simple and there
was no strong reason to assume that long loop reflexes played a
significant role in the electromyographic responses observed here.
More suitable tests can be developed if the functional role of such
a sensori-motor mechanism(s) becomes better defined.

Acknowledgement: Supported by the Social and Rehabilitation Services
Research and Training Centre, No. 8 Temple University. The author
wishes to thank Virginia Tierney and Janice Augenbach for their
assistance and interest. The Norwich Pharmacal Co. (Eaton Labor-
atoires) also provided financial support.

REFERENCES

Alnaes, E., 1967. Static and dynamic properties of Golgi tendon
    organs in the anterior tibial and soleus muscle of the cat. Acta
    Physiol. Scand. 70, 176–187.
Eccles, J.C., Eccles, R., and Lundberg, A., 1957. Synaptic action
    on motoneurons caused by impulses in Golgi tendon organ afferents.
    J. Physiol. 138, 227–252.
Evarts, E.V., 1968. Relation of pyramidal tract activity to force
    exerted during voluntary movement. J. Neurophysiol. 31, 14–27.
Evarts, E.V., Bizzi, E., Burke, R.E., Delong, M., and Thach, W.T.,
    1970. Central Control of Movement. Neurosci. Res. Prog. Bull.,
    Vol. 9, No. 1.
Granit, R., 1955. Receptors and Sensory Perception. Yale Univ.
    Press, New Haven, 369 pp.
Granit, R., 1968. The functional role of the muscle spindle's
    primary end organs. Proc. Roy. Soc. Med. 61, 69–78.
Granit, R., 1972. Constant errors in the execution and appreciation
    of movement. Brain 95, 649–660.
Hammond, P.H., Merton, P.A., and Sutton, G.G., 1956. Nervous grad-
    ation of muscular contraction. Brit. Med. Bull. 12, 214–218.
Henneman, E., Somjen, G., and Carpenter, D.O., 1965. Functional
    significance of cell size in spinal motoneurons. J. Neurophysiol.
    28, 560–580.
Hongo, T., Jankowska, E., and Lundberg, A., 1969. The rubrospinal
    tract II. Facilitation of interneuronal transmission in reflex
    paths to motoneurons. Brain Res. 7, 365–391.
Houk, J.C., Singer, J.J., and Goldman, M.R., 1970. An evaluation of
    length and force feedback to soleus muscles of decerebrate cats.
    J. Neurophysiol. 33, 784–811.
Houk, J.C., and Henneman, E., 1967. Responses of Golgi tendon organs
    to active contractions of the soleus muscle of the cat. J. Neuro-
    physiol. 30, 466–481.

Hultborn, H., Jankowska, E., and Lindström, S., 1968. Recurrent inhibition from motor axon collaterals in interneurones monosynaptically activated from Ia afferents. Brain Res. 9, 367–369.

Hunt, C.C., and Kuffler, S.W., 1951. Stretch receptor discharges during muscle contraction. J. Physiol. 113, 298–315.

Jansen, J.K.S., and Rudjord, T., 1964. On the silent period and Golgi tendon organs of the soleus muscle of the cat. Acta Physiol. Scand. 62, 364–379.

Kernell, D., 1965. The limits of firing frequency in cat lumbosacral motoneurons possessing different time course of afterhyperpolarization. Acta Physiol. Scand. 65, 87–100.

Koeze, T.H., Phillips, C.G., and Sheridan, J.D., 1968. Thresholds of cortical activation of muscle spindles and α motoneurons of the baboon's hand. J. Physiol. 195, 419–449.

Lennerstrand, G., and Thoden, Y., 1968. Muscle spindle responses to concomitant variations in length and in fusimotor activation. Acta Physiol. Scand. 74, 153–165.

Lundberg, A., 1970. The excitatory control of the Ia inhibitory pathway. In Excitatory Synaptic Mechanisms, Proc. 5th Int. Meeting Neurobiol., pp. 333–340.

Marsden, C.D., Merton, P.A., and Morton, H.B., 1973. Is the human stretch reflex cortical rather than spinal? The Lancet 759–761.

Matthews, P.B.C., and Rushworth, G., 1957a. The selective effect of procaine on the stretch reflex and tendon jerk of soleus muscle when applied to its nerve. J. Physiol. 135, 245–262.

Matthews, P.B.C. and Rushworth, G., 1957b. The relative sensitivity of muscle nerve fibres to procaine. J. Physiol. 135, 263–269.

Matthews, P.B.C. and Stein, R.B., 1969. The sensitivity of muscle spindle afferents to small sinusoidal changes in length. J. Physiol. 200, 723–743.

Matthews, P.B.C., 1972. Mammalian Muscle Receptors and Their Central Actions. Williams and Wilkins Co., Baltimore.

Merton, P.A., 1953. Speculations on the servo-control of movement. In The Spinal Cord (Ed. Worstenholme, G.E.W.) Churchill, Lond. pp. 247–255.

Monster, A.W., 1973a. Reflex responses in the human electrospinogram. Submitted for publication.

Monster, A.W., 1973b. Control of muscle contraction and the stability of myotatic reflexes. Proc. Int. Symp. on Dynamics and Control in Physiol. Systems. Rochester, N.Y.

Monster, A.W., 1973c. Effect of the peripheral and central sensory component in the calibration of position. In New Developments in Electromyography and Clinical Neurophysiology (Ed. Desmedt, J.E.) Karger, Basel, pp. 383–403.

Nichols, T.R., and Houk, J.C., 1973. Reflex compensation for variations in the mechanical properties of muscle. Science 181, 182–184.

Oscarsson, O., 1970. Functional organization of spinocerebellar paths. In Handbook of Sensory Physiology, Vol. II. (Ed. Iggo, A.) Springer, Berlin, pp. 121–127.

Phillips, C.G., 1969. Motor apparatus of the baboon's hand. Proc. Roy. Soc. Biol. 173, 141–174.

Rosén, I., and Sjölund, B., 1973. Organization of group I activated cells in the main and external cuneate nuclei of the cat: convergence patterns demonstrated by natural stimulation. Exp. Brain Res. 16, 238–246.

Sears, T.A., 1973. Servo control of the intercostal muscles. In New Development in Electromyography and Clinical Neurophysiology (Ed. Desmedt, J.E.) Karger, Basel, pp. 404–417.

Tokizane, T., and Shimazu, H., 1964. Functional Differentiation of Human Skeletal Muscle. Univ. Tokyo Press, Tokyo.

Vallbo, Å.B., 1970. Discharge patterns in human muscle spindle afferents during isometric contractions. Acta Physiol. Scand. 80, 552–566.

CONTROL OF POSTURAL REACTIONS IN MAN: THE INITIATION OF GAIT

R. Herman, T. Cook, B. Cozzens and W. Freedman

Department of Rehabilitation Medicine, Temple
University Health Sciences Centre, Philadelphia, Pa.
and Krusen Center for Research and Engineering,
Moss Rehabilitation Hospital, Philadelphia, Pa.

This study seeks to establish how locomotion is initiated and to
characterize the role of central and/or peripheral mechanisms
in the control of this behaviour. Initiation of gait is defined as
a series of postural reactions in both the swing and stance
limbs. Postural reactions of both lower limbs were assessed
after an auditory signal (AS) on a "walkway" (by recording myoelectric potentials from the TA, MG, S, RF, VM, MH, BiF,
G. Med., G. Max. muscles (the abbreviations are defined in
the Methods); joint position of ankle, knee and hip; amplitude
and position of vertical forces; and moments (torque) about the
ankle joints) through one complete stride of the swing leg and
through toe-off of the stance leg. The influence of muscle and
joint afferents was evaluated by differential suppression of the
tibial nerve with dilute solutions of Xylocaine, by inhibiting
the excitation-coupling reaction of muscle with a peroral administration of dantrolene sodium, and by restraining joint
motion with a below-knee orthosis. In both limbs, the gait
was initiated, before angular displacement, by a sudden
reduction in EMG activity of the MG and S muscles (e.g. 150
msec after AS) followed shortly by an intense discharge in the
TA muscle and to a lesser degree in the RF and G. Med. muscles. Sensory disturbances did not alter the reaction time from
the AS to the initial change in EMG activity. Pronounced TA
discharge led to dorsiflexion of the ankle joint and to a reduced
plantar-flexing moment about the ankle joint. During the yield
stage of the I phase (the phases of gait are defined in the Results),

363

separation of the line of vertical force from the line of the
centre of gravity in association with the discharge in the MG
and S muscles and the behaviour of the contractile and rheologic properties of muscle induced an increase in plantar-
flexing torque. During the I phase of both limbs and the subsequent E_2 and E_3 phases of the swing limb, fixed spatiotemporal ordering of both extensor and flexor activity was
observed. Among all subjects, alternate, reciprocal patterns
of EMG activity between agonists and antagonists were associated with routinized sequential responses of the ankle, knee,
and hip joints and with uniform ankle torque-ankle position
relationships. This stable response was virtually unchanged
by modifying sensory input. Partial narcotization of the tibial
nerve did not influence the periodicity or the magnitude of the
extensor MG and S muscles during the stance and pre-stance
(E_1) phases; the TA discharge, however, decreased reciprocally. The role of the inherent contractile properties of muscle during yield of the extensors was evident following dantrolene administration. To compensate for changes in muscle
stiffness, EMG activity increased five- to ten-fold. Neural
control of initiation of the stepping cycle appears to be pre-
programmed at the supraspinal (command) level. Inhibition
and excitation of postural muscles are most likely due to the
direct action of descending pathways on alpha motoneurones.
Command signals subsequently may "switch on" a stereotyped
repertoire of events, the function of a central program.
Alterations in reafferent information (result of performance)
lead to readjustment in the intensity of motor discharges, but
not to modification of the basic pattern of locomotion. A central program thus requires, at least to a certain degree,
supraspinal and peripheral modulating inputs to sustain fine
tuning of the step cycle.

INTRODUCTION

What central-peripheral arrangements emerge during evolution
of the step cycle? In both primates and man, it is unclear whether,
in the presence of stereotyped motor behaviour (e.g. quiet stance,
locomotion), sensory feedback of peripheral events is necessary
for optimal control of motor behaviour. Following bilateral deafferentation, according to Taub et al. (1965) and Taub and Berman
(1968), primates with no somatic sensation, vision or pre-operative
training can develop strength, co-ordination and reciprocation in

conditioned hand and locomotor activity. Compared to animals with intact somatic sensation, however, these primates require more time to learn a skilled task and demonstrate awkwardness in motor output form and pattern (Konorski, 1967). Taub feels that centrally induced motor outflow signals alone are capable of generating precise movements by means of either "central efferent monitoring" (an internal sensory representation of an intended movement) or a central engrammatic repertoire. Similarly, in man, there is evidence of a neural program controlling synergistic behaviour of muscles involved in co-ordinated shoulder-hand function (Finley, 1969).

Similarly, a number of Swedish (e.g. Jankowska et al., 1967a, b; Lundberg, 1969; Grillner, 1972b) and Russian (e.g. Shik et al., 1966; Orlovskii and Fel'dman, 1972) investigators have stressed that the basic features of the cat gait cycle are derived from an intraspinal (i.e. lumbosacral) program (see Grillner, this volume). It is difficult, however, to adhere exclusively to this central theory of motor control without considering certain significant functional limitations observed with such behavioural models (Evarts et al., 1971; Herman, 1973).

How is locomotion initiated? Considerable data exist concerning the synergistic and temporal behaviour of muscles and muscle mechanics during human locomotion (Eberhart et al., 1969; Morrison, 1970). In man, however, little information is available regarding the process of initiation of the gait cycle. In the mesencephalic preparation of the cat, the condition for onset of the stepping cycle is stimulation of the mid-brain (Grillner and Shik, 1973). The spinal "synergism of the stepping limb" is activated when the segmental reflex apparatus is brought to a state assuring, in the presence of existing alternation, step movements of the limb (Shik et al., 1966). The spinal program may be triggered by peripheral events such as hip movement (Grillner, 1972b; Grillner and Shik, 1973), but the role ascribed to hip afferents may be due to the action of treadmill induced motion and does not appear to be relevant to the initiation of the stepping cycle in man. In man, the stimulation of the gait cycle is apparently a function of the direct action of fast descending pathways influencing both extensor and flexor motor activity (see below). Reafferent information (e.g. information of magnitude and rate of loading of a limb), however, during the subsequent phase of initiation, appears to be an essential factor in attaining and sustaining optimal co-ordinated function (see Discussion and Herman, 1973).

METHODS

This investigation was designed to establish how human locomotion is initiated and to characterize the role of central and/or
peripheral mechanisms in the control of this behaviour. For the
purposes of this study, the initiation of gait on the swing or step-
off side is characterized by a series of events from the time when
a quietly standing subject responds to an auditory signal (AS)
through one complete step of the swing limb, until toe-off of the
stance limb (see Results for explanation). Beginning 1 second
prior to the AS the following parameters were monitored: (1)
floor reaction forces; (2) joint displacement of the hips, knees
and ankles; (3) myoelectrical activity of the tibialis anterior (TA),
medial gastrocnemius (MG), soleus (S), rectus femoris (RF),
vastus medialis (VM), medial hamstrings (MH), biceps femoris
(BiF), gluteus medius (G. Med.) and gluteus maximus (G. Max.)
muscles; (4) the position of the ankle joint in space; and (5)
torque about the ankle joint (see Fig. 1).

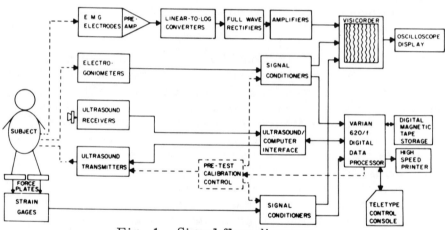

Fig. 1.   Signal flow diagram.

Floor Reaction Forces

The process of initiation of the stepping cycle was assessed on
a locomotion laboratory "walkway" which contained two 152.4 cm
x 30.8 cm strain-gauge force plates capable of measuring the vertical force as well as longitudinal and lateral shear forces under
each foot. Each plate was instrumented with 6 strain gauge bridges
whose outputs were fed into a Varian 620f computer which sampled

the data at a rate of 50 samples/sec. The computer analysis provided the location and magnitude of the vertical force under each foot and the magnitude of the longitudinal and lateral shear forces under each foot.

Joint Displacement

Angular displacements of the limb segments with respect to one another were monitored by the use of hip, knee, and ankle electrogoniometers (elgons) bilaterally. The elgon output was linear to within 0.5%. The knee elgon incorporated a "floating centre" which permitted the potentiometer to follow the polycentric motion of the knee joint. The signals from the elgons were recorded on an ultraviolet oscillograph (Honeywell 1612 Visicorder) concurrent with the electromyograms (see below) and were also recorded on magnetic tape for computer analysis.

Myoelectrical Activity

Myoelectrical activity was detected with surface electrode assemblies consisting of a high input impedance circuit mounted directly over silver/silver chloride discs which contacted the skin through a confined volume of electrode paste. A microminiature integrated circuit amplifier in the electrode assembly raised the signal level 100 times. The shielded cable from the preamplifier was coupled to a junction box mounted on an overhead, variable speed trolley. The EMG signal was processed before being recorded on the ultraviolet oscillograph. The logarithmic scale made it possible to detect and display signal changes within a dynamic range of from less than 3 μV to 4 mV.

Ankle Position

The force plate area of the walkway was within the field of a system of 6 ultrasound receivers, 3 on each side of the walkway. A small circular (2 cm dia) ultrasound transmitter (with an output signal of 100 pulses/sec of 40 kHz ultrasound), was fastened with double-sided adhesive over the lateral malleolus of each ankle. Given the fixed position of each receiver, a triangulation procedure was used to locate the spatial co-ordinates of the transmitter and, after adjusting for the distance from the transmitter to the centre

of the joint, the co-ordinates of the ankle joint axis were determined. The wave length of the 40 kHz ultrasound permitted calculation of the distance from the transmitter to each receiver to
an accurary of 0.4 cm. The values were calculated by the computer
which determined ankle position every 20 msec.

Ankle Torque

Torque about the ankle axis (in the sagittal plane) was calculated
by the formula:

$$F_V (X_F - X_A) + F_{LS} (Y_A) = \text{Torque},$$

where F_V is the vertical force, X_F is the distance from a reference
plane to the line of action of the vertical force, X_A is the distance
from the reference plane to the ankle axis, F_{LS} is the longitudinal
shear force, and Y_A is the vertical distance from the floor to the
ankle axis. Note that this formula assumes that the ankle axis is
perpendicular to the direction of walking.

General Procedure

The population consisted of 17 subjects, aged 18 to 28; 10 males
and 7 females. The subjects had no history or evidence of neuro-
motor dysfunction.

To determine the normal parameters of gait initiation, joint
displacement and force data were collected on all 17 subjects;
myoelectrical and ankle position data were collected on 12 of the
subjects. Additionally, 5 of the subjects were evaluated: (a)
following differential suppression of the tibial nerve with dilute
solutions of Xylocaine; (b) following peroral administration of
dantrolene sodium; and (c) while wearing a polypropylene ankle-
foot orthosis with an anterior shell designed to severely restrain
ankle motion.

Specific Procedure

Each subject wore his own, conventional-heeled shoes for the
procedure. Following instrumentation with electrodes, elgons
and ultrasound transmitters and the necessary calibration proced-

ures, the subject was asked to assume a comfortable standing position on the walkway force plates. Once the subject was satisfied that the stance was natural and "normal" for him, the outlines of both feet were traced on the paper which had previously been taped over the force plate area. During each trial the subject's feet were replaced on the tracings, thus assuring the reliability of the starting position. The subject was merely instructed to "begin walking" when he heard the electronic tone. He was not instructed regarding on which limb to step off, and, if he inquired he was told to step off on whichever limb felt most natural. The time from assumption of the quiet standing position to the AS was randomly varied so that there was no means of anticipating the signal.

Under each condition (control, dantrolene, nerve block and brace) data were collected, beginning 1 sec prior to the AS through the subsequent gait phases, for a minimum of 8 trials. During each of the trials, data (EMG, joint displacement, auditory signal, vertical forces) were continuously recorded using the ultraviolet recorder; during 4 of these trials, data (joint displacement, auditory signal, vertical and shear force magnitudes and locations, ankle positions, ankle torques) were collected using the computer.

RESULTS

A gait classification scheme similar to that described by Phillipson during his investigation of dog locomotion and used by several investigators (Engberg and Lundberg, 1969; Grillner, 1972a; Goslow and Stuart, 1973; Goslow et al., 1973) for descriptive analysis of locomotion in cats is utilized in this study to compare animal with human locomotor behaviour and to maintain consistency in reporting of data.

The initiation of the gait cycle is divided into five phases in the swing or "take-off" limb (Fig. 2): the I_{sw} phase from an auditory (or "go") signal to toe-off, a flexor (F) phase from toe-off to maximum knee flexion, the first extension phase (E_1) from maximum knee flexion to heel strike, the second extension phase (E_2) from heel strike to heel-off and the third extension phase (E_3) from heel-off to toe-off. The stance or support limb (during the I, F, E_1 and the beginning of E_2 phase of the swing limb) is designated as being in the I_{st} phase. The duration of the I_{st} phase is from the auditory signal to toe-off.

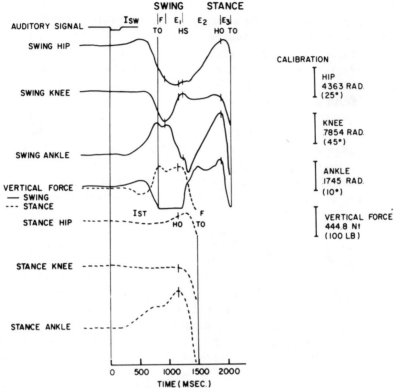

Fig. 2. Gait classification scheme based upon vertical force and angular displacements of the swing and stance limbs. Note the force increase on the swing limb and decrease on the stance limb during the I phase (downward deflection of hip and knee motion recording and upward deflection of ankle motion recording indicates a <u>flexor</u> direction). See text for description. (TO: toe-off; HS: heel strike; HO: heel-off; I_{sw}, F, E_1, E_2, E_3 and I_{st} are defined in text - see Results).

Joint Displacement

In all subjects, angular motion is sequentially determined, i.e. there is a definite ordering of angular displacement, with ankle leading knee and knee leading hip movement (cf in the cat, where hip motion lags behind both ankle and knee motion, which are in phase) (Engberg and Lundberg, 1969; Lundberg, 1969) (Fig. 3). In both I_{sw} and I_{st} peak ankle dorsiflexion (at heel-off) is reached

CONTROL

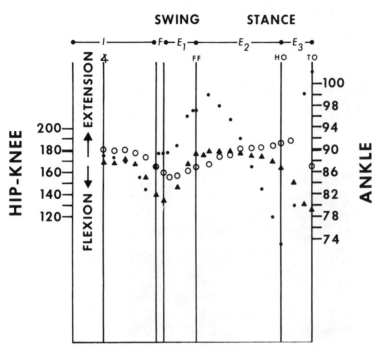

Fig. 3. Angular motion (in degrees) of the ankle (·), knee (▲), and hip (o) joints of the swing limb. All movements are calibrated from a standard anatomical position: hip and knee at 180° and ankle at 90°. See text for description. (ᶯ - initiation of ankle motion; FF - foot flat).

just prior to or concurrently with toe-off of that limb while peak flexion of the knee and hip occur at the end of the F phase and in the middle of the E_1 phase respectively. During the E_2 phase, i.e. following rapid plantar flexion to the foot flat position, the ankle dorsiflexes as the tibia rotates over the talus. During the foot flat stage of E_2, the knee flexes slightly; as the ankle dorsiflexes, the knee is maintained rigidly for 2/3 of this period and, then, commences flexion. Maximum dorsiflexion is observed at the end of the E_2 phase while knee flexion continues throughout E_3. The hip is fully extended in the mid-E_3 phase at which time hip flexion begins.

The pattern (as described above) is observed in all normal subjects. Further, the sequential pattern of joint motion is not dis-

turbed by differential block of the tibial nerve, by suppression of
excitation coupling with dantrolene administration, or by constraint of ankle joint motion with an ankle-foot orthosis.

EMG Recordings

During quiet stance, there is usually considerable EMG activity
in both the extensor soleus and medial gastrocnemius muscles
while the flexor tibialis anterior muscle shows relatively little
activity (Fig. 4-6).

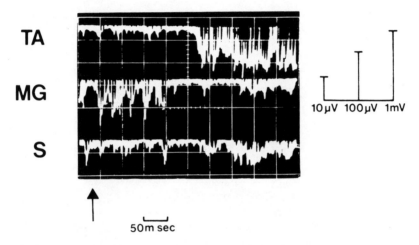

Fig. 4. EMG recordings from tibialis anterior (TA), medial
gastrocnemius (MG), and soleus (S) muscles of the swing limb
using a logarithmic amplification system. Note (1) the depression of EMG activity of the MG and S muscles, approximately
150 msec following an auditory signal (↑), (2) the increased
EMG activity of the TA muscle 50 msec later, and (3) the
reciprocal arrangement between the MG-S and the TA muscles
during quiet stance, i.e. prior to alterations in EMG activity
as described in (1) and (2) above.

I_{SW} Phase

During the I_{SW} phase, the sudden <u>decrease</u> in EMG activity in the
soleus and medial gastrocnemius muscles occurs following the
auditory signal (Fig. 4). The reaction time from the auditory signal to suppression of EMG activity ranges from 130-210 msec with

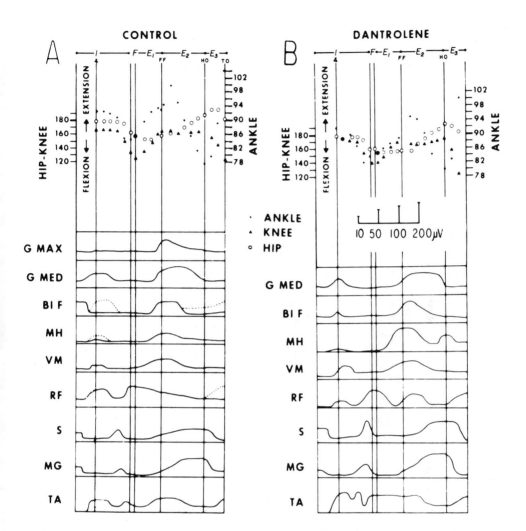

Fig. 5. (A) Envelope of log amplified EMG activity of the gluteus maximum (G. Max.), gluteus medius (G. Med.), biceps femoris (BiF), medial hamstring (MH), vastus medialis (VM), rectus femoris (RF), soleus (S), medial gastrocnemius (MG), and tibialis anterior (TA) muscles of the swing limb during the initial step cycle (i. e. I through E_3 phase) with angular motion of the hip, knee, and ankle joints (upper graph). Dotted lines indicate commonly observed variations. Note the temporal sequencing of the S, MG, and TA muscles (see also Fig. 6). Further discussion in text. (B) Similar recordings following Dantrolene administration.

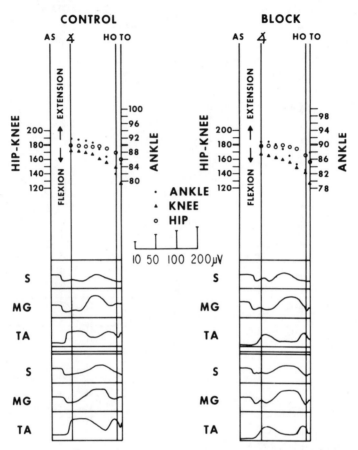

Fig. 6. Envelope of log amplified EMG (Control) activity of the S, MG, and TA muscles prior to and following a differential block of the tibial nerve with 0.5% Xylocaine solution (Block) during the I_{SW} phase (from the auditory signal (AS) to toe-off). Two sets of control and block data are demonstrated. Joint motion is relatively unchanged following the block. See text for description.

a mean of 150 msec. This alteration in motor discharges is followed (within 20-60 msec) by a rapidly rising and intense EMG discharge in the tibialis anterior (Figs. 4-6) and by a more slowly rising discharge in both the rectus femoris and gluteus medius muscles. Infrequently, the medial gastrocnemius, soleus, vastus medialis, and biceps femoris muscles will fire concurrently with the tibialis anterior, rectus femoris, and gluteus medius. The yield stage (i. e. extension of the calf musculature during ankle dorsiflexion) of the I_{SW} phase commences 80-140 msec following the initiation of the tibialis anterior burst. During this stage both the soleus and medial gastrocnemius muscles increase their firing levels considerably while the antagonist tibialis anterior demonstrates reciprocal reduction in its discharge level. At the completion of yield (approximately 50-100 msec prior to toe-off) activity in both the medial gastrocnemius and soleus muscles decreases while the activity in the tibialis anterior increases markedly. At the end of the I phase, there is some reduction of tibialis anterior firing, which continues into the F phase. Thus, from quiet stance to toe-off there are four periods in which the agonist gastrocnemius-soleus and antagonist tibialis anterior muscle groups demonstrate an alternating EMG pattern (Figs. 5a, 6).

F Phase

All EMG activity is at a low level, aside from the discharge in the rectus femoris muscle which begins firing just prior to the F phase.

E_1 Phase

Both flexors and extensors of the knee and ankle demonstrate motor discharges during this phase. As in the cat (Engberg and Lundberg, 1969), the gastrocnemius and soleus muscles begin firing near the termination of this period; discharges are, however, more pronounced and appear earlier in the tibialis anterior, most likely to prepare the lower limb for heel strike, to guide the lengthening contraction of the tibialis anterior during rapid plantar flexion to foot flat in the E_2 phase, and to assist tibial rotation on the talus during the early part of the yield portion of the E_2 phase.

E_2 and E_3 Phases

During the first half of the E_2 phase, both the gastrocnemius and soleus muscles demonstrate an increasing level of EMG activity; during the second half, the firing level of the gastrocnemius increases abruptly while the soleus demonstrates more gradual rise, reaching a peak at a time similar to the gastrocnemius

(Fig. 5A). Both muscles are at peak levels at or near the end of the yield (i. e. at maximum dorsiflexion). Increased EMG activity in the gastrocnemius and soleus muscles is accompanied by depression of EMG discharges in the tibialis anterior; during E_3, medial gastrocnemius and soleus activity decreases while the intensity of the tibialis anterior discharge reciprocally increases.

I_{st} Phase

In the stance limb, depression of postural EMG activity in the gastrocnemius and soleus muscles following the auditory signal is also observed. Compared to the swing limb, however, the reaction time from the AS to suppression of the gastrocnemius and soleus muscles and to activation of the tibialis anterior muscles if often of longer duration (e.g. 190 msec). As in the E_3 phase of the swing limb, the yield stage demonstrates a gradual build-up of EMG activity in the soleus and a pronounced discharge in the medial gastrocnemius. Both discharges reach a peak prior to heel off (see EMG insert, Fig. 9'A). This is accompanied by reciprocal inhibition of the tibialis anterior muscle. At heel off there is a rapid decline of activity in the gastrocnemius and soleus muscles with a subsequent rise in EMG activity in the tibialis anterior. Thus, as in the I_{sw} phase, the I_{st} phase demonstrates four periods of alternation (see above).

Biomechanical Measurements

Data derived from recordings of vertical force, location of force under each foot, resolution of the positions of forces between the two lower limbs, the lever arm (i. e. perpendicular distance from the line of action of the vertical force to the ankle axis), and moments or torque about the ankle joint are depicted in Fig. 7. In all subjects, during the I_{sw} phase, the results of biomechanical measurements can be correlated with the four periods of alternation of agonist and antagonist EMG activity; hence, four biomechanical stages are delineated.

(1) Stage of Balance - During quiet stance, dorsiflexing torque resulting from the vertical projection of the centre of mass is encountered by a plantar flexing torque maintained by excitation of the extensor and inhibition of the flexor muscles and by the inherent properties of muscle (see below);

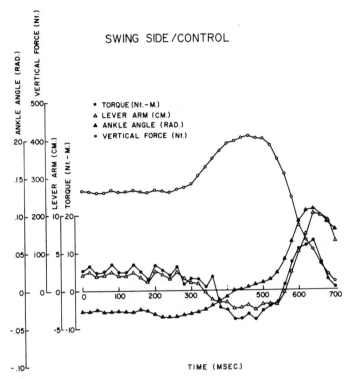

Fig. 7. Data derived from recordings of vertical force, lever arm, ankle angle, and ankle torque in a control subject during the I_{SW} phase. Upward deflection of the ankle angle recordings indicates movement in dorsiflexion (0 Rad. is equivalent to 90° ankle angle); positive torque values designate a plantar flexing movement and negative values a dorsiflexing movement. Lever arm values reveal the distance from the line of action of the vertical force to the ankle axis: positive and negative values are related to the vertical force falling in front of and behind the ankle axis respectively.

(2) Stage of Imbalance - Following EMG activation of the tibialis anterior muscle (Figs. 5a, 6) and suppression of the gastrocnemius and soleus muscles (leading to angular displacement), the counteracting plantar flexing torque is decreased, despite the increase in vertical force on that limb. This alteration is attributed to the EMG discharge in the tibialis anterior and to the shortening of the lever arm (see Methods). As the vertical projection of

the centre of force under the foot moves closer to the ankle axis, an imbalance is developed, creating a tendency to fall forward;

(3) Stage of Reaction - This falling tendency, associated with continuing dorsiflexion, is limited by an increase in plantar flexing torque, a function of the lengthening contraction of the extensor muscles of the calf (Figs. 5a, 6). The force of the lengthening contraction is derived from both the inherent passive and active (e.g. torque-position, torque-velocity) properties of muscle and the frequently observed increase in EMG activity in the gastrocnemius and soleus muscles during the yield stage. The force associated with the EMG response is related to the dynamics of the movement, i.e. force is considerably higher, at any one angular position, during the lengthening contraction than during either an isometric (cf stage 1) or shortening contraction (Joyce et al., 1969; Freedman, 1971; Grillner, 1972a).

(4) Stage of Preswing - At the termination of ankle dorsiflexion and during the brief period of plantar flexion prior to toe-off, plantar flexing torque decreases, due primarily to the rapidly falling vertical force. The EMG discharge in the gastrocnemius and soleus muscles is maximum at peak dorsiflexion and, as a result of the lag in electromechanical coupling of muscle, should effect a development of torque during the subsequent plantar flexion; however, this is not observed due, in part, to the differences in torque derived from lengthening and shortening contractions (see above). EMG activity in the tibialis anterior, occurring late in the I_{sw} phase, will most likely have its effect during both the subsequent F and E_1 phases principally due to the time delays in the development of muscle force (see above).

Similar reasoning can be applied to the I_{st} phase (Fig. 9a); in the stage of imbalance, however, the reduced plantar flexing moment occurs due to both the shortening of the lever arm and a decrease in the vertical force. Further, in the stage of reaction, higher plantar flexing torques are the result of an increase in both the lever arm and the vertical force.

Differential Nerve Block

The tibial nerve was differentially blocked by a perineural infiltration of 0.5% Xylocaine solution (3-5 cc). During recovery, a gamma block was inferred in the presence of (1) normal motor

power (subject could support body weight with plantar flexion of the
foot); (2) suppression of temperature and pain sensation; (3) normal tactile and joint position sense; and (4) absent or markedly
suppressed response to a tap of the Achilles tendon (Smith et al.,
1972).

In the cat, it appears that muscle spindles, during the stance
phase, are cyclically modulated by fusimotor neurones (Severin
et al., 1967). Differential narcotization of the tibial nerve leads
to a marked diminution in EMG discharge in the E_2 phase, but to
no change in the basic temporal pattern of EMG discharges
(Severin, 1970). It is pointed out, nevertheless, that direct
excitatory influences arriving at the alpha motoneurone play an
important role at the end of the E_1 phase (i. e. prior to heel
contact) and during the yield phase of E_2 (Lundberg, 1969; Severin,
1970). In man, application of dilute solutions of Xylocaine to the
tibial nerve does not interfere with the temporal patterns of EMG
discharge to the extensor gastrocnemius and soleus muscles and
to the flexor tibialis anterior muscles, with the magnitude of the
discharges of the extensor muscles, or with the alternating be-
heaviour between the motor groups during the yield stages of I_{sw},
I_{st}, and E_2 (Fig. 6, 8). There is however a frequently observed
decrease in the magnitude of the motor discharge to the tibialis
anterior muscle during stance (i. e. of I_{st}, I_{sw}, and E_2 phases).
As expected, such changes in tibialis anterior activity lead to a
reduction in the magnitude of the dorsiflexing moment about the
ankle joint, thereby creating a relative increase in plantar flexing
moment in each of the four stages during the I_{st} and I_{sw} (see
biomechanical measurements above). This disturbance, however,
does not alter the basic pattern of joint motion (Fig. 6) and of torque
development.

Mechanical Properties of Muscle

The significance of the rheologic and contractile properties of
muscle in the control of posture and locomotion has recently been
emphasized in both animal and man (Joyce et al., 1969; Rack,
1970; Freedman, 1971; Grillner, 1972a; Goslow and Stuart, 1973;
Herman et al., 1973).

Freedman (1971) and Herman et al. (1973) observed in man,
that muscle properties can stabilize the myotatic reflex system
(by adequately compensating for disturbances in position and/or
load of a limb without undue time delays), a function often ascribed

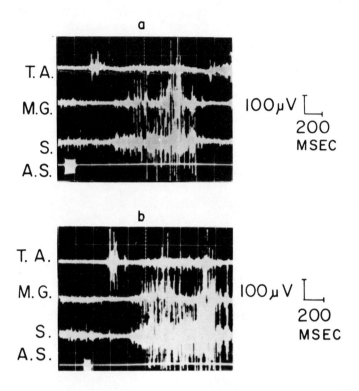

Fig. 8. EMG recordings from the TA, MG and S muscles
using a linear amplification system prior to (a) and following
(b) a differential block of the tibial nerve with 0.5% Xylocaine
solution during the I_{st} phase. Following the block, the EMG
of the extensor muscles of the calf either is unchanged or
shows enhanced activity. Note that the block does not alter
the reaction time from the auditory signal (AS) to depression
of the MG and S signals and to excitation of the TA signal.

only to the primary endings of the muscle spindle.

It is suggested that the changes in stiffness (i.e. torque developed per unit of angular displacement) during the yield stage of
I_{st}, I_{sw} and E_2 may be attributed not only to an increase in the
motor discharge pattern to the gastrocnemius and soleus muscles,

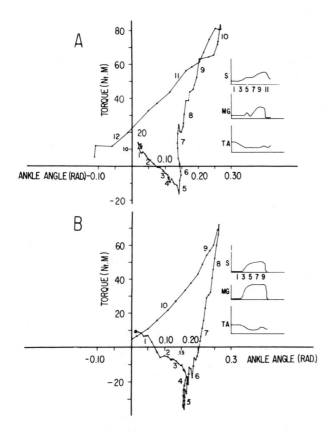

Fig. 9. Ankle torque-angular position curves during the I
phase prior to (a) and following (b) administration of Dantrolene Sodium. Each number (e.g. 1-12 in a) represents a
time course of 100 msec or an accumulation of five points
along the curve. (a) 1-4 demonstrated a decreasing plantar
flexing torque during the initial stage of dorsiflexion (positive
values in radians); this is the Stage of Imbalance. Numbers
5-10 indicate a change in direction of torque development,
i.e. an increasing plantar flexing torque, during further
dorsiflexion of the ankle; this is the Stage of Reaction. At
the termination of dorsiflexion, the heel rises from the floor;
plantar flexing torque decreases during the brief period of
ankle plantar flexion; this is the Stage of Preswing. The EMG
related to these changes is shown to the right of the curve.
(b) The torque-position curve following Dantrolene treatment
is virtually unchanged; note, however, the degree of dorsi-

Fig. 9, continued: flexing torque (1-4) as angular displacement
(dorsiflexion) commences during the Stage of Imbalance and a
delay in counteracting this tendency (4-6) during the Stage of
Reaction. A pronounced increase in EMG activity is required
to stabilize motor performance.

but also to the inherent mechanical properties of muscle such as
tension-length and force-velocity relationships, and lengthening
of the series-elastic tissue (Herman, 1970a; Herman et al., 1973).

In order to evaluate the role of muscle stiffness in control of
initiation of locomotion, dantrolene sodium (2 mg/kg) was administered perorally to 5 subjects. In man, at this dose level, dantrolene suppresses the excitation-coupling reaction of muscle, as
evidenced by reduction of both the magnitude (e.g. twitch contractions are reduced by 50-70% while tetanus contractions at 20 pps
are reduced by 30-40%) and rate of rise of force when a controlled
stimulus is applied to a chemically denervated muscle or group of
muscles (Herman et al., 1972; Monster et al., 1973; Mayer, 1973).

Each subject was studied on the walkway 2 hours following the
administration of dantrolene sodium. Clinically, the gait pattern
was not altered. The data, however, reveal pronounced changes
in the EMG activity in both flexors and extensors. In general, the
intensity and duration of motor activity are enhanced (usually a
five- to ten-fold increase is observed); the temporal sequencing of
discharges in any one muscle, however, remains unchanged;
likewise, the alternate behaviour between flexor and extensor
discharges is not disturbed. For example, during the stage of
imbalance, interference with the contractile machinery is manifested by a more intense tibialis anterior discharge (Fig. 5b)
which is required to initiate angular displacement. The resulting
dorsiflexing moment cannot be sufficiently counteracted (see Stage
of Reaction) due to the reduced effectiveness of the inherent properties of the extensor muscles. To overcome this tendency, the
extensor muscles react with an intense, rapidly rising discharge
(Figs. 5b, 9b). These results suggest that the contractile state
of muscle is an extremely important feature of the control system
and that changes in the inherent properties can bring about a compensatory "rearrangement" with respect to increased motoneurone
output. Such compensatory behaviour of the nervous system leads
to a stable performance, as judged by the observed torque-time,
torque-position, and angular motion relationships (Figs. 5b, 9).

DISCUSSION

The results of this investigation suggest that both central and peripheral factors are related to the initiation of the stepping cycle: (1) Presumably, the initiation of the stepping cycle is triggered by direct action of descending pathways on both the extensor and flexor motoneurone pools. According to information derived from animal investigations (Orlovskii, 1970, 1972a, b, c; Grillner et al., 1971), the change in postural EMG activity between the gastrocnemius-soleus and tibialis anterior muscles following the auditory signal can be attributed to decreased excitation of the vestibulospinal pathway and an increased excitation of the reticulospinal,rubrospinal, and/or pyramidal tract pathways. The failure of a gamma block to modify the reaction time (e.g. 150 msec to the gastrocnemius-soleus activity and approximately 200 msec to tibialis anterior activity) is further evidence of central excitation of the alpha motoneurones of both extensors and flexors. These findings are also consistent with other investigations in man which showed that (a) a block of vestibular afferents causes a reduction of tonic innervation and hence of stretch reflexes in the extensor muscles, while the presence of the "unloading reflex" (presumably due to fusimotor activity) is unaltered (Struppler et al., 1973); and (b) voluntary contraction is initiated by direct activation of alpha motoneurones rather than by a follow-up servo through participation of the fusimotor system (Vallbo, 1971).

(2) The role of the muscle spindle receptors was evaluated by assessing EMG patterns during each phase and following a differential block of the tibial nerve. The firing pattern of the extensor muscles of the calf prior to heel-strike during the E_1 stage (presumably preparing the limb for floor contact) (Lundberg, 1969; Jones and Watt, 1971), and the unchanged activity in these muscles during stance (including quiet stance) following the block suggests that the patterns of discharge (temporal ordering and alternating character of the discharges), the magnitude of the discharge and the uniform sequence of angular displacement are not influenced substantially by a reduction in the spindle afferent output and presumably, therefore, by a facilitatory reflex motoneurone discharge. Further, the extensor muscles of the calf do not demonstrate an unloading reflex during the period of rapid shortening between heel-strike and foot-flat of E_2. Both the lack of an unloading reflex and a frequently observed reduction in tibialis anterior activity following a fusimotor block, suggest that direct excitation of alpha motor fibres with or without concomitant static

fusimotor activity can be operative functionally. Despite these results, it is difficult to assess the role of spindle afferents when other central and peripheral pathways can readily compensate for disturbance in fusimotor drive. Various afferents, including the muscle spindles, can serve to modulate supraspinal centres (via spino-cerebellar pathways and the cerebellum), eliciting information of the phase of the step and the level of locomotor activity (Orlovskii, 1970; Arshavskii et al., 1972). It is conceivable, then, that suppression of some afferents (as in this study, suppression of muscle spindle discharges following a differential block and perhaps Golgi tendon organ discharges following dantrolene administration) is compensated for by the presence of a dynamic response in many of the undisturbed afferents (skin, joint, etc) and/or by the cerebellum modifying its tonic and phasic influence on descending pathways. Such changes would lead to altered intensity of motoneurone discharges. By varying the intensity of the motoneurone discharge during each phase, a neural program can presumably control the rhythmicity and duration of the stepping cycle.

This does not imply that spindle afferents do not participate in organized movements. Fusimotor activity coactivated with alpha motor activity has been observed during respiration and locomotion in cats (Euler, 1966; Sears, 1966; Perret and Busser, 1972) and during volitional skilled activities in man (Vallbo, 1971). During the stance phase of the cat stepping cycle, muscle spindle afferents which are phasically excited by fusimotor modulation (Severin et al., 1967), can in turn modulate supraspinal systems such as the vestibulospinal and reticulospinal pathways (via cerebellum) and the pyramidal tract pathways (via sensorimotor cortex) (Orlovskii, 1970, 1972b; Evarts, 1973).

(3) Whether the motor discharges to muscles are induced directly or indirectly across the gamma loop, a critical factor in the development of force is the inherent properties of muscle (see Results). When muscle's ability to develop force during lengthening and shortening (e.g. tension-length, force-velocity characteristics) is reduced, the nervous system provides an increase in motoneurone discharge to maintain adequately the rhythm and periodicity of the stepping cycle. Such adjustments are most likely controlled by supraspinal centres which presumably receive information of the magnitude and rate of change of muscle force from sensors such as the Golgi tendon organs and tactile receptors.

(4) In the absence of postural disturbances (e.g. change in character of the terrain, imposed perturbance of the substrate or bodily segment), a sophisticated supraspinal (or intraspinal) program can control certain aspects of the stepping cycle, i.e. reciprocal behaviour between agonist and antagonist (e.g. the four stages of EMG alternation of I_{sw} and I_{st}) and the temporal pattern of motor discharges in any one muscle (Lundberg, 1969; Grillner, 1972b). Somatic afferentation is required, most likely, to modulate suprasegmental structures (e.g. cerebellum, sensori-motor cortex) (a) to sustain a highly tuned co-ordinated loco-motor system (see above), (b) to provide information during skilled maneouvres by distinguishing finer levels of motor outflow discharges, and (c) to elicit, as rapidly as possible, compensatory changes in the presence of postural disturbances (a "safety factor"). In man, the value of such a safety factor is limited by the delays in setup time of muscle receptors, transmission time across the myotatic loop, and electromechanical coupling of muscle. Sudden changes in position and load can be counteracted, however, without significant time delays by the inherent passive and active properties of muscle. These adjustments may be followed by spinal reflex activity providing further stabilizing effects until the supraspinal centres (e.g. somatosensory cortex, cerebellum) can adjust the actual movement to the intended movement (Phillips, 1969; Herman, 1970b; Brooks, 1971; Evarts, 1973).

Acknowledgement: This study was supported, in part, by grants No. 23P-55115 and 16P 56804 from the Social and Rehabilitation Services, Department of Health, Education and Welfare, Washington, D.C., U.S.A. and by a grant from Eaton Laboratories, Norwich, New York.

REFERENCES

Arshavskii, Iu. I., Berkinblit, M.B., Fukson, O.I., Gel'fand, I.M., and Orlovskii, G.N., 1972. Recordings of neurones of the dorsal spinocerebellar tract during evoked locomotion. Brain Res. 43, 272-275.

Brooks, V.B., 1971. Tight input-output coupling. Neurosci. Res. Prog. Bull. 9, 51-59.

Eberhart, H.D., Inman, V.T., and Bresler, B., 1969. The principal elements in human locomotion. In Human Limbs and their Substitutes. Hafner, N.Y. pp. 437-471.

Engberg, I., and Lundberg, A., 1969. An electromyographic analysis of muscular activity in the hindlimb of the cat during unrestrained locomotion. Acta Physiol. Scand. 75, 614-630.

Euler, C. von 1966. Proprioceptive control in respiration. In
Nobel Symposium. I. Muscle Afferents and Motor Control. Almqvist
and Wiksells, Stockholm. pp. 197-208.

Evarts, E.V., 1973. Motor cortex reflexes associated with learned
movement. Science 179, 501-503.

Evarts, E.V., Bizzi, E., Burke, R.E., Delong, M., Thach, W.T. Jr.,
1971. Central control of movement. Neurosci. Res. Progr. Bull.
9, 1-170.

Finley, F.R., 1969. Pattern recognition of myoelectric signals in
the control of an arm prosthesis. J. Can. Phys. Therap. Assoc.
21, 19-24.

Freedman, W., 1971. Systems Analysis of the Myotatic Reflex in
Normal, Hemiplegic and Paraplegic Man. Ph.D. Thesis, Drexel Univ.
Phila.

Goslow, G.E. Jr., Stauffer, E.K., Kemeth, W.C., and Stuart, D.G.,
1973. The cat step cycle: Responses of muscle spindles and tendon
organs to passive stretch within the locomotor range. Brain Res.
In press.

Goslow, G.E. Jr., and Stuart, D.G., 1973. The cat step cycle. I.
Joint angles and muscle lengths during unrestrained locomotion.
J. Morphol. In press.

Grillner, S., 1972a. The role of muscle stiffness in meeting the
changing postural and locomotor requirements for force development by the ankle extensors. Acta Physiol. Scand. 86, 92-108.

Grillner, S., 1972b. On the spinal generation of locomotion. In
Sensory Organization of Movements. Leningrad.

Grillner, S., Hongo, T., and Lund, S., 1971. Convergent effects on
alpha motoneurones from the vestibulospinal tract and a pathway
descending in the medial longitudinal fasciculus. Exp. Brain Res.
12, 457-479.

Grillner, S., and Shik, M.L., 1973. On the descending control of
the lumbosacral spinal cord from the "mesencephalic locomotor
region". Acta Physiol. Scand. 87, 320-333.

Herman, R., 1970a. The myotatic reflex. Brain 93, 273-312.

Herman, R., 1970b. Electromyographic evidence of some control
factors involved in the acquisition of skilled performance. Amer.
J. Phys. Med. 49, 177-191.

Herman, R., 1973. Augmented sensory feedback in the control of limb
movement. In Proceedings of Houston Neurological Symposium. In
press.

Herman, R., Freedman, W., Monster, A.W., and Tamai, Y., 1973. A
systematic analysis of myotatic reflex activity in human spastic
muscle. In New Developments in Electromyography and Clinical
Neurophysiology. S. Karger, Basel. pp. 556-578.

Herman, R., Mayer, N., and Mecomber, S., 1972. Clinical pharmaco-
physiology of dantrolene sodium. Amer. J. Phys. Med. 51, 296-311.

Jankowska, E., Jukes, M.G.M., Lund, S., and Lundberg, A., 1967a.
The effect of DOPA on the spinal cord. 5. Reciprocal organization of pathways transmitting excitatory action to alpha
motoneurones of flexors and extensors. Acta Physiol. Scand.
70, 369-388.

Jankowska, E., Jukes, M.G,M., Lund, S., and Lundberg, A., 1967b.
The effect of DOPA On the spinal cord. 6. Half-centre organization of inter-neurones transmitting effects from the flexor
reflex afferents. Acta Physiol. Scand. 70, 389-402.

Jones, G.M., and Watt, D.G.D., 1971. Observations on the control
of stepping and hopping movements in man. J. Physiol. 219,
709-727.

Joyce, G.C., Rack, P.M.H., and Westbury, D.R., 1969. The mechanical
properties of cat soleus muscle during controlled lengthening
and shortening movements. J. Physiol. 204, 461-474.

Konorski, J., 1967. Integration Activity of the Brain. Univ. of
Chicago Press, Chicago.

Lundberg, A., 1969. Reflex control of stepping. The Nansen
Memorial Lecture. V. Universitetsforlaget, Oslo.

Mayer, N., 1973. A necessary method for determining the force-
velocity relation of human muscle. Submitted as M.S. Thesis
to Drexel Univ. Phila.

Monster, A.W., Tamai, Y., and McHenry, J., 1973. Dantrolene sodium:
its effect on extrafusal muscle fibers. Arch. Phys. Med. In press.

Morrison, J.B.,1970. The mechanics of muscle function in locomotion.
J. Biomechanics 3, 431-451.

Orlovskii, G.N., 1970. Influence of the cerebellum on the reticulospinal neurones during locomotion. Biophysics 15, 928-936.

Orlovskii, G.N., 1972a. The effect of different descending systems
on flexor and extensor activity during locomotion. Brain Res. 40,
359-371.

Orlovskii, G.N., 1972b. Activity of vestibulospinal neurons during
locomotion. Brain Res. 46, 85-98.

Orlovskii, G.N., 1972c. Activity of rubrospinal neurons during
locomotion. Brain Res. 46, 99-112.

Orlovskii. G.N., and Fel'dman, A.G., 1972. Role of afferent activity
in the generation of stepping movements. Neirofiziologiya 4,
401-409.

Perret, C., and Buser, P., 1972. Static and dynamic fusimotor activity during locomotor movements in the cat. Brain Res. 40, 165-169.

Phillips, C.G., 1969. Motor apparatus of the baboon's hand. Proc.
Roy. Soc. B 173, 141-174.

Rack, P.M.H., 1970. The significance of mechanical properties of
muscle in the reflex control of posture. In Excitatory Synaptic
Mechanisms. Universitetsforlaget, Oslo. pp. 317-322.

Sears, T.A., 1966. Pathways of supra-spinal origin regulating the
activity of respiratory motoneurones. In Nobel Symposium I. Muscle
afferents and motor control. Almqvist and Wiksells, Stockholm.
pp. 187-196.

Severin, F.V., 1970. The role of the gamma motor system in the activation of the extensor alpha motor neurones during controlled locomotion. Biophysics 15, 1138-1145.

Severin, F.V., Orlovskii, G.N., and Shik, M.L., 1967. Work of the muscle receptors during controlled locomotion. Biophysics 12, 575-586.

Shik, M.L., Orlovskii, G.N., and Severin, F.V., 1966. Organization of the locomotor synergism. Biophysics 11, 1011-1019.

Smith, J.L., Roberts, E.M., and Atkins, E., 1972. Fusimotor neuron block and voluntary arm movements in man. Amer. J. Phys. Med. 51, 225-239.

Struppler, A., Burg, D., and Erbel, F., 1973. The unloading reflex under normal and pathological conditions in man. In New Developments in EMG and Clinical Neurophysiology. S. Karger, Basel. pp. 603-617.

Taub, E., Bacon, R.C., Berman, A.J., 1965. Acquisition of a trace-conditioned avoidance response after deafferentation of the responding limb. J. Comp. Physiol. Psychol. 59, 275-279.

Taub, E., and Berman, A.J., 1968. Movement and learning in the absence of sensory feedback. In The Neuropsychology of Spatially oriented behavior. The Dorsey Press, Homewood, Ill. pp. 173-192.

Vallbo, A.B., 1971. Muscle spindle response at the onset of isometric voluntary contractions in man. Time difference between fusimotor and skeletomotor effects. J. Physiol. 218, 405-431.

DISCUSSION SUMMARY

J. V. Basmajian

Emory University School of Medicine and Yerkes
Regional Primate Research Center, Atlanta, Georgia

The discussion periods during the morning of the second day were filled with enthusiasm, rapid repartee, humour and cordial partisanship, all of which is difficult to summarize faithfully. Bearing upon the paper by Vallbo, Emilio Bizzi of the Department of Psychology at the Massachusetts Institute of Technology, offered a short report on the lack of evidence for servo-assistance of centrally programmed head movements in monkeys. In an elegant set of experiments done with F. Bertora and J. Dichgans, they tested the effectiveness of sensory feedback in the compensation for differing loads by contracting muscles. They applied inertial loads to the head of normal monkeys during randomly selected trials and compared normal and loaded horizontal movement before and after surgical section of the cervical dorsal roots. Their results indicated that visually-triggered head movements are accomplished without servo-assistance.

Other comments on Vallbo's paper came from Melvill Jones and Houk. Melvill Jones asked about possible studies on the role of spindles in spasticity and was told that these were going on at Uppsala. Houk questioned Vallbo's definition of "primary" and "secondary": Vallbo's definition depends completely on the dynamic responses. Kennedy asked whether subjects were doing peculiar movements, but in reply, he was assured that the movements appeared natural and gave a stable steady-state response.

The paper by Matthews released the most vigorous debate of the session - perhaps of the symposium - with many speakers demanding their say. In addition, Grillner, Nichols and Rymer gave formal short reports as follow-ups.

The contribution of the secondary endings caused considerable disagreement. The question was raised from several sides as to the confidence one might have that the effects of primary endings could be excluded. In reply to a question by Gilman about which elements are paralyzed by procaine at various intervals after application, Matthews replied that gammas are affected rapidly, alphas and Ia's are affected last, and group II's fall between. The early fall in the stretch reflex is a gamma block. Gilman and Grillner both emphasized that the responses are not clearcut.

Wiesendanger asked whether the extra stretch induced tension superimposed on vibration could be accounted for by a long pathway. Matthews replied that the latencies are not known but certainly in the decerebrate cat the cortex is excluded.

R. Stein asked for reactions to Rymer's hypothesis from proponents of various views. Matthews believes that it beautifully extends the work of David Westbury (University of Birmingham, England), whose findings were in general agreement with Rymer's. Granit emphasized that the secondaries may have very different roles to play in different muscles and during different complex postures. Abrahams agreed and drew attention to the concept of the intention to produce a movement; what you are doing at the moment influences how you perform a new movement. Thus, a major influence lies above the spinal cord. In response to questions by Houk as to differences between the conditions of the Nichols and Matthews experiments, Matthews responded that he used similar velocities but larger amplitudes.

Following the paper by Rack, Melvill Jones commented that Rack's reported 50 msec corresponded to the late reflex since the monosynaptic reflex was more in the order of 16 msec. Rack replied that the shorter time did not include the time for muscular contraction. Paul Stein commented that there was a possibility that a cerebral route was involved and that the response was 2 or 3 cycles "back"; Rack felt that this was extremely unlikely. In reply to a series of questions by Houk, Rack agreed that the resonance frequencies of 10 Hz that he had obtained in his work could well be related to clonus.

The paper by Brooks led Padsha to ask whether the 3 Hz

frequency might be a harmonic of the heart beat; however, Brooks believed that it was independent. R. Stein questioned Brooks' concept of an on-going clock. Gottlieb reported records very similar to Brooks' in his experiments with the human ankle. Both velocity and acceleration are highly correlated with the EMGs in the protagonist muscle group. Because of decoupling between the load and the muscle due to series elasticity, oscillation of the loop itself is a likelier explanation. Houk drew attention to earlier work by Lippold (confirmed by him in unpublished work in cat) that cooling the muscle slows down the frequency of oscillation and that this is correlated with the slowing of the twitch contraction.

Following Padsha's short report, questions arose as to technique. He pointed out that subjects were not aware of the effects of respiration. Also, no study has yet been made of varying rates of breathing and the effects of limb immobilization.

F. J. Kottke (University of Minnesota, Minneapolis) gave a short report from the clinical point of view. Clinicians believe that stretch reflex responses initiated by the primary sensory fibres have been well defined. There are other stretch reflexes in muscle of poorly defined origin and distribution. Kottke suggested that these are initiated by stretch of the endings of the secondary sensory fibres of muscle spindles. In response to a question by W. D. Chapple (University of Connecticut, Storrs, Connecticut), Kottke was unable to cite evidence for eliciting of long reflexes in neurological patients by using vibration. Gilman questioned whether secondary afferents are responsible for the various components of the Sherringtonian reflexes mentioned by Kottke. Kottke reiterated that from the clinician's viewpoint extensor thrust cannot be caused by the primaries.

Granit summed up the discussion by re-emphasizing the complexities of human behaviour. He offered the example of the human hand: its activities are very elaborate and one cannot really extrapolate research results from one particular digit to the total functional control of the hand.

DISCUSSION SUMMARY

J. C. Houk

Department of Physiology, Johns Hopkins Medical
School, Baltimore, Maryland

In summarizing the discussion from the afternoon session
on the control of posture, I shall include only those points which
I feel may be of most general interest to the people participating
in the conference. The first discussion concerned Talbott's
paper. Stephens asked Talbott to indicate what he thought the
dog was trying to control when standing on the platform. Talbott
responded by pointing out that the coefficients describing the
body and head in space had very small variances whereas those
describing other variables such as the angle of the knee had
large variances. He therefore presumed that the position of the
body and head in space were being controlled. Melvill Jones
pointed out that the unpredictable modes of behaviour could not
be studied with the sinusoidal inputs they had used; he also asked
whether or not there was some frequency above which the dog
broke down on the platform. Talbott indicated that above 4 Hz
the dog would no longer perform. Talbott also discussed variation
in his results, stressing that during one day's performance the
variance in a given set of coefficients was extremely small. The
chairman then asked whether or not the forces expected if the
dog were a rigid body had been calculated. Talbott said they had
not been, although there were some situations when it was clear
that more than the body weight was being supported. Dr. H.
Hemami from Ohio State University (Columbis, Ohio) indicated
that he had attempted to solve a similar problem and in setting
up the problem came out with ten non-linear differential equations.
Following Nashner's paper, Melvill Jones pointed out that he
had recorded from vestibular neurones which responded to linear
acceleration but not tilt and felt that this might lend support to
Nashner's division of vestibular information into high frequency

and low frequency components. In response to other questions, Nashner indicated that no discomfort was associated with standing on his platform with stabilized ankle joint and that the responses to galvanic stimulation were not asummetrical but were recorded simultaneously in both gastrocnemius muscles. Dr. Herman was unable to attend the conference due to pressing family problems. However, his paper was presented by his colleague, T. Cook, and a further paper was presented by Dr. V. Monster, also from Herman's laboratory. In studies of the initiation of gait described by Cook, dantrolene sodium was studied for its possible disturbing effects. Drs. Basmajian and Monster pointed out to the audience that dantrolene fairly specifically blocked excitation-contraction coupling in muscle and was suitable for use in human subjects. Dantrolene had been in use for some time on an experimental basis for the relief of spasticity. Dantrolene thus reduces the force resulting from any given level of EMG. This knowledge of the site of action of dantrolene was needed to resolve some of the issues which arose in the discussion of load compensation that occurred also at this time (below). Dr. B. Ritchie (Yale University, New Haven, Connecticut) questioned Cook about the use of a logarithmic scale for expressing EMG responses. Cook replied that the same effects could be seen with a linear scale. Nashner suggested that the subject may initiate gait with a free fall following which cues for subsequent reactions might come from the vestibular system.

Stein asked for a discussion of whether or not the results presented in this and previous sessions supported the hypothesis that stretch reflexes provided effective load compensation. He suggested that Cook's studies with dantrolene and with procaine block, and the responses to ankle rotation presented by Nashner, argued against effective load compensation. Vigorous discussion followed. Nashner said that he could not presently judge the relative contributions of muscle properties, spinal reflexes and more central reactions based on vestibular and visual cues. Dr. E. Eldred (U.C.L.A., Los Angeles) added cues based on foot pressure to Nashner's list of unknown components. With regard to Cook's studies, it was pointed out that procaine block did not represent a variation in load but rather an interference with feedback that might otherwise compensate for a variation in load. The fact that patterns of torque were quite normal after dantrolene administration indicated that there was compensation, evidenced by increased EMG signals, for the weakening of muscle

produced by this drug. Although this point did not come up in the
discussion, it should be mentioned that dantrolene creates a
variation in the properties of skeletal muscle rather than a
variation in load. It was suggested that the dantrolene and procaine block experiments might be combined to test for differences in compensation of muscular weakness before and after
interfering with peripheral feedback. It was also pointed out,
however, that the relatively slow action of these procedures
would permit any result to be explained by central adaptive
mechanisms.

In reviewing these various arguments, it seems clear that
the hypothesis for load compensation is neither proven nor refuted
by the data presented. Only Bizzi's experiment, which was presented in an earlier session, actually tests the hypothesis.

Stephens asked whether any of the participants could estimate
the relative importance of the various cues in postural stabilization.
Nashner said that any of several systems could provide sufficient
feedback for postural stabilization. Performance deteriorated
significantly only when all low-frequency, or all high-frequency,
sources of feedback were eliminated. Brookhart gave further
examples where sensory cues were eliminated with little effect
on standing behaviour in dogs. The technique of blocking feedback
is difficult to interpret since rather large reductions in gain
would be expected, on theoretical grounds, to have relatively
minor effects on performance until the loop gain of the system is
reduced to unity.

In response to Gilman's paper, Granit mentioned that
K. E. Hagbarth at the University of Uppsala, Sweden, had noted
unusually high discharge rates of spindle receptors in Parkinsonian
patients. Matthews reminded the audience that a change in spindle
activity need not necessarily be related to a modification of reflex
tonus since the lesions might also modulate interneuronal pathways
that would have independent effects on tonus.

Following Wiesendanger's presentation, Grillner noted that
the stimulus currents were rather strong, suggesting that underlying structures might have been activated rather than supplementary
motor neurones. Smith mentioned recent evidence indicating that
the radioactive tracing technique labelled afferent fibres as well
as efferent fibres. Gilman commented on the difficulty of producing
precentral lesions without interfering with the blood supply to the

supplementary motor area.

The afternoon session ended with some general comments by Brookhart. He emphasized the need to relate our rather impressive knowledge concerning neurophysiological mechanisms to situations involving normal motor reactions in intact animals and man.

A CONSIDERATION OF STRETCH AND VIBRATION DATA IN RELATION TO THE TONIC STRETCH REFLEX

S. Grillner

Department of Physiology, University of Göteborg, Göteborg, Sweden

The primary endings of the muscle spindle have for a long period of time been regarded as the main source of autogenetic excitation in tonic and phasic stretch reflexes. This idea has been questioned since 1969, and it has been suggested that the secondaries play the main role in tonic reflexes. An account is given of the different arguments for and against the secondary endings being the main source for excitation in the stretch reflex.

In 1969, P. B. C. Matthews postulated that the secondary endings of the spindle would have a powerful excitatory effect being responsible for 80% or more of the stretch evoked excitation in the tonic stretch reflex of the decerebrate cat whereas the primary endings only would contribute the smaller remaining part.

This was based on a comparison of the increase of tension with vibration at different muscle lengths (0-7 mm from maximum extension) as compared to that of stretching the soleus muscle in the same length range. It was found that vibration (which in soleus is a reasonably selective tool for activating primary endings) at each length increased the muscle tension only moderately, whereas a stretch of the same muscle increased the tension to a much larger extent. The stretch of soleus will not increase the discharge in the primary endings nearly as much as the vibration.

Hence it must be concluded that the increase of tension during stretching cannot depend only on the activation of the primary ending. The two alternative explanations for these findings are that this additional increase depends on (a) activation of a different receptor system which causes the additional increase in tension; (b) that the properties of the actively contracting muscle fibres are such that the tension increases as the muscle is stretched all the way to its maximal value (i. e. the muscle stiffness).

CAN MUSCLE PROPERTIES BE INVOLVED?

At the time of Matthews' original report, the discharge rate of the stretch reflex activated alpha motor neurones supplying soleus was not known. Grillner and Udo (1971a) reported that motor units at maximal extension were firing in a quite narrow frequency range (7. 8 $\pm$ 1. 0; S. D.) and that except for the initial recruitment of the individual units, virtually no change in frequency occurred as the muscle was stretched to different muscle lengths (Fig. 2; see below for modulation of the discharge during each period of phasic stretch). It is important to note that these are recordings from motor units recorded in the actively contracting muscle with the different inhibitory and excitatory reflexes intact as well as the efferent supply giving normal activation of the different receptors located in the muscle.

With this knowledge of the discharge rate, we can estimate the muscle properties by stretching the actively contracting muscle in order to estimate the stiffness. On stimulation of different ventral rootlets in a distributed way (Rack and Westbury, 1969) at similar frequencies (Fig. 1A; see also Grillner, 1971; Grillner and Udo, 1971a), it can be seen that the active muscle tension increases monotonically as the muscle is stretched to maximum extension. Similar results were obtained also by Joyce et al. (1969). From their Fig. 3 it can be estimated that the active tension increases up to maximal extension at both 10 imp/sec (60 g. wt/mm) and 5 imp/sec (90 g. wt/mm) if the tension is measured after the initial give in the muscle during each stretch. On the other hand, if the muscle is taken to different levels of extension and then stimulated rather little change in tension has been found (Rack and Westbury, 1969) in this particular length range. The fact that the

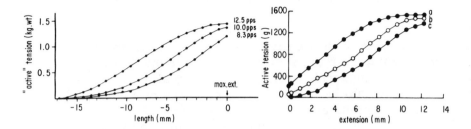

Fig. 1. Muscle stiffness of a soleus nerve-muscle preparation compared with the tonic stretch reflex during stretch
with and without concomitant reflex stimulation. The left
graph shows the length tension diagram of a soleus muscle
stimulated by means of distributed stimulation of five fascicles
of the ventral roots at the frequency indicated to the right of
each nerve (from Grillner, 1972). The ordinate shows the
active tension at different lengths which means that the
tension contributed by passive factors has been subtracted
from the total tension. For comparison the right graph shows
Fig. 8 from Matthews (1959b) in which C shows a normal
soleus stretch reflex, whereas in the other curves the effect
of electrical stimulation of the nerve to medial gastrocnemius
at 90 c/s (A) and 55 c/s (B) is shown.

muscle as during the tonic stretch reflex is extended to its new
length each time would be expected to result in larger tensions
under the subsequent phase of maintained stretch than in the
tension that could be obtained if the same number of motor units
were brought into action during isometric conditions (Cavagna
et al., 1968). Furthermore, since the frequency during extension
is somewhat higher (see below) than during the subsequent phase
at a given length, the tension will for a long period of time
remain higher as compared to what it would have been if the
muscle had had the same frequency all the time (cf. Burke et
al., 1970). In view of the greater efficacy of distributed
stimulation as compared to synchronous stimulation in this low
frequency region (Rack and Westbury, 1969, Figs. 5 and 7), it
seems desirable to use distributed stimulation when trying to
estimate the role of the muscle properties but it should be noted
that also during synchronous nerve stimulation at 10/sec the
stiffness can be approximately 80 g.wt/mm during the last

7 mm of stretch as deduced from Fig. 8 of Matthews (1959a).

All in all, the present available evidence indicates that the role of the stiffness of the contracting muscle fibres appear to play a considerable role in generating the increase in force observed in the tonic stretch reflex and during slow velocity (stretch) and it should be noted that the stiffness of a good tonic stretch reflex of soleus as described by Matthews (1959a, 1969) is in the order of 100 g. wt/mm which is near to the values observed with the pure muscle (Grillner, 1972; cf. above). Hence, it seems reasonable at present to infer that the discrepancy between stretch and vibration observed by Matthews (1969) is to a large extent explained by pure muscle properties (cf. Grillner, 1970, 1972; Grillner and Udo, 1971a, b).

HOW EFFECTIVE ARE THE PRIMARY ENDINGS?

When motor units are recorded as described above with the afferent and efferent nerve supply intact, the majority of the soleus motor units are recruited already at a relatively short muscle length and only few motor units are recruited close to maximal extension during a slow velocity stretch (Grillner and Udo, 1971b). Nichol's results (this Symposium) indicate that during the maintained stretch at different levels (i. e. the tonic stretch reflex), most of the motor units are recruited already at a short muscle length (70% of the muscle force).

Individual motor units do not increase their firing rate except during the first few intervals when they are recruited but do then stay at a maintained level during a slow extension only to drop in rate 1-2 imp/sec at the termination of stretch (Fig. 2A). If a motor unit is stretched in 1 mm steps, one can during each phasic stretch see an acceleration of the unit with about 1.5 imp/sec but at the termination of each stretch it falls back to the previous discharge rate (Fig. 2C). If another excitatory input is added one can well get an even higher discharge rate (Fig. 2B).

These data imply that the units are quite sensitive even to very slow phasic stretches and the only endings that seem to have the adequate phase sensitivity to give this response are the primary endings. Hence, the primary endings seem to be quite potent in enhancing the discharge rate during the stretch reflex

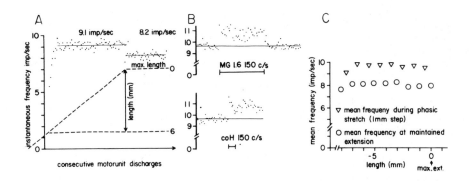

Fig. 2. The instantaneous discharge rate of motor units
during slow constant muscle stretch, interrupted muscle
stretch and during reflex activation superimposed on muscle
stretch. A shows the discharge of a motor unit recorded
with an electrode in the soleus muscle during slow extension
of the muscle (0.8 mm/sec). For the first few intervals
after recruitment the discharge rate increased, but thereafter the level is quite constant throughout the extension, but
decreased somewhat when the muscle was held at maximal
extension. C is recorded from another motor unit during
intermittent extension of 1 mm at a time. Note the remarkable
constancy of the motor unit discharge rate to maintained
extension at different levels of extension, which indicates
that no net excitation is added during 8 mm of muscle stretch.
Note also the constancy of the size of the dynamic response of
the motor unit. B is recorded from a motor unit discharging
during maintained muscle stretch, when the nerve to medial
gastrocnemius is stimulated repetitively at a strength including
the Ia fibres giving heteronymous excitation. The rate is
enhanced during exactly the period stimulated whereas similar
stimulation of the nerve to the contralateral hamstring muscles
gives a similar increase in discharge rate which outlasts the
stimulus (Grillner and Udo, unpublished., Methods in
1971a, b).

conditions, which would not be expected with the original group II hypothesis. Another interesting feature is that the discharge rate during maintained stretch as well as during each phasic stretch stays at the same level throughout the last 7 mm of stretch. This implies that in already discharging motor units there appears to be virtually no change in net excitation during this period of stretch in the region where Matthews (1969) suggests a very powerful excitation for the secondary endings. This presumably reflects that in this region the excitatory and inhibitory stretch evoked effects on the discharging motor units cancel each other.

Hence these data imply that primary endings can exert a comparatively powerful effect under stretch reflex conditions (Fig. 2A, C).

VIBRATION AS A SELECTIVE TOOL FOR ACTIVATION OF PRIMARY ENDINGS

Brown et al. (1967) showed that for soleus, vibration appears to be selective and to effectively activate each primary ending. But some caution must be used when using other muscles as the entire triceps surae of the gastrocnemii since Brown et al. (1967, p. 796) note for medial gastrocnemius that "mechanical resonances in the muscle appeared to be influencing the transmission of the vibration from the tendon to the receptors".

INTRACELLULAR STUDIES USING VIBRATION AND STRETCH

Westbury (1972) has recorded triceps surae motoneurones intracellularly in anaesthetized cats without tonic stretch reflexes and Rymer (this Symposium) medial gastrocnemius motoneurones in decerebrate cats. Both found a lack of occlusion between stretch and vibration indicating that some additional process takes place.

It should be noted that in many of the motoneurones recorded by Westbury (1972), a quite small depolarization is obtained by vibration as compared with the size of the monosynaptic EPSP obtained on single electrical stimulation (triceps surae). The EPSPs averaged between 8-10 mV for these motoneurones

(Eccles et al. , 1957). This indicates most likely either that
vibration of the entire triceps surae is not effective in activating
all spindle afferents or that a powerful presynaptic inhibition of
the primaries takes place. The synchronous excitation of the
primary endings during vibration very effectively evoked presynaptic inhibition between the Ia afferents to the triceps surae
(Pompeiano, personal communication), whereas the asynchronous
stretch evoked activity might be less effective in this respect.
One probable effect of stretching would be that the secondaries
block some of this presynaptic inhibition between the primaries
(Pompeiano, personal communication). It seems at present very
difficult to estimate if and to what extent this probable effect of
the secondaries is significant during ordinary stretch reflex
conditions as opposed to vibration.

If one accepts Westbury's (1972) experiments as indicating
an indirect effect of group II, it follows that this postulated
effect cannot affect the Golgi tendon organ pathways, since in
this preparation there is no muscle activity and hence no autogenetic Ib activity.

THE EFFECT OF VIBRATION AFTER PROCAINE BLOCK

An indirect approach used by McGrath and Matthews (1970)
compares the effect of vibration before and after paralyzing
small fibres in the muscle nerve such as group II and III afferents
and gamma efferents. The effect of vibration is reduced after
procaine, which would be expected if the group II afferents were
excitatory in the stretch reflex (see also preceding paragraph).
It should be considered, however, that the procaine block
reduces tonically the afferent activity from Ia, group II and III
afferents. This could well influence the long term resting
excitability of the alpha motoneurones through spinal as well as
supraspinal circuits regulating the long term excitability of alpha
and gamma motoneurones via descending systems (cf. Partridge,
1960).

CONCLUDING REMARKS

As discussed above, it appears that the large part of the motor
units have been recruited during the last 7 mm before maximal
extension. The effect of the vibration would be to recruit the

remaining motoneurones and to increase the frequency of already
discharging motor units (see Brown et al., 1968), which is also
accomplished by repetitively stimulating heteronymous excitatory
afferents (Grillner and Udo, 1971a). The main effect would be
to move from one length tension curve to another, as in Fig. 1A.

Stretching would, in addition, cause an increase of tension
due to the muscle stiffness, whereas vibration at the new length
would be expected to give a rather similar effect at the new
length. The graph (Fig. 1B) is from Matthews (1959a) and shows
the effect of a slow extension of soleus with and without concomitant stimulation of the synergistic medial gastrocnemius at
group I strength. This will result in an increased discharge
rate and a movement from one length tension curve to another.
Note the marked similarities between the muscle properties
in Fig. 1A and the stretch reflex in Fig. 1B.

Although the intracellular studies suggest an indirect effect of
the secondary endings, it is at present not possible to assess the
relative importance of this effect demonstrated with vibration.
The lack of frequency modulation of motor units as discussed
above strongly suggests that little net excitation is added during
the last part of a good stretch reflex (cf. above and Fig. 2), and
hence the strong group II contribution postulated by Matthews
(1969) appears unlikely. The available evidence indicates that
the primary endings of the spindle are the main channel for
excitation in tonic and phasic stretch reflexes, whereas transmission in the direct inhibitory pathways from the secondaries
to the alpha motoneurones is depressed as compared to the acute
spinal preparation (Grillner and Udo, 1970a; Holmquist and
Lundberg, 1961).

REFERENCES

Brown, M.C., Engberg, J., and Matthews, P.B.C., 1967. The relative
    sensitivity to vibration of muscle receptors of the cat. J.
    Physiol. 192, 773-800.
Brown, M.L., Lawrence, D.G., and Matthews, P.B.C., 1968. Reflex
    inhibition by Ia afferent input of spontaneously discharging
    gamma motoneurones in the decerebrate cat. J. Physiol. 198,
    5-7P.
Burke, R.E., Rudomin, P., and Zajac, F.E., III., 1970. Catch
    property in single mammalian motor units. Science 168, 122-124.

Cavagna, G.A., Dusman, B., and Margaria, R., 1960. Positive work
    done by a previously stretched muscle. J. Appl. Physiol. 24,
    21-32.
Eccles, J.L., Eccles, R.M., and Lundberg, A., 1957. The conver-
    gence of monosynaptic excitatory afferents onto many different
    species of alpha motoneurones. J. Physiol. 137, 22-56.
Grillner, S., 1970. Is the tonic stretch reflex dependent upon
    group II excitation? Acta Physiol. Scand. 78, 431-432.
Grillner, S., 1972. The role of muscle stiffness in meeting the
    changing postural and locomotor requirements for force develop-
    ment by the ankle extensors. Acta Physiol. Scand. 86, 92-108.
Grillner, S., and Udo, M., 1970. Is the tonic stretch reflex
    dependent on suppression of autogenetic inhibitory reflexes?
    Acta Physiol. Scand. 79, 13-14A.
Grillner, S., and Udo, M., 1971a. Motor unit activity and stiff-
    ness of the contracting muscle fibres in the tonic stretch
    reflex. Acta Physiol. Scand. 81, 422-424.
Grillner, S., and Udo, M., 1971b. Recruitment in the tonic stretch
    reflex. Acta Physiol. Scand. 81, 571-573.
Higgins, D.L., Partridge, L.D., and Glaser, G.H., 1962. A trans-
    ient cerebellar influence on stretch responses. J. Neurophysiol.
    25, 684-692.
Holmquist, B., and Lundberg, A., 1961. Differential supraspinal
    control of synaptic actions evoked by volleys in the flexion
    reflex in alpha motoneurones. Acta Physiol. Scand. Suppl. 54,
    1-51.
Joyce, G.L., Rack, P.M.H., and Westbury, D.R., 1969. Properties of
    cat soleus muscle during controlled lengthening and shortening
    movements. J. Physiol. 204, 461-474.
Matthews, P.B.C., 1959a. The dependence of tension upon extension
    in the stretch reflex of the soleus muscle of the decerebrate
    cat. J. Physiol. 147, 521-546.
Matthews, P.B.C., 1959b. A study of certain factors influencing
    the stretch reflex of the decerebrate cat. J. Physiol. 147,
    547-564.
Matthews, P.B.C., 1969. Evidence that the secondary as well as the
    primary endings of the muscle spindles may be responsible for
    the tonic stretch reflex of the decerebrate cat. J. Physiol.
    204, 365-393.
McGrath, G.J., and Matthews, P.B.C., 1970. Support for an auto-
    genetic excitatory reflex action of the spindle secondaries
    from the effect of gamma blockade by procaine. J. Physiol.
    210, 176-177P.
Rack, P.M.H., and Westbury, D.R., 1969. The effects of length and
    stimulus rate on tension in the isometric cat soleus muscle.
    J. Physiol. 204, 443-460.
Westbury, D., 1972. A study of stretch and vibration reflexes of
    the cat by intracellular recording from motoneurones. J.
    Physiol. 226, 37-56.

REFLEX AND NON-REFLEX STIFFNESS OF SOLEUS MUSCLE IN THE CAT

T. R. Nichols

Department of Physiology, Harvard Medical School
Boston, Massachusetts

The apparent mechanical properties of the soleus muscle in the cat are significantly modified when autogenetic reflex connections around the muscle are intact. The apparent steady-state stiffness of the muscle is increased when a fraction of its motor units are activated. In the transient response to muscle stretch, autogenetic reflexes not only increase the apparent stiffness of the muscle, but also mask sudden reductions in force which occur in the absence of reflexes. The reflexes are fast enough to mask these reductions up to stretch velocities of at least 85 mm/sec.

A matter of current debate is the extent to which the tonic stretch reflex can be accounted for by the stiffness of already recruited motor units (Grillner and Udo, 1971). This question can be asked from a different perspective: What modifications in the mechanical properties of a muscle occur if autogenetic reflexes are present? I would like to present two results which illustrate such modifications. The first shows that feedback from muscle receptors is important in determining the spring-like characteristic of the tonic stretch reflex over the entire physiological range of the muscle. The second shows that the transient response of activated muscle to imposed length changes is significantly modified when autogenetic reflexes are present.

For example, part A of Fig. 1 shows the length-tension curve of a stretch reflex in the soleus muscle of a decerebrate cat as

407

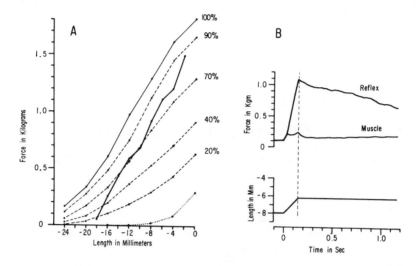

Fig. 1. Modification of the mechanical properties of a muscle by autogenetic reflexes in the steady state (A) and in the transient phase (B). A - Length-tension curve of the stretch reflex in the soleus muscle of a decerebrate cat (heavy line). The muscle was stretched in 2 mm increments and held at each length for 30 sec. Also shown are the length-tension curve of the entire muscle stimulated at a rate of 8 per sec (light solid line) and the length-tension curves of four fixed populations of motor units obtained by stimulating portions of ventral root at 8 per sec (dashed lines). The percentages of the total force exerted by each portion are indicated. In the cases of stimulated muscle, the muscle was allowed to rest at each length for 30 sec before stimulation. The passive length-tension curve is indicated by the dotted line.

In order to directly compare transient responses of activated muscle and of reflexes, the operating point (operating length, operating force) must be matched in the two cases. Matched operating points are illustrated in part A by the intersections of reflex and muscle length-tension curves. B - Comparison of reflex and activated muscle responses to a 1.8 mm ramp stretch of 140 msec in duration. The response of the activated muscle in the absence of reflexes was obtained after cutting the dorsal roots and using a crossed extensor reflex response. Data in part B are from a different experiment than the data in part A.

well as the length-tension curve of the same muscle stimulated
at 8 per sec after the ventral roots were cut. In the reflex experiment, the muscle was held at each length for 30 sec. In the
muscle experiment, the muscle was allowed to rest at each
length for 30 sec before stimulation. The dashed lines are the
length-tension curves of four fixed populations of motor units
obtained by stimulating portions of the L7 and S1 ventral roots.
The light solid line is the length-tension curve of the entire
muscle stimulated through the muscle nerve, and the heavy line
is the length-tension curve of the stretch reflex. If motor units
in the reflex are limited in the steady-state to a firing rate of
about 8 per sec, then the fact that the reflex length-tension
curve cuts across the muscle curves suggests that the process of
recruitment takes place over the entire range of the reflex.
The possibility for some frequency modulation has not been
excluded, however. The length thresholds of the reflexes may
vary considerably from experiment to experiment, but the
stiffnesses are often similar. It is apparent from these facts
that autogenetic reflexes can endow the muscle with a high
apparent stiffness without activating all of the motor units.

The stiffness of the stretch reflex is even higher during a
transient response to a rapidly applied length change than it is
in the steady-state. In contrast, activated soleus muscle in the
absence of reflexes exhibits a phase of decreased stiffness
transiently (Nichols and Houk, 1973). Part B of the Fig. shows
the response of an active soleus muscle to a 1.8 mm ramp
stretch before and after reflex connections were cut. The stiffness of the reflex expressed as change in force divided by
change in length 1 sec after initiation of the ramp is 170 gm/mm
compared to a slope of 80 gm/mm in the steady-state curve
shown in part A. The response of the active muscle in the absence of the reflex was obtained in the same preparation by
cutting the dorsal roots and then using a crossed-extensor reflex
to adjust the baseline or operating force to match that of the
reflex response. Note that the transient response is similar to
that described by Joyce et al. (1969), in that force "gives way"
suddenly during and at the completion of the ramp stretch. The
stiffness of this response after 1 sec is 20 gm/mm. The reflex
has not only produced a higher stiffness than the muscle, but it
has also effectively compensated for the sudden reduction in
force of the previously activated muscle, as predicted by Rack
(1970), and discussed in more detail by Nichols and Houk (1973).

Finally, there is the question as to whether the reflex is fast
enough to compensate for the sudden reductions in muscular
force which might occur when the muscle is stretched as rapidly
as it is when the animal is trotting or running (Rack, 1970). The
fastest ramps that I have tried were 40 msec in duration and
85 mm/sec in velocity. In these cases, the "gives" in force
were masked. EMG studies during these experiments
showed reflex latencies as short as 15 msec. The latency from
EMG to contractile force was approximately 5 msec.

REFERENCES

Grillner, S. and Udo, M., 1971.   Recruitment in the tonic stretch
   reflex.   Acta Physiol. Scand. 81, 571-573
Joyce, G.C., Rack, P.M.H. and Westbury, D.R., 1969.   The mechanical properties of cat soleus muscle during controlled lengthening and shortening movements.   J. Physiol. 204, 461-474.
Nichols, T.R. and Houk, J.C., 1973.   Reflex compensation for
   variations in the mechanical properties of a muscle.   Science
   181, 182-184.
Rack, P.M.H., 1970.   The significance of   mechanical properties
   of muscle in the reflex control of posture.   In   Excitatory
   Synaptic Mechanisms.   (Ed. Andersen, P. and Jansen, J.K.S.).
   Universitetsforlaget, Oslo.

EFFECTS OF SECONDARY MUSCLE SPINDLE AFFERENT DISCHARGE ON EXTENSOR MOTO- NEURONES IN THE DECEREBRATE CAT

W. Z. Rymer and J. V. Walsh

Laboratory of Neural Control, National Institute of
Neurological Diseases and Stroke, National Institutes
of Health, Bethesda, Maryland

High frequency longitudinal vibration of the medial gastroc-nemius tendon in the decerebrate cat is known to produce phase-locked discharge of virtually all the primary spindle endings in the muscle (Matthews, 1966). When low frequency sinusoidal stretch is superimposed the resulting excitatory effects on homonymous motoneurones are probably produced by secondary muscle spindle afferent discharge. Using standard intracellular recording techniques, it was found that motoneurones showing maintained discharge in response to tendon vibration alone also demonstrated increased dis-charge frequency in response to superimposed muscle stretch. All motoneurones investigated showed sinusoidal membrane potential variation during combined sinusoidal stretch and vibration of the muscle tendon. This potential swing was approximately in phase with the slow stretch and proportional to it in amplitude. The EPSPs induced by vibration showed considerable size variation in the course of the slow stretch. They were largest when the muscle length was maximal, often showing a two-fold increase in amplitude. Rectangular current pulses were used to measure membrane resistance at successive stages of the slow stretch, but these measurements did not indicate any significant variations. As well, prolonged intra-cellular chloride injection and membrane hyperpolarization did not decrease the size of the slow sinusoidal potential

411

swing. These observations suggest that somatic IPSPs do not contribute to the slow potential change. It seems possible that the secondary effect is mediated, at least in part, via the 1a afferent system, and may act by presynaptic dis-inhibition.

Recently, Matthews (1969) has suggested that secondary muscle spindle afferent input from gastrocnemius and soleus muscles in the decerebrate cat is excitatory to homonymous motoneurones. This hypothesis was based in part on the observation that increasing muscle stretch did not occlude the reflex increase in muscle tension induced by vibrating the muscle tendon. Grillner (1970) has objected to this approach on the grounds that the apparent lack of occlusion could have occurred simply as a result of increased muscle length. The debate centres on the slope of the length tension curve for active muscle. Matthews has argued that at the muscle lengths used, the curve is flat, whereas Grillner has provided evidence that the slope is still steep. A possible solution to this controversy is to examine the frequency of motoneuronal discharge for various combinations of muscle stretch and vibration.

It is known that under specified conditions, longitudinal vibration of a muscle tendon produces phase-locked discharge of virtually all the primary muscle spindle endings in the muscle (Matthews, 1966). If we superimpose a slow sinusoidal stretch, then, provided that primary spindle afferent input remains constant, any observed excitatory effects accompanying this stretch are probably a result of secondary spindle afferent discharge. Our investigation of primary ending responses during tendon vibration has shown that superimposed slow sinusoidal stretch does not allow spindle "unloading" as long as the stretch frequency is less than 0.5 Hz and its amplitude is less than 1 mm. In addition, the mean muscle length must be sufficient to induce a significant tonic reflex response. Spindle "unloading" is detected by dropped impulses and by widening of the interval histogram which is normally extremely sharp for vibration induced impulse trains. It is necessary that the vibration amplitude be in a range of 80-110 μm at a frequency of 140-150 Hz to insure consistent primary ending response.

The frequency of motoneuronal discharge may be monitored at a number of sites. Fine tungsten microelectrodes provide reasonably selective EMG recordings from muscle, and the frequency of neuronal discharge may be measured using spike amplitude and shape discrimination techniques. In addition, recordings were made from dissected ventral root filaments and directly from motoneurones with micropipettes. Motoneurones which showed sustained discharge in response to tendon vibration alone, also demonstrated increased discharge during added muscle stretch. When this stretch was sinusoidal in form, the curves of instantaneous frequency were sinusoidal in shape, as was the shape of a post stimulus histogram initiated at the onset of the slow muscle stretch.

As anticipated, this discharge frequency variation produced by sinusoidal muscle stretch was associated with varying membrane depolarization. These membrane potential changes were not induced exclusively by sinusoidal stretch. Maintained changes in muscle length were also associated with sustained depolarization. Our observations are essentially similar to those of Westbury (1972), but our preparations were unanaesthetized, decerebrate and demonstrated considerable muscle rigidity, implying sustained fusimotor tone. This tone may have helped to prevent muscle spindle unloading as muscle length varies, a factor difficult to eliminate in anaesthetized preparations.

The EPSPs induced by vibration showed considerable variation in size throughout the slow sinusoidal stretch. EPSP size increased with increasing muscle length, and sometimes showed a two-fold size variation. This relationship between EPSP size and muscle length was also demonstrated for maintained muscle displacement, which suggests that the EPSP changes could not have been caused by spindle unloading in the course of sinusoidal muscle stretch.

Matthews has suggested that secondary afferent input to motoneurones may act indirectly by disinhibition. It is conceivable that IPSPs which were inhibited by secondary spindle afferent discharge could produce both the slow membrane potential swing and the variation in EPSP size. However, membrane resistance measurements using rectangular current pulses at various stages of the slow stretch did not indicate any significant variations, implying that there were no major somatic conductance changes induced. In addition, prolonged intracellular chloride injection and membrane hyperpolarization (using citrate microelectrodes) did not decrease the size of the slow potential swing or influence the variation in EPSP size. These observations indicate that somatic

IPSPs are probably not responsible for the described effects, although involvement of remote dendritic IPSPs can not be excluded.

The other major alternative is that this disinhibition is presynaptic, i. e. secondary afferent discharge inhibits the interneurones responsible for presynaptic inhibition. This hypothesis would account for the variation of EPSP size and possibly for the slow membrane potential changes as well, although this has not yet been investigated. The possibility of some polysynaptic excitatory input to motoneurones from secondary afferent fibres is not eliminated by these observations.

It seems possible that the effects of secondary muscle spindle afferent discharge on motoneurones is mediated at least in part via the Ia afferent input and the mechanism used may be presynaptic disinhibition.

REFERENCES

Grillner, S., 1970. Is the tonic stretch reflex dependent upon Group II excitation? Acta. Physiol. Scand. 78, 431-432.
Matthews, P.B.C., 1966. The reflex excitation of the soleus muscle of the decerebrate cat caused by vibration applied to its tendon. J. Physiol. 184, 450-472.
Matthews, P.B.C., 1969. Evidence that the secondary as well as the primary endings of the muscle spindles may be responsible for the tonic stretch reflex of the decerebrate cat. J. Physiol. 204, 365-393.
Westbury, D.R., 1972. A study of stretch and vibration reflexes of the cat by intracellular recording from motoneurons. J. Physiol. 226, 37-56.

THE BASES OF TREMOR DURING A MAINTAINED POSTURE

S. M. Padsha and R. B. Stein

Department of Physiology, University of Alberta
Edmonton, Canada

Characteristics of the finger tremor in normal human subjects
were studied. Spectral analysis shows (i) a major peak at about
0. 3 Hz, (ii) a secondary peak at about 1 Hz, and (iii) a broad
peak at about 10 Hz. The peak at 0. 3 Hz correlates well with
respiration, the 1 Hz peak with the electrocardiogram and the
10 Hz peaks with the electromyogram from finger extensors.
The relative contributions of these three factors in generating
normal physiological tremor were measured and the previously
undescribed contribution of respiration proved to be the largest.
The time delays in generating each component of normal tremor
were measured and possible mechanisms are suggested.

Recording the finger tremor is a routine clinical test in neurology
and the tremor is classified by a variety of names and yet the basis
of the physiological tremor in healthy subjects is not fully understood. A number of factors have been attributed to the origin of
the physiological tremor, e. g. the influence of the heart beat
(Brumlik, 1962), stretch reflex (Lippold, 1970). However, the
major peak in the spectrum of physiological tremor occurs at a
frequency too low to be accounted for by these factors and may be
related to respiration (Sutton and Sykes, 1967). This work estimates the relative contributions of the various factors producing
the physiological tremor. The physiological finger tremor in
healthy human subjects is defined here as the involuntary fluctuations
in force that occur during an effort to maintain posture.

The subject sat on a chair with his or her elbow resting on a
table and the hand and wrist elevated above the table and the fingers

outstretched. The nail of the right middle finger lifted a strain-
gauge with a force of 50-100 g. The strain gauge was a part of a
D. C. Wheatstone bridge circuit. The bridge output was amplified
and monitored by a microammeter which the subject could see and
it was recorded on a tape recorder. Simultaneously, the electrocardiogram, the respiratory air flow, and the surface electromyogram from the extensors of the finger were recorded. The subjects
kept their eyes closed during the recording, only occasionally
opening to see if the tension was well maintained. Each recording
session lasted about 5 min.

Power spectral analysis was performed on the records of the
finger tremor tension oscillations, the analog signal of the respiratory air flow, the time interval between successive R waves
of the electrocardiogram and the rectified and filtered surface
electromyogram by the methods described by French and Holden
(1971) and Milner-Brown et al. (1973a).

Fig. 1 illustrates the average of 28 power spectra of the right
middle finger tremor, the respiration, the cardiac pulse and the
surface EMG from one subject. The power spectrum of the tremor
had a peak at about 0. 25 Hz and this corresponds to the peak in
the spectrum of the respiration. There are secondary peaks at
about 0. 5 Hz (1st harmonic) in both spectra. There is also a
peak at about 1 Hz in the tremor spectrum and this corresponds
to the peak in the spectrum of the cardiac pulse. There are two
secondary peaks at about 2 and 3 Hz in the tremor and the cardiac
spectra, which are due to the harmonics of the cardiac pulse
frequency. The third prominent peak in the tremor spectrum is
at about 8 Hz and this is close to the peak in the EMG spectrum.
Similar results were obtained from 7 healthy adults (4 males and
3 females).

From the power spectra of the respiration ($G_x(f)$), the tremor,
($G_y(f)$) and the cross-spectrum of the respiration and the tremor
($G_{xy}(f)$), a quantitative estimate of the linear contribution of the
respiration to the finger tremor was calculated by the coherence
function ($|G_{xy}(f)|^2$)/($G_x(f)$ $G_y(f)$). Similar estimates were made
for the contributions of the cardiac pulse and the EMG to the
finger tremor.

The effect of the respiration was the largest and accounted for
about 23% of the finger tremor. The electrocardiogram and the
electromyogram accounted for 10% and 11% of the tremor respec-

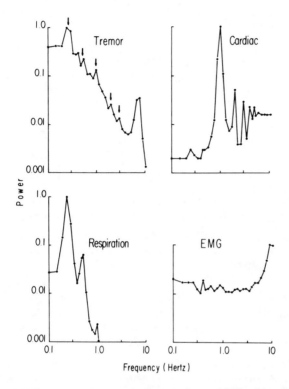

Fig. 1. Power spectra of the right middle finger tremor, the respiratory air flow, the cardiac pulse and the rectified surface electromyogram in one subject. Each trace is the average of 28 spectra and is normalized to its primary peak and plotted on a log-log scale. The arrows on the tremor spectrum indicate the primary and the secondary peaks in the cardiac and the respiratory spectra.

tively. The remaining 58% was due to non-linear effects of these causes or to other causes.

The time delay between the respiration and the finger tremor was measured by the cross-correlation function, which is the inverse Fourier transform of the cross-spectral function between respiration and tremor. In Fig. 2 there was a delay of 320 msec between the peak of respiratory airflow and the peak of the finger tremor. The delay in 5 subjects was 56 $\pm$ 227 msec (mean $\pm$ S. D.) which is not significantly different from 0. The auto-correlation function is also shown in Fig. 2. The close relationship

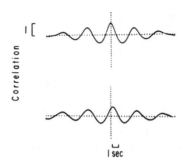

<u>Fig. 2.</u> Top trace: autocorrelation of the respiration indicating
a rhythmic rate of about 15/min. Bottom trace: cross-correlation
between the respiration and the finger tremor shows the close
relationship between the two events. The delay between the
peak of the respiratory air flow and the peak of the finger
tremor is 320 msec in this example. The cross-correlation has
not been normalized.

between the autocorrelation function for respiratory air flow and
the cross-correlation function suggests that the force required
to move the air is the direct cause of the respiratory component
of normal tremor. Similar estimates between the R wave of the
electrocardiogram and the peak of the tremor wave gave a delay
of 343 + 55 msec (mean + S. D.). This is close to the time required
for the pressure wave from the heart to reach the fingers (Carrie
and Bickford, 1969). The delay between the peaks in the EMG
and the tremor was between 50 and 60 msec. This is approximately
equal to the contraction time for the motor units in finger muscles
(Milner-Brown et al., 1973b).

REFERENCES

Brumlik, J., 1962. On the nature of normal tremor. Neurology
    (Minn.) <u>12</u>, 159-179.
Carrie, J.R.G., and Bickford, R.G., 1969. Cardiovascular factors
    in limb tremor. Neurology <u>19</u>, 116-127.
French, A.S., and Holden, A.V., 1971. Frequency domain analysis of
    neurophysiological data. Comp. Progr. Biomed. <u>1</u>, 219-234.
Lippold, O.C.J., 1970. Oscillations in the stretch reflex arc and
    the origin of the rhythmical 8-12 c/s component of physiological
    tremor. J. Physiol. <u>206</u>, 359-382.

Milner-Brown, H.S., Stein, R.B., and Yemm, R., 1973a. The contractile properties of human motor units during voluntary isometric
contractions. J. Physiol. 228, 285-306.
Milner-Brown, H.S., Stein, R.B., and Yemm, R., 1973b. The orderly
recruitment of human motor units during voluntary isometric
contractions. J. Physiol. 230, 359-370.
Sutton, C.G., and Sykes, K., 1967. The variations of hand tremor
with force in healthy subjects. J. Physiol. 191, 699-711.

COMPENSATION OF POSTURAL CONTROL BY SQUIRREL MONKEYS FOLLOWING DORSAL COLUMN LESIONS

C. H. M. Beck

Department of Psychology, University of Alberta, Edmonton, Canada

The impairment in postural adjustment seen by Melzack in dorsal column cats while jumping to a moving platform was observed in squirrel monkeys with similar lesions when tested 2 weeks postoperatively. However, as Brookhart's group has found with dogs, if the squirrel monkey is permitted to reach a stable chronic state by delaying testing until 2 months postoperatively, effective compensation of postural control occurs. Extreme reliance on visual information by dorsal column animals as suggested by Dubrovsky was not observed in limb control during locomotion but was seen in other experiments on control of the hands in reaching.

Cats exhibit postural deficits in turning on a narrow beam and in jumping to a moving surface when tested 2 weeks after dorsal column section (Melzack and Bridges, 1971). However, dogs effectively compensate posturally to a sudden change of support to one leg in tests administered 2 months after dorsal column lesions (Reynolds et al., 1972). The possibility that differences in the delay between the operation and the time of testing could account for these conflicting findings is one hypothesis examined in the present study. Dubrovsky et al. (1971) suggested that dorsal column section in cats produced a kinesthetic deficit and as a consequence the experimental animals were more reliant on visual cues. This hypothesis was tested in the present study by observing dorsal column monkeys' postural adjustment to a rotating surface compared to one which appeared visually to be rotating.

Twelve squirrel monkeys were tested preoperatively, 2 weeks postoperatively and again 2 months postoperatively on their ability to jump onto and off of a 55 cm diameter turntable from a small perch 55 cm above the turntable. The time from the dropping of a raisin on the floor to the monkey's jumping from the perch to the floor was referred to as the 'down time'. The time from the monkey's touching the raisin on the floor to the animal's jumping back upon the perch was referred to as the 'up time'. In the first 3 or 4 test conditions an Archimedes spiral covered the floor of the turntable. The test conditions were: (1) a spiral pattern on a stationary floor; (2) a spiral pattern on a rotating floor; (3) a rotating spiral pattern overlain by a stationary floor of clear plastic; (4) a concentric ring pattern on a rotating floor. The floor rotated at 1.2 revolutions/sec. The monkeys were tested in a counterbalanced order across conditions. Testing preoperatively continued for 2 sessions per condition at 20 trials per session or until the animal achieved up and down times of less than 1.0 sec. At 2 weeks and again at 2 months following intended bilateral dorsal column section to 9 animals and sham operations on 3 animals, the monkeys were tested for 2 sessions on each condition. Of the lesioned animals, only number 15 achieved preoperative jump times at 2 weeks postoperatively. Table 1 compares the actual extent of the lesions in different monkeys. Monkey 15 has twice as much dorsal column intact as any other monkey. The other 8 operates were unable to perform the tests. The animals exhibited slippage of limbs, hesitancy and fear of jumping, and a wide based gait. In the home cage they sat on the cage floor rather than on their perches. At 2 months postoperatively, however, all animals reached preoperative levels of performance except for monkey number 3, who was slow on the up times on the two conditions with rotating floors. This animal suffered extensive dorsolateral column injury (Table 1). Thus, the data on time of postoperative testing support the hypothesized significance of this variable in resolving the conflicting observations of Melzack and Bridges (1971) and Reynolds et al. (1972). The findings also provide for generalizations of Melzack and Bridges (1971) observations of the postural effects of dorsal column lesions in cats to monkeys. No support was obtained for the hypothesis that extreme reliance on visual cues would impair postural control on a surface which appeared visually to be moving but actually was stationary. Postoperative asymptotic up times were the same on all 4 tests (see Fig. 1 for up times), except for monkey number 3. Possibly the apparent movement induced by the rotating spiral was not as effective a visual illusion for squirrel monkeys as it was for the experimenter. Evidence from unpublished experiments with these animals indicates an extreme reliance on visual as opposed to somatic information in control of the hands during reaching rather than in control of the limbs during locomotion.

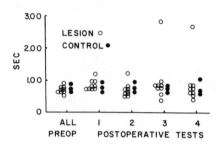

Fig. 1. Final session median 'up times' for each monkey preoperatively for all 4 test conditions combined and 2 months postoperatively for each test condition separately. Test conditions: (1) spiral pattern on stationary floor; (2) spiral pattern on rotating floor; (3) rotating spiral overlain by stationary clear plastic floor; (4) concentric ring pattern on rotating floor.

Brain Damage	Lesioned Monkeys								
	M9	M3	M4	M7	M10	M11	M12	M14	M15
DC Spared	4%	12%	0%	0%	15%	18%	13%	22%	45%
LCST Damaged	L+	R+++	L+R+	L+					

Note: DC = Dorsal Columns; LCST = Lateral Corticospinal Tract; L = Left; R = Right; + = slight damage; +++ = severe damage.

TABLE 1

Brain Damage Summary

Acknowledgement: This research was supported by a grant from the Medical Research Council.

REFERENCES

Dubrovsky, G., Davelaar, E. and Garcia-Rill, E., 1971.   The role of dorsal columns in serial order acts.   Exp. Neurol. 33, 93–102.

Melzack, R. and Bridges, J.A., 1971.   Dorsal column contributions to motor behaviour.   Exp. Neurol. 33, 53–68.

Reynolds, P.J., Talbott, R.E. and Brookhart, J.M., 1972.   Control of postural reactions in the dog: the role of the dorsal column feedback pathway.   Brain Res. 40, 159–164.

PROPOSAL FOR MODE OF ACTION OF

ANTICHOLINERGIC DRUGS USED IN

PARKINSON'S DISEASE

K. C. Marshall

Department of Physiology, University of Ottawa
Canada

Anticholinergic drugs have been used for relief of Parkinsonism and Duvoisin (1967) has shown that the anticholinesterase agent physostigmine exacerbates the condition. Because it has been reported that atropine can block transmission in the cerebello-thalamic pathway (see Marshall and McLennan, 1972 for references), it seemed possible that anticholinergic therapy for Parkinson's disease might owe some of its effects to interference with synaptic transmission in the ventrolateral nucleus of the thalamus (VL). We have just started to test this idea by studying the effects of various drugs on synaptic activity in VL.

The experimental subjects were cats lightly anaesthetized with a halothane-nitrous oxide mixture. Our first tests were to determine the minimum doses of anticholinergics which can block cerebello-thalamic transmission, and we have found that as little as 0.2 mg/Kg of atropine sulphate I.V. can cause a marked blocking of the postsynaptic component of the response evoked in VL after stimulation of the superior cerebellar peduncle; and a small reduction can be seen with a dose of 0.1 mg/Kg. In addition, we have seen that 0.25 mg/Kg of physostigmine I.V. markedly enhances the postsynaptic response in VL, but we have not yet tested the minimal dose for this effect. That the atropine effects have some specificity for VL is seen by comparison with the experiments of David et al. (1963) in which 5-10 mg/Kg of atropine did not alter the postsynaptic potential in the lateral geniculate nucleus after stimulation of the optic nerve.

Dr. Gilman's work now indicates that a depression of activity in VL can depress fusimotor activity, and perhaps, by extrapolation, limb rigidity in humans. It is interesting that the anticholinergic drugs used for Parkinson's disease are best known for their improvement of rigidity.

I feel, therefore, that we must add to the existing ideas on the subject, the possibility that anticholinergic drugs exert at least some of their anti-Parkinsonian effects by reducing excitability of VL neurones.

REFERENCES

David, J.P., Murayama, S., Machne, Z., and Unna, K.R., 1963.
    Evidence supporting cholinergic transmission at the lateral
    geniculate body of the cat. Int. J. Neuropharmacol. 2,
    113-125.
Duvoisin, R.C., 1967. Cholinergic-anticholinergic antagonism in
    Parkinsonism. Arch. Neurol. 17, 124-136.
Marshall, K.C., and McLennan, H., 1972. The synaptic activation
    of neurones of the feline ventrolateral thalamic nucleus:
    possible cholinergic mechanisms. Exp. Brain Res. 15, 472-483.

PART III: CONTROL OF LOCOMOTION

CONTROL OF MOTOR OUTPUT

D. Kennedy

Stanford University, Stanford, California

Considerable evidence indicates that proprioceptive feedback from moving limbs does not contribute information used
by the central nervous system in generating locomotor patterns.
The basic motor score is determined by patterned activity in
central neurons, or by the inhibitory and/or excitatory connections between them; such scores are usually genetic, but could
in principle result from autogenetic interactions between the
CNS and the environment or the body periphery. Separate
centers for the production of cyclic output (as, for example,
in different limb-bearing segments) are held in particular
phase relations by interconnections that carry replicas of
the motor output from one center to another. These messages
formally resemble the 'efference copy' of von Holst. The output of the ensemble is commanded by neurons that trigger the
pattern but do not contribute to its structure.

What role remains for proprioceptive feedback? The muscle
length- and tension-detecting and regulating circuits that have
been most carefully worked out to date (those involving intercostal spindles in mammalian respiration, and muscle receptor
organs in arthropod postural control) suggest that the primary
function is in load compensation. A central command can, if
a proprioceptive servo with the proper gain exists, produce a
movement that will be of identical amplitude under a variety
of unpredictable load conditions. This concept can be extended
to explain the function of a variety of 'positive feedback' re-

429

flexes, in which proprioceptive or exteroreceptive return
appears to amplify the motor discharge producing an active
movement.

Movements that an animal executes in stereotyped, repetitive
sequences - locomotion and ventilation, for example - are
characterized by fixed temporal and spatial relations between
the discharges in different motor pathways. This kind of co-
ordination presumably reflects the properties of a neural pattern
generator. Over the past few years, work on relatively simple
nervous systems has resulted in a number of models (or at least
metaphors) that attempt to account for pattern generation. The
central question they attempt to answer is the following: How do
central nervous circuits develop and distribute information about
the moment-to-moment status of the various subroutines they
are controlling?

MODELS FOR PATTERN GENERATION

In the 1940's and early 1950's (see, e.g., Gray, 1950) it was
widely believed that such information was returned from the
periphery, and then used by the central nervous system to
initiate the next subroutine. According to this view, motor
sequences depend for their phasing upon sensory feedback, and
the sequence unfolds in the manner of a reflex chain.

We know of no motor systems that actually use this method,
and of a great many that do not. The appendages of crustaceans
employed in locomotion and ventilation, those of insects in flight
and singing and those of some vertebrates in walking, all produce the
appropriate pattern when each possible route of peripheral feedback has been cut - as long as adequate unpatterned excitation is
fed to the CNS. There are one or two interesting cases in which
altering the sensory feedback alters the cycle period, and in
which,therefore, a phasic role for the sensory input is possible.
Mellon (1969), for example, has shown that feedback from proprioceptors can influence the frequency of swimming in scallops. The
feedback may, however, merely be manipulating a central oscillator within a limited range, in which case we would still have to
attribute most of the patterning to the center.

A slightly less peripheralist position is represented by the notion of a sensory template or, as it was called by Hoyle (1964), a sensory tape. In this formulation, the pattern of sensory feedback is compared with a centrally-stored version of what the feedback should look like. Real-time versions of this model are not very persuasive; first, they require alarmingly rapid midcourse corrections on the part of reflex systems which frequently have rather long loop times; second, they predict substantial variation in the execution of a given behavior pattern, since any number of different combinations of muscle activity might, in principle, yield the same proprioceptive return. Neither of these features has been observed in the motor systems studied so far.

Sensory templates might, however, be useful in the development of a motor pattern. In one case, that of song development in certain passerine birds, they are known to be involved in exactly that way (see Nottebohm, 1970, for review). Young white-crowned sparrows develop the characteristic song provided that they have heard a male of the same species sing in their first summer, and provided they can then hear their own efforts to sing. It appears that feedback is being compared with a centrally stored version of the 'song'. But once it is developed feedback is unnecessary: Deafening an adult white-crown does not affect its song at all. The song sparrow lacks the early sensitivity of the templates to environmental influence; but, like the white-crown, the deafened song sparrow cannot perfect its own song. Sensory feedback is thus employed to transfer a stored pattern from the sensory to the motor side of the central nervous system.

A motor program that is independent of contemporaneous information from the periphery is called a motor score or program. As the above example shows, motor scores are not necessarily genetically wired. They could be, but, alternatively, they could be established by environmental influences during development. These influences might, in principle, act in any of the following ways:

1) by modulating the properties of a sensory template, which in turn applies its pattern to the motor score;
2) by programming central connections directly, through meeting the stimulus requirements of a cell that rejects input unless it is activated by the right spatiotemporal pattern of arriving activity (cf Stent, 1973).

3) by patterning connections according to myotypic influence, that is, by allowing a peripheral genetic map to exert a secondary influence over the making of central connections. Although in fact this is a variant of genetic wiring, it would be called 'epigenetic' in the classical terminology of developmental biology.

Evidence from a number of systems favors the most straightforward hypothesis of genetic control. Many motor scores are actually elaborated long before they are used (Bentley and Hoy, 1972) - indeed, before the peripheral apparatus required for their expression has developed. In such cases, it is improbable that the central circuitry is influenced by sensory feedback. Some locomotor rhythms can be expressed even though (1) the motor nerves have been prevented from reaching the structures they normally innervate, and (2) no sensory connections have been allowed to form between the moving parts and the CNS (Davis and Davis, 1973). It is difficult to avoid the conclusion that the genome is sufficient for the elaboration of motor scores.

This conclusion poses two further questions: First, if the momentary state of a movement is not communicated to other parts of the pattern generator by sensory feedback, what does distribute that kind of information? Second, if proprioceptors are not required for the phasing of motor output, what are they good for?

It appears that the first requirement is met by phase-coordinating elements that have some (thought not all) of the properties of efference copy neurones. The basic cycle of a motor program is distributed to other control centers involved in related subroutines; this co-ordinating signal affects the second output in such a way that the phase relation between the two is constant despite variations in cycle period. Such elements, though not described until recently (Stein, 1971; Davis, et al., 1973), are critical components of pattern-generating circuits. The definition of efference copy (von Holst, 1954) was developed in connection with perceptual problems, and hence traditionally required that the copy be returned to the sensorium. Since the function of phase co-ordination is probably a widespread and important use of the basic principle of motor return, the definition should be broadened to include it.

ROLE OF PROPRIOCEPTION

A variety of receptors - not all of them associated with tendons, joints or muscles - have the basic function of determining whether a movement is being completed on schedule. They accomplish this by measuring external inertial forces that retard muscles from reaching their commanded length. In principle, such 'load compensation' could be accomplished by any receptor in series with a muscle (located in the tendon, for example) that could respond to passive loading as well as to active contraction. In this case, a given motor command would excite the receptor more if the system were loaded than if it were unloaded. If the afferent signals then excite motoneurones that innervate the muscles from which they come, extra excitation will be supplied to the movement. The difficulty is that tendon receptors report a sum and not a difference: The system has no reference level without some independent register of its own efferent activity. This may be why series-arranged tendon organs are used for quite different purposes in vertebrates, though perhaps not in invertebrates.

Co-activated parallel receptor muscles avoid this difficulty. They receive the same commands as the working muscle, and ideally they shorten at a somewhat higher rate in an unloaded movement: that is, the receptor muscle is said to 'lead' the working muscle. This condition is called 'alpha-gamma linkage' when it occurs in the mammalian muscle spindle, and results from the fact that central commands impinge jointly on the large alpha motoneurones innervating working muscles and small gamma motoneurones innervating their spindles. The smaller cells have lower thresholds, presumably owing to the 'size principle' (Henneman, et al., 1965), and loading of the parallel working muscles retards their shortening and increases the afferent discharge from the receptor. This kind of arrangement has evolved at least twice: in the crustacean MRO (Fields, 1966; Fields al., 1967) and in the mammalian muscle spindle (Kuffler, et al., 1951). In the former case, coactivation occurs because the same neurones innervate receptor and working muscles; a parallel excitatory input of the kind involved in gamma bias is unnecessary. Von Euler's group has shown that in the mammalian respiratory system this kind of arrangement accomplishes load compensation (Corda et al., 1965; Critchlow and von Euler, 1963), and similar evidence for the MRO has been gathered in our laboratory at Stanford (Fields et al., 1967; Page and Sokolove, 1972; Sokolove, 1973).

An important extension of this view holds that any receptor capable of detecting relative movement between organism and environment can function in a load-compensating circuit. In the abdominal appendages of crustaceans, for example, a cyclic locomotor movement programmed in the central nervous system is employed to generate forward thrust (Hughes and Wiersma, 1960; Wiersma and Ikeda, 1964). The appendages themselves are fringed with fine hairs; as the appendage moves through the water during the powerstroke, the hairs bend in relation to it. Davis (1969a, b) showed that this bending in turn excites the powerstroke motoneurones. If one looks at the relative movement of the organism and the water, this reflex can be interpreted in terms of load compensation. Consider the limiting case in which the rate of forward movement of the organism equals the velocity of the powerstroke. Under these conditions the medium exerts no restoring force against the moving appendage, and the hairs are not bent. At all lower velocities of locomotion, the appendage is doing work on the medium, and the bending of the hairs is proportional to the force exerted. The value is maximum when the organism lies 'dead in the water'. Just as in the case of the MRO or muscle spindle, the incremental excitation supplied by the load-compensating circuit is proportional to the load.

At what point in the chain of motor command should load-compensating feedback be supplied? Two principles seem quite general, and make good theoretical sense.

1. The feedback should not be self-reexciting. MRO afferents do not innervate the motoneurones that go to the receptor muscle; spindle afferents do not excite fusimotor neurones. If these connections were made, additional receptor excitation would occur, and the proportionality between load and sensory return would be lost.

2. The feedback should be supplied at the lowest level in the motor control circuit. In most cyclic motor programs, the neurones or networks comprising the oscillator are presynaptic to themotoneurones. In several of the systems that have been intensively studied there is a fixed relationship between the period of the oscillator and the amplitude of the oscillation: in other words, the motor output is stronger at short cycle lengths (Davis and Kennedy, 1972). The output amplitude can be manipulated independently

only at a point in the circuit downstream from that at which this proportionality is established.

The basic program for stereotyped, cyclic behaviours is thus viewed as a central phenomenon, modulated in strength but not in frequency by peripheral input. Phase co-ordination is accomplished by links between neurones or networks, whose nature we do not know except that they produce a temporally modulated output and may therefore be called oscillators. But what is a segmental oscillator? We do not know how much of the output pattern is conferred by connectivity between neurones, and how much by the endogenous properties of single cells. Conventional wisdom holds that most output patterning is an emergent property, dependent upon connectivity for its basic structure. Models like that proposed by Wilson and Waldron (1968) for insect flight, which depends upon reciprocal inhibition, have dominated our view of pattern-generating circuits up to now. But, in a variety of systems, recent results (eg. Maynard, 1972) suggest instead that oscillatory properties inherent in single neurones may be adequate to determine the basic cycle timing.

REFERENCES

Bentley, D.R., and Hoy, R.R., 1972. Genetic control of the neural network generating cricket (Teleogryllus gryllus) song patterns. Anim. Behav. 20, 478-492.

Corda, M., Eklund, G., and von Euler, C., 1965. External intercostal and phrenic α motor responses to changes in respiratory load. Acta Physiol. Scand. 63, 391-400.

Critchlow, V., and von Euler, C., 1963. Intercostal muscle spindle activity and its gamma motor control. J. Physiol. 168, 820-847.

Davis, W.J., 1969a. Reflex organization in the swimmeret system of the lobster. I. Intrasegmental reflexes. J. Exp. Biol. 51, 547-563.

Davis, W.J., 1969b. Reflex organization in the swimmeret system of the lobster. II. Reflex dynamics. J. Exp. Biol. 51, 565-573.

Davis, W.J., and Davis, K.B., 1973. Ontogeny of a simple locomotor system: role of the periphery in the development of central nervous circuitry. Amer. Zool. 13, 409-426.

Davis, W.J., and Kennedy, D., 1972. Command interneurons controlling swimmeret movements in the lobster. I. Types of effects on motoneurons. J. Neurophysiol. 35, 1-12.

Davis, W.J., Siegler, M.V.S., and Mpitsos, G.J., 1973. Distributed neuronal oscillators and efference copy in the feeding system of Pleurobranchaea . J. Neurophysiol. 36, 258-274.

Fields, H.L., 1966. Proprioceptive control of posture in the crayfish abdomen. J. Exp. Biol. 44, 455-468.

Fields, H.L., Evoy, W.H. and Kennedy, D., 1967. Reflex role
  played by efferent control of an invertebrate stretch receptor.
  J. Neurophysiol. 30, 859-874.
Gray, J., 1950. The role of peripheral sense organs during
  locomotion in the vertebrates. Symp. Soc. Exp. Biol. 4, 112-126.
Henneman, E., Somjen, G. and Carpenter, D.O., 1965. Functional
  significance of cell size in spinal motoneurons. J. Neurophysiol.
  28, 560-580.
Holst, E. von., 1954. Relations between the central nervous system
  and the peripheral organs. Brit. J. Anim. Behav. 2, 89-94.
Hoyle, G., 1964. Exploration of neuronal mechanisms underlying
  behavior in insects. In Neural Theory and Modeling. Stanford
  Univ. Press. pp. 346-376.
Hughes, G.M., and Wiersma, C.A.G., 1960. The coordination of
  swimmeret movements in the crayfish, Procambarus clarkii
  (Girard). J. Exp. Biol. 37, 657-670.
Kuffler, S.W., Hunt, C.C. and Quilliam, J.P., 1951. Function
  of medullated small nerve fibers in mammalian ventral roots:
  efferent muscle spindle innervation. J. Neurophysiol. 14, 29-54.
Maynard, D.M., 1972. Simpler networks. Ann. N.Y. Acad. Sci.
  193, 59-72.
Mellon, DeF., 1969. The reflex control of rhythmic motor output
  during swimming in the scallop. Z. Vergl. Physiol. 62, 318-336.
Nottebohm, F., 1970. Ontogeny of bird song. Science 167, 950-956.
Page, C.H. and Sokolove, P.G., 1972. Crayfish muscle receptor
  organ: role in regulation of postural flexion. Science 175 647-650.
Sokolove, P.G., 1973. Crayfish stretch receptor and motor unit
  behavior during abdominal extension. J. Comp. Physiol. In press.
Stein, P.G., 1971. Intersegmental coordination of swimmeret
  motoneuron activity in crayfish. J. Neurophysiol. 34, 310-318.
Stent, G.S., 1973. A physiological mechanism for Hebbs'
  postualte of learning. Proc. Nat. Acad. Sci. U.S. 70, 997-1001.
Wiersma, C.A.G. and Ikeda, K., 1964. Interneurons commanding
  swimmeret movements in the crayfish, Procambarus clarkii
  (Girard). Comp. Biochem. Physiol. 12, 509-525.
Wilson, D.M., and Waldron, I., 1968. Models for the generation
  of the motor output pattern in flying locusts. Proc. Inst.
  Elec. Electron. Eng. 56, 1058-1064.

NEURONAL ORGANIZATION AND ONTOGENY IN THE LOBSTER SWIMMERET SYSTEM

W. J. Davis

The Thimann Laboratories, University of California
Santa Cruz, California

General principles of neuronal organization and ontogeny in locomotor systems are explored, using the lobster swimmeret system as a model. Centrally, this motor system consists of command interneurones that activate segmental ganglionic oscillators that in turn drive the swimmeret motoneurones. Several sensory receptors excite the command interneurones, and in some cases the corresponding receptive fields have been mapped on the periphery. Swimmeret motoneurones are normally recruited in order of increasing size. The motoneurones follow this size principle also in their effects on muscles (smaller motoneurones have less effect) and in their normal discharge patterns (smaller motoneurones show less adaptation).

Strong intra- and intersegmental swimmeret reflexes are organized so that cyclic proprioceptive feedback from the appendages is routed to the motoneurones but not to the central oscillators. By this arrangement, the sensory feedback phasically amplifies the central motor program without fundamentally influencing its internal temporal structure.

During ontogeny, the swimmeret system develops postembryonically in several discrete developmental stages. To test the hypothesis of peripheral specification of central nervous circuitry, presumptive swimmeret sense organs and muscles were ablated prior to their differentiation. The corresponding swimmeret motoneurones nevertheless grew and formed central connections, as evidenced by the appearance of normal patterns of rhythmic locomotor discharge and normal reflexes at the usual times. Therefore, neither sensory nor myotypic specification of the central circuitry occurs in the ontogeny of this locomotor program; instead, the genetic "blueprint" for the motor program is stored entirely within the central nervous system.

Findings from the swimmeret system are compared with analogous findings from vertebrate motor systems.

INTRODUCTION

A lobster has upon its tail four pairs of ventral appendages, the abdominal pleopods, or swimmerets. These appendages undergo rhythmic, metachronal movements that participate in locomotion, respiration, reproduction, righting and optomotor responses. The swimmeret system has been extensively studied as a general model of locomotor systems (Hughes and Wiersma, 1960; Wiersma and Ikeda, 1964; Ikeda and Wiersma, 1964; Davis, 1968a, b, c, 1969a, b, c, 1970, 1971, 1973; Davis and Murphey, 1969; Davis and Ayers, 1972; Davis and Kennedy, 1972a, b, c; Davis and Davis, 1973; Stein, 1971). My purpose here is to review the major conclusions of these studies and to present some new data, with the aim of highlighting those general principles of neuronal organization that the swimmeret system shares in common with other motor systems in invertebrates and vertebrates alike.

CENTRAL ORGANIZATION

Command Interneurones

Wiersma and his colleagues first showed that the swimmeret rhythm can be elicited from the isolated, deafferented abdomen by electrically stimulating central nerve cells (Hughes and Wiersma, 1960; Wiersma and Ikeda, 1964; Ikeda and Wiersma, 1964). This pioneering work not only provided the first rigorous proof that motor programs are endogenous to the central nervous system; it also showed that such programs are under the control of central command neurones. More detailed studies on swimmeret command neurones disclosed that they have broadly-distributed

peripheral receptive fields (Davis and Kennedy, 1972a; Fig. 1A),
and thus that these cells are interneurones rather than primary
sensory neurones known to project intersegmentally (Wiersma
and Hughes, 1961). Stimulation of tactile receptors on the ventral
and lateral surfaces of the tail readily induces swimmeret beating
in an isolated abdomen, and the same stimulus has a potent excitatory influence on the discharge of swimmeret command interneurones (Fig. 1B). Presumably these afferent receptors mediate
positive feedback reinforcement of forward locomotion, e.g.
swimming in the larvae, much as wind receptors on the head of a
locust mediate positive feedback reinforcement of flight (Weis-Fogh,
1949). Additional sensory organs also activate swimmeret beating,
e.g. the statocyst receptors (Davis, 1968c), and the eyes (Davis
and Ayers, 1972), presumably by means of the command interneurones. Direct evidence in support of this proposal is lacking,
for recordings of command fibre activity in semi-intact animals
have not yet been made.

The principal conclusions of studies on the central organization
of swimmeret command interneurones concern the issue of redun-
dancy. At least five swimmeret command cells exist on each side
of the ventral nerve cord, but none of these has precisely the same
effect on motor output. Moreover, none can alone elicit the full
range of output seen in intact lobsters (Davis and Kennedy, 1972a).
Instead, each command cell is specialized to control a different,
and in some cases highly restricted, fraction of the output range,
suggesting that the overt behaviour results from the concerted
action of more than one command interneurone. Indeed, stimulation
of command interneurones in pairs has shown that the simultaneous
activity can, by excitatory summation, produce the full range of
efferent output seen in intact lobsters (Davis and Kennedy, 1972b).
We are reminded that in mammals, the details of motor performance can be predicted more accurately from measures of activity
in several pyramidal cells than from activity in only one cell
(Humphrey et al., 1970). Proof that swimmeret beating in intact
lobsters normally results from the combined action of several
command interneurones, however, must await recording from these
cells during voluntary behaviour - a technically difficult feat at
best.

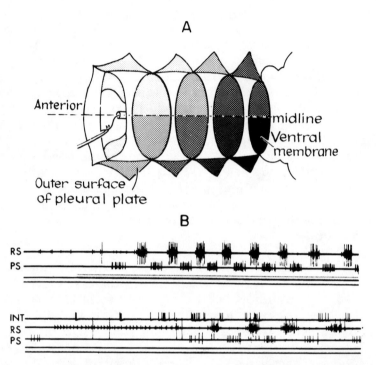

Fig. 1. Receptive field and efferent effects of a single swimmeret command interneurone. A. Schematic ventral surface of
a lobster's abdomen (swimmerets absent), showing areas that
effectively excite the command interneurone whose effects are
shown below. Stronger effects are designated by darker stiple.
Note bilateral effects (but strongest ipsilaterally), and decline
in efficacy from rear to front. (From Davis and Kennedy, unpublished data). B. Input and output of a single command fibre.
Upper record, recording of motor output from the power stroke
(PS) and return stroke (RS) motoneurones of a single deafferented swimmeret during electrical stimulation of a single command fibre. The third and fourth traces are a stimulus monitor
and a time base (1 mark/10 msec). Lower record, recording
from the command interneurone (INT) during tactile stimulation
of the ventral membrane. Note discharge of the command fibre
and simultaneous motor output. (From Davis and Kennedy, 1972a).

Oscillators

The unpatterned activity of command interneurones is translated into rhythmic motor discharge by central nervous oscillators. Although nothing is known about the composition of the swimmeret oscillators, some of their major properties have been inferred from careful examination of the efferent output that they cause. First, each abdominal ganglion - perhaps each hemi-ganglion - has its own oscillator, since an individual ganglion can produce rhythmic output in isolation from its neighbours. Second, each oscillator produces an approximately sinusoidal signal whose amplitude varies inversely with period (Fig. 2; Davis, 1968a,

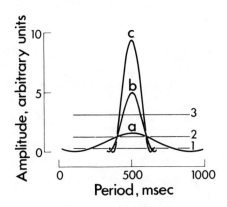

Fig. 2. Schematization of a hypothetical model to account for rhythmic motor output in the swimmeret system. The sine waves (a-c) represent excitatory input to motoneurones having different thresholds (1-3). The chief features of the model are: (1) the excitation is sinusoidal; (2) the amplitude of the excitation is inversely related to period; and (3) the details of motor activity are determined by differences in motoneurone threshold that are related to motoneurone size (from Davis, 1971).

1969a, 1971; Davis and Murphey, 1969; Davis and Kennedy, 1972c). As a result of this relationship, the strength of the swimmeret movements increases with the frequency of the rhythm. Third, the sinusoidal signal is received simultaneously by synergic motoneurones supplying a given swimmeret (Davis and Kennedy, 1972c) with the detailed pattern of efferent impulses generated at the motoneurone level according to functional properties associated

with motoneurone size (see below). Fourth, the oscillator probably
simultaneously excites synergists and inhibits antagonists (Davis
and Kennedy, 1972c), as found also in the crustacean ventilatory
system (Mendelson, 1971), but direct evidence in support of this
proposal is lacking.

Size Principle

The relative simplicity of invertebrate preparations in general
has permitted a detailed examination of the functional implications
of motoneurone size in the swimmeret system. As the frequency of
stimulation of single swimmeret command interneurones is increased, the motoneurones are recruited in order of increasing
size (Davis, 1971), as found also in vertebrates (Henneman, 1957;
Granit et al., 1957; Henneman et al., 1965a, b; Somjen et al.,
1965; Burke, 1968; Fedde et al., 1969). Motoneurones are also
recruited by size within each cycle of motor output (Davis and
Kennedy, 1972c). This "size principle" has further implications
(Fig. 3); increasing motoneurone size, determined by measuring
soma diameter and axonal conduction velocity, is associated with:
(1) greater adaptation by the motoneurones to injected current;
(2) less tendency to discharge repetively; (3) larger excitatory
junctional potentials (ejp's) in the muscle fibres they innervate;
and (4) less facilitation of the ejp during repetitive stimulation.
Findings analogous to these have been reported for vertebrate
motoneurones (Granit et al., 1957; Bradley and Somjen, 1961;
Sasaki and Otani, 1961; Ushiyama et al., 1966; Burke, 1967;
Burke et al., 1971) and recently for locust flight (Hinkle and
Camhi, 1972) and walking (Burrows and Hoyle, 1973) motoneurones.
It seems fair to conclude that size principle is a general feature
of both invertebrate and vertebrate motor systems, although
exceptions are known (Granit and Burke, 1973).

Intersegmental Coupling

The existence of independent ganglionic oscillators in the
swimmeret system implies the need for coupling between them
during co-ordinated swimmeret beating. The work of Wiersma
and his colleagues (Hughes and Wiersma, 1960; Wiersma and Ikeda,
1964; Ikeda and Wiersma, 1964) and Stein (1971) has shown that this
coupling is accomplished by a specific class of ascending and descending interneurones. These intersegmental coupling neurones

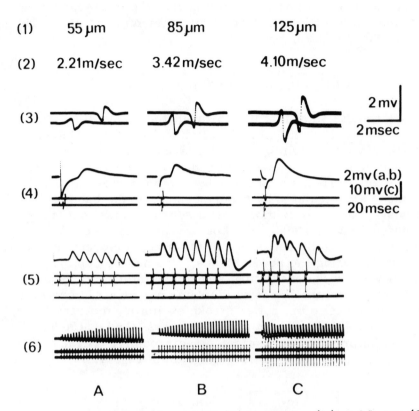

Fig. 3. Properties of a small (A), medium (B) and large (C) motoneurone innervating the main power stroke muscle. (1) soma diameters; (2) axonal conduction velocities; (3) amplitudes of action potentials recorded with two extracellular electrodes at different positions on the motor nerve; (4) amplitudes of excitatory junctional potentials (ejp's) recorded from a single muscle fibre (upper trace in each record); (5) adaptation to a maintained intracellular depolarizing current; and (6) facilitation properties of extracellular ejp's (upper trace in each record) during 50 Hz stimulation. Note anti-facilitation produced by the largest motoneurone. Time marks in (5) (lowest trace), 1/10 msec (from Davis, 1971).

carry a corollary of motor output from one abdominal segment to the next, resulting in the co-ordination of adjacent limbs. Antidromic stimulation of small bundles that contain these coupling

interneurones resets the burst rhythm (Stein, personnal communication), raising the interesting possibility that these interneurones
not only couple the oscillators of adjacent segments, but also form
part or all of the oscillator pool.

REFLEX ORGANIZATION

The above results show that the co-ordinated locomotor output
underlying swimmeret beating can be elicited from the isolated,
deafferented nervous system by stimulation of command interneurones, and thus that the swimmeret rhythm is centrally programmed. Strong reflexes also contribute to the motor output;
however, these are mediated by proprioceptors in the base of
each appendage, and also by more distal sensory setae that fringe
each appendage (Davis, 1969b, c). Both the proprioceptors and
the setae are activated by retraction of the limb, a movement that
occurs naturally during the power stroke. The proprioceptors
excite both power stroke and return stroke excitatory motoneurones,
but silence peripheral inhibitors to the same muscles. In contrast,
the sensory setae excite the power stroke excitatory motoneurones,
but profoundly inhibit the return stroke exciters (Davis, 1969b, c);
peripheral inhibitors are again affected reciprocally. These findings
are summarized in the reflex wiring diagram of Fig. 4.

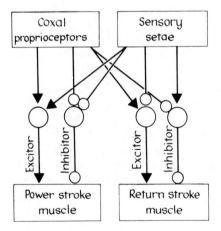

Fig. 4. Reflex organization in the swimmeret system. Filled
arrowheads designate excitatory connections, while open circles
designate inhibitory connections. See text for further description
(After Davis, 1969b).

From the above data one may infer that both the proprioceptors and the sensory setae reinforce the power stroke movement by means of positive feedback. During the power stroke the excitation provided by the proprioceptors to return stroke motoneurones is completely cancelled by inhibition from the setae. At the end of the power stroke, however, as the limb velocity necessarily decreases, the inhibitory feedback from the setae to the return stroke motoneurones is correspondingly reduced. Hence the return stroke motoneurones are released so that they may respond to the excitatory influence of the proprioceptors that are now maximally stretched.

Although the intrasegmental swimmeret reflexes reinforce the power stroke and also help to initiate the return stroke, both of these features of the motor program occur in absence of sensory feedback. Hence the reflexes must at most play a supplementary role. Furthermore, no reflex is available to initiate the power stroke of each movement cycle, which must therefore originate centrally. We are led to the most important corollary of the above interpretation; namely, the swimmeret reflexes are incapable of contributing to the periodicity seen in the normal locomotor program.

What then is the relative role of the swimmeret reflexes? An answer is provided by experimentally conflicting the sensory feedback from the swimmeret with the activity of the endogenous central oscillators. Such an artificial competition between reflex and central mechanisms was implemented in detached abdomens by forcibly moving a swimmeret to different positions while recording the cyclic motor output to the return stroke motoneurones of the same appendage. Retracting the swimmeret, which stretches the excitatory proprioceptors, increases the number of impulses in each return stroke burst and also increases the average discharge frequency of individual motoneurones (Fig. 5). The frequency of the rhythm, however, is unchanged (Figs. 5, 6). Activation of the inhibitory setae reduces both the number of impulses in each burst and also the discharge frequency, but again the frequency of the rhythm is unchanged (Fig. 7). In other words, sensory feedback from the swimmeret movements influences the amplitude of motoneurone bursts, but not the period of the rhythm. These results indicate that the feedback is returned to the motoneurones rather than to the neuronal oscillator that drives them. By this arrangement, the sensory feedback amplifies the central motor score, but does not control its timing. This and other features of the swimmeret

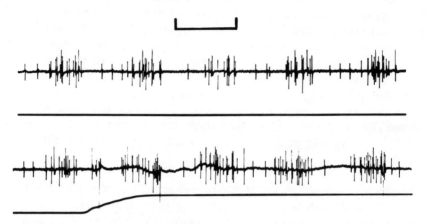

Fig. 5. Activation of the swimmeret reflexes during spontaneous,
rhythmic motor output. Upper trace in each record, extracellular
recording from the return stroke motoneurones of one swimmeret;
lower trace, position of the appendage (upward deflection corresponds to forced limb retraction). Continuous records. Limb retraction causes more intense bursts but no change in frequency
of the rhythm. Time mark, 500 msec.

system are incorporated in the general wiring diagram of Fig. 8.

Intersegmental swimmeret reflexes also contribute to the motor
output programs. These are organized exactly like the intrasegmental reflexes, except they extend between segments (Davis, unpublished observations). Moreover, the intersegmental reflexes are
polarized; anterior-going reflexes are strong, but posterior-going
ones are absent. By this arrangement they presumably reinforce
the rear-to-front metachrony that characterizes the normal swimmeret movements. The intersegmental reflexes may utilize the
same central pathways as the intersegmental coupling information
described above, but this possibility has not been tested.

ONTOGENY

The data reviewed above provide sufficient background for experimental rather than purely descriptive studies on the swimmeret
system. This system is especially amenable to ontogenetic studies,
because most of its development occurs in a series of post-

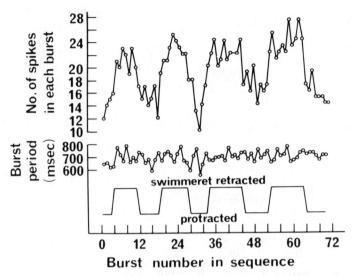

Fig. 6. Graph of data like that shown in Fig. 5. Alternately retracting and protracting the swimmeret changes the number of spikes/burst but does not alter the burst period (time between the initiation of successive bursts).

embryonic stages. When the larvae hatch, the swimmerets are represented externally by four pairs of undifferentiated limb buds. Light and electron microscopy has confirmed that the swimmeret muscles and sense organs are not yet formed at this time, but recordings from the ventral nerve cord show rhythmic bursts of action potentials that recur with the same period as swimmeret movements in more advanced stages (Davis and Davis, 1973). These results suggest that the central oscillators and the intersegmental coupling interneurones are operative when the laevae hatch, but simply not yet connected to a differentiated motor apparatus. By the end of the first larval stage, 2-3 days after hatching, the appendages are partially differentiated and undergo spontaneous, twitching movements. The swimmerets are not fully developed and capable of rhythmic, co-ordinated movements, however, until the end of the third larval stage, nearly 3 weeks after hatching.

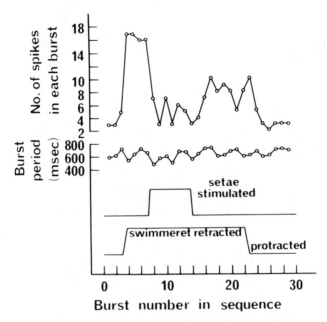

Fig. 7. Effect of swimmeret retraction (excitatory) and setae stimulation (inhibitory) on spontaneous, rhythmic bursts in return stroke motoneurones. Swimmeret retraction increases the number of spikes/burst, while setae stimulation markedly reduces the number of spikes/burst. Neither sensory input alters the burst period.

The above developmental scheme enabled us to test a hypothesis that has been studied and debated for nearly a century, namely, the hypothesis that peripheral structures specify the central nervous connections of motor systems during ontogeny. Peripheral sense organs could, in principle, help to designate central connections by furnishing essential feedback from movements in a developing motor system (e.g. Hamburger, 1970; Jacobson, 1970; Gaze, 1970). Muscles could play an analogous role in establishing central circuitry by the well-known hypothesis of myotypic specification (Weiss, 1936, 1937, 1941; Jacobson, 1970; Gaze, 1970).

To test the hypothesis of peripheral specification in the swimmeret system, presumptive swimmeret sense organs and muscles were destroyed immediately after the larvae hatched (Davis, 1973; Davis and Davis, 1973). The swimmeret motoneurones nevertheless

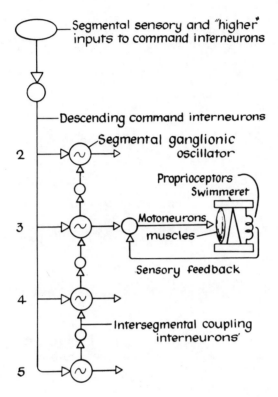

Fig. 8. Summary of the neuronal organization of the swimmeret system. Numbers on the left designate abdominal segments. A schematic swimmeret is shown only for the third segment. See text for further description.

grew normally, terminating blindly in undifferentiated "scar" tissue at the site of the ablation. Electrophysiological recordings made from such motoneurones in fourth stage and older larvae showed that normal swimmeret reflexes and normal cyclic motor programs were acquired at the usual time (Fig. 9; Davis, 1973; Davis and Davis, 1973). In other words, depriving the swimmeret motoneurones of feedback from their normal sense organs and of

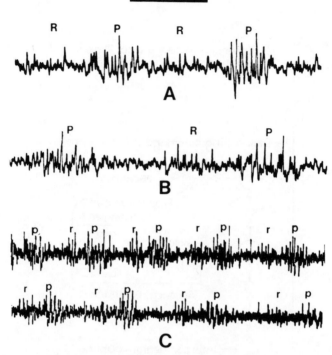

Fig. 9. Extracellular recordings from a swimmeret nerve of sixth-stage larvae during "voluntary" swimmeret beating. A. normal (unoperated) specimens, B and C. Presumptive swimmeret destroyed in the early first stage. P and R, power stroke and return stroke discharge, respectively. The two traces in C are continuous. Time mark, 50 msec in A and B, 100 msec in C (from Davis, 1973).

contact with their normal target muscles did not interfere with the normal developmental sequence or timetable of the central apparatus. We are forced to the conclusion that in this simple invertebrate locomotor system, at least, specification of central nervous connections by peripheral structures does not occur. Independence between the periphery and the central nervous system apparently characterizes not only the generation of the adult motor program but also its formation during ontogeny. The genetic "blueprint" for this motor system must be stored entirely in the central nervous system - a feature which certainly complicates further analysis.

COMPARISON WITH VERTEBRATE MOTOR SYSTEMS

To what extent do the studies reviewed above furnish general principles of neuronal organization, applicable also to the more complicated and less accessible motor systems of mammals? Recent studies on cat locomotion have revealed several fundamental similtarities with the lobster swimmeret system (Arshavsky et al., 1972a, b; Engberg and Lundberg, 1969; Lundberg, 1971; Lundberg and Weight, 1971; Orlovsky, 1969, 1972a, b, c; Orlovsky and Pavolva, 1972; Shik et al., 1966a, b). First, the major features of the locomotor output in the cat are programmed centrally; their expression does not require intact intrasegmental reflexes. Second, the oscillators that underlie cat locomotion are distributed widely in the central nervous system. In fact, it appears that, as in the swimmeret system, each limb has its own pattern generating machinery. Third, the central oscillators underlying cat locomotion are apparently interconnected by neurones in the ventral spinocerebellar tract that transmit a corollary of motor discharge. These cells, presumably interneurones, carry bursts of impulses that occur at the same time as motor bursts and ascend from lower to higher centres (Arshavsky et al., 1972b), exactly as found in the swimmeret system and also in other invertebrate motor systems (Davis, Siegler and Mpitsos, 1973). Fourth, size principle, with all of its implications for motoneurone recruitment patterns and physiology, applies equally well to lobsters and to cats. Finally, complex patterns of neuronal activity develop in cultured spinal cords of rodents, suggesting that here also the formation of central circuitry is independent of feedback from peripheral structures (Crain, 1966; Coner and Crain, 1972). This hypothesis requires more definitive testing, however, perhaps by means of experiments similar in design to those performed on larval lobsters.

Invertebrates and vertebrates are, of course, constructed along much different lines, and it may prove simplistic to expect exact parallels in neuronal organization. The identification of so many common denominators, however, suggests fundamental similarities in the underlying organizational principles. In this case, we may expect that extrapolation of generalities from lower to higher organisms will prove as beneficial to neurophysiology as it has to genetics and molecular biology.

Acknowledgment. Supported by NIH Research Grant NS-09050.

REFERENCES

Arshavsky, Ju.J., Berkinblitt, M.B., Fuxon, O.J., Gelfand, J.M.
   and Orlovsky, G.N., 1972a. Recordings of neurons of the dorsal
   spino-cerebellar tract during locomotion. Brain Res. 43, 272-275.
Arshavsky, Ju.J., Berkinblitt, M.B., Fuxon, O.J., Gelfand, J.M.
   and Orlovsky, G.N., 1972b. Origin of modulation in neurons of
   the ventral spino-cerebellar tract during locomotion. Brain
   Res. 43, 276-279.
Bradley, K. and Somjen, G., 1961. Accommodation in motoneurones
   of the rat and the cat. J. Physiol. 156, 75-92.
Burke, R.E., 1967. Motor unit types of cat triceps surae muscle.
   J. Physiol. 193, 141-160.
Burke, R.E., 1968. Firing patterns of gastrocnemius motor units
   in the decerebrate cat. J. Physiol. 196, 631-654.
Burke, R.E., Levine, D.N., Zajac, F.E., III, Tsairis, P. and
   Engel, W.K., 1971. Mammalian motor units: Physiological-
   histochemical correlation in three types in cat gastrocnemius.
   Science 174, 709-712.
Burrows, M. and Hoyle, G., 1973. Neural mechanisms underlying
   behavior in the locust Schistocerca gregaria. III. Topography
   of limb motoneurons in the metathoracic ganglion. J. Neurobiol.
   4, 167-186.
Corner, M.A. and Crain, S.M., 1972. Patterns of spontaneous
   bioelectric activity during maturation in culture of fetal
   rodent medulla and spinal cord tissues. J. Neurobiol. 3, 25-45.
Crain, S.M., 1966. Development of "organotypic" bioelectric
   activities in central nervous tissues during maturation in
   culture. Int. Rev. Neurobiol. 9, 1-43.
Davis, W.J., 1968a. Quantitative analysis of swimmeret beating
   in the lobster. J. Exp. Biol. 48, 643-662.
Davis, W.J., 1968b. The neuromuscular basis of lobster swimmeret
   beating. J. Exp. Zool. 168, 363-378.
Davis, W.J., 1968c. Lobster righting responses and their neural
   control. Proc. Roy. Soc. B 170, 435-456.
Davis, W.J., 1969a. The neural control of swimmeret beating in
   the lobster. J. Exp. Biol. 50, 99-118.
Davis, W.J., 1969b. Reflex organization in the swimmeret system
   of the lobster. I. Intrasegmental reflexes. J. Exp. Biol.
   51, 547-563.
Davis, W.J., 1969c. Reflex organization in the swimmeret system
   of the lobster. II. Reflex dynamics. J. Exp. Biol. 51, 565-573.
Davis, W.J., 1970. Motoneuron morphology and synaptic contacts:
   Determination by intracellular dye injection. Science 168,
   1358-1360.
Davis, W.J., 1971. Functional significance of motoneuron size and
   soma position in swimmeret system of the lobster. J. Neurophysiol.
   34, 274-288.

Davis, W.J., 1973. Development of locomotor patterns in absence of peripheral sense organs and muscles. Proc. Nat. Acad. Sci. 70, 954-958.

Davis, W.J. and Ayers, J.L., 1972. Locomotion: Control by positive feedback optokinetic responses. Science 177, 183-185.

Davis, W.J. and Davis, K.B., 1973. Ontogeny of a simple locomotor system: Role of the periphery in specifying the development of the central nervous system. Amer. Zool. 13, 409-425.

Davis, W.J. and Murphey, R.K., 1969. Bursting patterns of swimmeret motoneurons in the lobster, simulated with a digital computer. J. Exp. Biol. 50, 119-128.

Davis, W.J. and Kennedy, D., 1972a. Command interneurons controlling swimmeret movements in the lobster. I. Types of effects on motoneurons. J. Neurophysiol. 35, 1-12.

Davis, W.J. and Kennedy, D., 1972b. Command interneurons controlling swimmeret movements in the lobster. II. Interaction of effects on motoneurons. J. Neurophysiol. 35, 13-19.

Davis, W.J. and Kennedy, D., 1972c. Command interneurons controlling swimmeret movements in the lobster. III. Temporal relationships among bursts in different motoneurons. J. Neurophysiol. 35, 20-29.

Davis, W.J., Siegler, M.V.S. and Mpitsos, G.J., 1973. Distributed neuronal oscillators and efference copy in the feeding system of Pleurobranchaea. J. Neurophysiol. 36, 258-274.

Engberg, I. and Lundberg, A., 1969. An electromyographic analysis of muscular activity in the hindlimb of the cat during unrestrained locomotion. Acta Physiol. Scand. 75, 614-630.

Fedde, M.R., De Wet, P.D. and Kitchell, R.L., 1969. Motor unit recruitment pattern and tonic activity in respiratory muscles of Gallus domesticus. J. Neurophysiol. 32, 995-1004.

Gaze, R.M., 1970. The Formation of Nerve Connections. Academic Press, N.Y.

Granit, R. and Burke, R.E., 1973. The control of movement and posture. Brain Res. 53, 1-28.

Granit, R., Phillips, C.G., Skoglund, S. and Steg, G., 1957. Differentiation of tonic from phasic alpha ventral horn cells by stretch, pinna and crossed extensor reflexes. J. Neurophysiol. 20, 470-481.

Hamburger, V., 1970. Embryonic motility in vertebrates. In The Neurosciences: Second Study Program, (Ed. Schmitt, F.O.) The Rockefeller Univ. Press, N.Y., pp. 141-151.

Henneman, E., 1957. Relation between size of neurons and their susceptibility to discharge. Science 126, 1345-1347.

Henneman, E., Somjen, G. and Carpenter, D.O., 1965a. Functional significance of cell size in spinal motoneurons. J. Neurophysiol. 28, 560-580.

Henneman, E., Somjen, G. and Carpenter, D.O., 1965b. Excitability and inhibitability of motoneurons of different sizes. J. Neurophysiol. 28, 599-620.

Hinkle, M. and Camhi, J.M., 1972. Locust motoneurons: Bursting activity correlated with axon diameter. Science 175, 553-556.

Hughes, G.M. and Wiersma, C.A.G., 1960. The co-ordination of swimmeret movements in the crayfish, Procambarus clarkii (Girard). J. Exp. Biol. 37, 657-670.

Humphrey, D.K., Schmidt, E.M. and Thompson, W.D., 1970. Predicting measures of motor performance from multiple cortical spike trains. Science 170, 758-762.

Ikeda, K. and Wiersma, C.A.G., 1964. Autogenic rhythmicity in the abdominal ganglia of the crayfish: The control of swimmeret movements. Comp. Biochem. Physiol. 12, 107-115.

Jacobson, M., 1970. Developmental Neurobiology. Holt, Rinehart and Winston, N.Y.

Lundberg, A., 1971. Function of the ventral spinocerebellar tract: A new hypothesis. Exp. Brain Res. 12, 317-330.

Lundberg, A. and Weight, F., 1971. Functional organization of connections to the ventral spinocerebellar tract. Exp. Brain Res. 12, 295-316.

Mendelson, M., 1971. Oscillator neurons in crustacean ganglia. Science 171, 1170-1173.

Orlovsky, G.N., 1969. Spontaneous and induced locomotion of the thalamic cat. Biofiz. 14, 1095-1102.

Orlovsky, G.N., 1972a. The effect of different descending systems on flexor and extensor activity during locomotion. Brain Res. 40, 359-372.

Orlovsky, G.N., 1972b. Activity of vestibulo-spinal neurons during locomotion. Brain Res. 46, 85-98.

Orlovsky, G.N., 1972c. Activity of rubrospinal neurons during locomotion. Brain Res. 46, 99-112.

Orlovsky, G.N. and Pavlova, G.A., 1972. Response of Deiter's neurons to tilt during locomotion. Brain Res. 42, 212-214.

Sasaki, K. and Otani, T., 1961. Accommodation in spinal motoneurons of the cat. Jap. J. Physiol. 11, 443-456.

Shik, M.L., Orlovsky, G.N. and Severin, F.V., 1966a. Organization of locomotor synergism. Biofiz. 11, 879-886.

Shik, M.L., Severin, F.V. and Orlovsky, G.N., 1966b. Control of walking and running by means of electrical stimulation of the midbrain. Biofiz. 11, 659-666.

Somjen, G., Carpenter, D.O. and Henneman, E., 1965. Responses of motoneurons of different sizes to graded stimulation of supra-spinal centers of the brain. J. Neurophysiol. 28, 958-965.

Stein, P.G.S., 1971. Intersegmental coordination of swimmeret motoneuron activity in crayfish. J. Neurophysiol. 34, 310-318.

Ushiyama, J., Koizumi, K. and Brooks, C. McC., 1966. Accommodative reactions of neuronal elements in the spinal cord. J. Neurophysiol. 29, 1028-1045.

Weis-Fogh, T., 1949. An aerodynamic sense organ stimulating and regulating flight in locusts. Nature 163, 873-874.

Weiss, P., 1936. Selectivity controlling the central-peripheral relations in the nervous system. Biol. Rev. 11, 494-531.

Weiss, P., 1937. Further experimental investigations on the
  phenomenon of homologous response in transplanted amphibian
  limbs. III. Homologous response in absence of sensory innervation. J. Comp. Neurol. 66, 537-548.
Weiss, P., 1941. Self-differentiation of the basic patterns of
  coordination. Comp. Psychol. Monogr. 17, 1-96.
Wiersma, C.A.G. and Hughes, G.M., 1961. On the functional anatomy
  of neuronal units in the abdominal cord of the crayfish,
  Procambarus clarkii (Girard). J. Comp. Neurol. 116, 209-228.
Wiersma, C.A.G. and Ikeda, K., 1964. Interneurons commanding
  swimmeret movements in the crayfish, Procambarus clarkii
  (Girard). Comp. Biochem. Physiol. 12, 509-525.

BURSTING MECHANISMS IN MOLLUSKAN LOCOMOTION

A. O. D. Willows, P. A. Getting and S. Thompson

Friday Harbor Laboratories, Washington and Department of Zoology, University of Washington, Seattle, Washington

Locomotion in animals almost invariably involves recurring bursts of impulses in motor neurones. In addition to the unsolved problems of mechanisms of patterning, and co-ordination, there remains the more fundamental issue of the origin of the membrane oscillations and the bursts themselves.

Numerous neurone types show spontaneous or elicitable bursting patterns in gastropod mollusks. The functions of some of these bursters in locomotion are known. The size and accessibility of these neurones permit analysis of features of the underlying mechanisms. We tested three bursting neurone types under four conditions to establish the effects of (i) wide variations in ambient temperature, (ii) bathing media containing high concentrations of Mg^{++}, to block synaptic interactions, (iii) direct injection of hyperpolarizing currents to reveal reversal potentials where possible, and (iv) ionic and drug agents supposed to interfere with Na^+-K^+ electrogenic pumping.

Bursting activity in each neurone type was found to respond differently to this set of tests. It was concluded that distinct mechanisms are involved in the generation of bursts in each of the three neurone types, and these are most likely: (i) chemically mediated synaptic interactions, (ii) cyclic electrogenic pumping or conductance changes, and (iii) electrically conducting junction interactions.

457

Apart from the flagellar or ciliary activity of single celled organisms, virtually every known form of locomotion in animals involves the generation of recurring co-ordinated bursts of impulses somewhere in the nervous system. It is evident from even superficial observation of locomotion in annelids, mollusks, arthropods, echinoderms and chordates, that the fundamental processes of locomotion, whether they be swimming, flying, crawling, hopping or perambulation, must involve the regular cyclic movement of body parts with respect to one another. It is likewise evident that where muscular contractions are involved in locomotion (and they are in the vast majority of cases) there must be an underlying neuronal basis for the observed cyclic, co-ordinated activity. A question which has never been satisfactorily and completely answered for any system involved in locomotory behaviour is how such patterns are generated and co-ordinated at the level of neurone-neurone interactions.

The question can be sub-divided into several interrelated parts. For any locomotory pattern one would like to know (i) how are individual bursts in single motor neurones generated? (ii) how are bursts in synergistic motor neurones co-ordinated both temporally and spatially? (iii) how are bursts in antagonistic motor neurones co-ordinated temporally and spatially? (iv) how is the overall sequence or pattern turned on, maintained, and then turned off at the appropriate times? Partial answers to some of these questions are becoming clear, particularly for invertebrate animals where the unit-level processes can be studied either centrally or peripherally in re-identifiable neurones. Thus, it has been found that flight and stridulation in insects (Kendig, 1968; Bentley, 1969), tail-flicking (Zucker et al., 1971) and cardiac activity (Watanabe, 1958) in crustacea, and swimming in opisthobranch mollusks (Willows et al., 1973) all involve synergistic neurones that interact positively one with another either through electrical interconnections or through chemically mediated synapses. In a few cells, antagonistic motor neurones have been proposed to interact through mutual inhibition (Bentley, 1969; Wilson, 1966; Willows et al., 1973). The events leading to initiation, maintenance and termination of locomotory patterns have also been studied in a few invertebrate examples. In insects (Elsner, 1969) and crustacea (Wiersma and Ikeda, 1964; Kennedy et al., 1966) and mollusks (Willows and Hoyle, 1969; Willows et al., 1973), it is known, for instance, that "decisions" about the initiation of rhythmic activity are made in particular neurones or neurone groups. Furthermore, the role of peripheral feedback in the generation and maintenance of these patterns has been found to be either tonic (Wilson, 1968) or unimportant (Dorsett et al., 1969, 1973).

On the other hand, the most fundamental question of all, viz. the first one relating to the mechanisms of cyclic burst formation in individual neurones, has received the least attention. With the exception of the observations of Wilson (1968) and Mendelson (1971), there is very little that can be said about the details of the burst generation process itself. This point is further emphasized by the frequent references to generalized diagrammatic representation of "central oscillators" that recur in the literature (Davis, 1968, 1969; Davis et al., 1973; Hoyle, 1970; Miller, 1967; Burrows and Willows, 1969).

Neurones having either spontaneous or elicitable bursting patterns are commonly encountered in the central ganglia of opisthobranch mollusks. In most cases, the bursts can be routinely recorded from re-identifiable neurones in different preparations of the same species and, even across species. The bursts take many forms (Fig. 1).

For some bursting neurone types in mollusks, the functional role of the bursts in the motor activities of the intact animal have been determined. Some drive withdrawal movements and initiation of swimming (TGN's, Fig. 1c), others are known to drive the flexion movements of swimming (flexion neurones, FN's, Fig. 1a), and still others drive movements of the buccal mass that are a part of the feeding process (Fig. 1e). Several other bursting neurone types have not yet been implicated in controlling any particular form of motor activity (e.g. the pleural ganglion neurones LP12, LP13 and RP12, Fig. 1b).

For many obvious reasons, including some implicit in what is outlined above, these neurones are useful experimental model systems for analysis of basic bursting mechanisms. The preliminary results presented in what follows argue that several fundamentally different mechanisms are involved in the generation of bursts in the different bursting types and conclusions can only be drawn as a result of the combination of several indirect tests. Fortunately, many gastropod neurones are sufficiently large (100-1000 μm in soma diameter) to permit simultaneous multiple intracellular electrode penetrations so that current and voltage

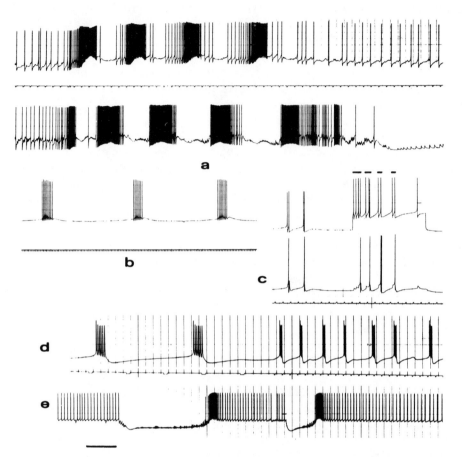

Fig. 1. Bursting patterns in neurones recorded intracellularly
from ganglia of Tritonia. (a) Two neurones recorded simultaneously on the left pedal ganglia drive ventral and dorsal flexions
of swimming recorded in an intact animal preparation during
swimming elicited by skin contact with starfish. Upper trace -
a ventral flexion neurone. Lower trace - a dorsal flexion neurone.
(b) Neurone on the left pleural ganglion (LP12) bursting spontaneously, recorded from an isolated ganglion. Neurones LP13 and
RP12 have been found to produce similar burst patterns. (c) Two
trigger group neurones recorded simultaneously on the left
pleural ganglion. Note near synchrony of short impulse bursts
in both cells. First two bursts in upper trace composed of 2
impulses each are accompanied by single impulses in neurone
of lower trace. Midway through record, depolarizing current
was injected for 10 sec into upper neurone causing series of 4

short bursts (marked by bars). Each burst accompanied by one or more impulses in lower trace. Each impulse in upper neurone produces depolarizing PSP in lower trace. (d) Neurone of isolated right pedal ganglion bursting spontaneously after 20 min exposure to 2% Metrazol (pentylenetetrazol). Note change in chart speed midway through record. Before and after exposure to this epileptogenic agent, firing in this neurone consisted of occasional impulses. (e) Neurone of isolated left buccal ganglion known to drive feeding movements of buccal apparatus. Four, 5 msec shocks delivered to right cerebral buccal connective cause hyperpolarizing PSP's seen at beginning of prolonged hyperpolarizing wave. Ensuing bursting occurred spontaneously. Calibration: a-d, marks indicate seconds; e, bar indicates 50 sec. Vertical bar - 50 mV.

changes taking place during bursts may be monitored or manipulated. The neurones may be exposed to drugs, metabolic inhibitors, alterations of temperature and other manipulative conditions which permit inference about bursting mechanisms.

EXPERIMENTAL METHODS

In all of our experiments, either isolated ganglia or intact animal preparations of the nudibranch Tritonia diomedia were used and standard intracellular stimulating and recording techniques were involved. Details of these preparations and techniques are provided elsewhere (Willows and Hoyle, 1969; Willows et al., 1973; Getting and Willows, 1973). Temperature changes, ion substitutions and drug exposures were made by exchanging the perfusion medium in the chamber containing the ganglia with at least 10 volumes of solution.

Three categories of bursting mechanisms or some combination of these three were considered as reasonable alternatives for study in these experiments. In principle, neurones might generate bursts by either (i) intrinsic oscillations developed in particular neurones through voltage or ion dependent electrogenic pumps or conductance changes occurring spontaneously or elicited in the first instance by appropriate synaptic inputs, (ii) through neurone to neurone interactions mediated by chemical synapses, or (iii) neurone to neurone interactions mediated by electrical synapses.

The conditions used to separate bursting processes into distinct categories were as follows: (i) Effect of alteration of temperature, to discriminate between mechanisms having substantially different temperature dependencies. It was assumed that neurone bursts relying primarily upon electrical junction interactions would be less sensitive to temperature change than would be chemical synapse mediated interactions, or metabolically driven pumps. Although there is evidence (Payton et al., 1969) that the electrical coupling factors between cells are altered by temperature change, this alteration (approximately 5X increase in junctional resistance with a temperature reduction from 25º - 5º C) is not confirmed in direct tests of known coupled neurones in Tritonia (Getting and Willows, unpublished observations). (ii) Effect of high magnesium concentrations (100-150 mM) in the fluid perfusing the brain, to discriminate bursting mechanisms that depend upon chemically mediated synaptic interactions from those that are neither endogenous to neurones or rely upon electrical synapses. (iii) Effect of hyperpolarization, to look for mechanisms involving ionic movements brought on by conductance changes. Thus, for instance, it is expected that (a) oscillations dependent upon excitatory, chemically mediated synaptic volleys would increase in amplitude with hyperpolarization, (b) electrical synapse mediated oscillations would be substantially unaffected, (c) if conductance changes to specific ions (e.g. K^+ or Cl^-) were involved in generating the oscillations, then the waves might decrease and then reverse as the equilibrium potential was crossed. (iv) Effects of exposure to chemical agents that interfere with Na^+-K^+ pump mechanisms, e.g. ouabain, DNP, reduced extracellular K^+ or replacement of Na^+ by Li^+. Such agents could be expected to interfere directly with metabolically driven electrogenic pumps that might underlie bursting phenomena whilst having indirect or longer term effects on synaptically mediated processes. These agents might be expected to produce effects similar to temperature reduction where metabolically driven pumping is involved.

Of the several neurone types having spontaneous or elicitable bursting properties, we chose three for study in the context of the above tests. These included the pedal ganglion neurones that show bursting activity during escape swimming (Fig. 1a), neurones on the pleural ganglia that apparently spontaneously produce bursts (LP12, LP13 and RP12) (Fig. 1b) and the trigger group neurones (Fig. 1c) that produce accelerating impulse bursts and elicit swimming behaviour.

PEDAL GANGLION, FLEXION NEURONES

Flexion neurones (FN's) are distributed on dorsal and ventral surfaces of both pedal ganglia (Willows et al., 1973). When stimulated individually in intact animal preparations at 10-20/sec, FN's elicit weak, but well-defined movements in longitudinal musculature that result in slight dorsal or ventral flexions. During swimming, these same neurones produce bursts of impulses 15-30/sec in phase with either dorsal, ventral or both flexion components of the behaviour (Fig. 1a). The bursts continue until swimming ends and are stereotyped in overall pattern and in terms of distribution of impulses in each particular burst.

As indicated by monitoring swimming in the whole intact animal and also the electrophysiological correlates of swimming in individual flexion neurones it is apparent that bursting in these neurones is not blocked, nor is it disorganized in any significant way by exposure to temperatures between 5^0 - 15^0 C. Co-ordination of antagonists is also unaffected by temperature changes over this range. However, the rate of bursting is markedly reduced as temperature is reduced. A semi-log plot of swim rate vs temperature (6^0 - 12.5^0C) has a straight line relationship (the slope is such that a 2.5 fold change in swim rate would occur for a 10^0 change in temperature, Fig. 2a).

A similar reduction in bursting rate with temperature reduction occurs whether measurement is made of (i) swim rate in a whole animal, (ii) burst rate in an intact animal preparation or (iii) burst rate in an isolated ganglion triggered by 10/sec shocks delivered for 0.5-1.5 sec to cerebral nerve trunk 2 (Fig. 2a). As expected, action potential durations are also prolonged by temperature reduction, increasing from 7-10 msec at 12^0C to 25-30 msec at 6^0C.

A partial or complete block of observable synaptic inputs to flexion neurones can be established by bathing an isolated ganglion in an artificial blood made by raising the Mg^{++} concentration to 100 mM by addition of isotonic $MgCl_2$. When an isolated preparation bathed in normal sea water is stimulated as described above (and see also Dorsett et al., 1969, 1973), normal swimming bursts are elicited. If the magnesium ion concentration is elevated to 150 mM and the ganglion is re-stimulated in the same way, the bursting is apparently completely blocked (Fig. 2b). Return to normal sea water perfusion leads to a reappearance of bursting. This observation is corroborated by the fact that bathing the entire animal in

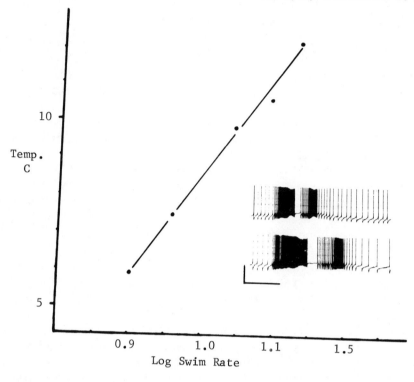

a

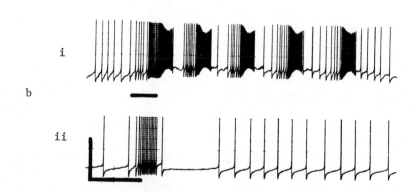

i

b

ii

Fig. 2. Effects of temperature and high Mg^{++} on flexion neurone bursting and swimming. (a) Swimming rate, plotted as a logarithm of the average rate for 12 animals (arbitrary units) as temperature was lowered from 12.5-6° C. Inset - two recordings from the same neurone, on the same time scale from flexion neurone bursting elicited in an isolated brain at 12° C (upper trace) and 5.5° C (lower trace). Both interburst intervals and burst durations show normal general pattern but are greatly prolonged at lower temperature. Co-ordination with antagonists (not shown) was also unaffected by temperature alteration. (b) (i) Flexion neurone bursting elicited in an isolated ganglion by brief (during bar, 10/sec, 5 msec duration shocks) stimulation of peripheral nerve trunk LCN2. Ganglion in normal sea water. (ii) After 20 min exposure to 150 mM Mg^{++} in isotonic sea water, same stimulation fails to elicit bursting, although it can be seen that the stimulation is still directly exciting the neurone. Calibration: (a) inset and (b) 5 sec and 50 mV.

isotonic $MgCl_2$ or injecting its body cavity with approximately 25% of its volume of isotonic $MgCl_2$ also eliminates swimming activity.

Hyperpolarization of single flexion neurones during the execution of a normal swim sequence in intact animal preparations can be carried to the point of virtually total block of impulse activity in the hyperpolarized neurone. However, despite the block, the directly observable swimming motor activity proceeds apparently unaffected. This is understandable in view of the fact that the withdrawl of one neurone from the relatively large (at least 30-50 neurones) pool controlling the overall response has only a negligible affect. However, examination of the subthreshold electrical activity reveals that although spiking is partially or completely blocked during hyperpolarization, the underlying volleys of excitatory postsynaptic potentials are enhanced in amplitude and the waves recur at the usual frequency (Fig. 3a). During the periods between bursts, impulses do not usually occur and instead, hyperpolarizing waves drive the membrane potential strongly to the negative side of threshold. The amplitudes of the hyperpolarizing waves decrease with increased applied hyperpolarizing currents. In extreme cases the hyperpolarizing wave can be reversed (H. Martin, unpublished observation). Thus, hyperpolarization of flexion neurones suggests that volleys of EPSPs underlie bursts and that IPSPs which can be reversed underlie the periods of inactivity between bursts.

Bathing the brains of intact preparations of Tritonia in 2×10^{-4} M ouabain in sea water for 5 min had little effect upon the ability of the animal to swim. Although peak spike frequencies were slightly reduced and some impulses were truncated, the overall pattern, duration and frequency of bursts was not seriously

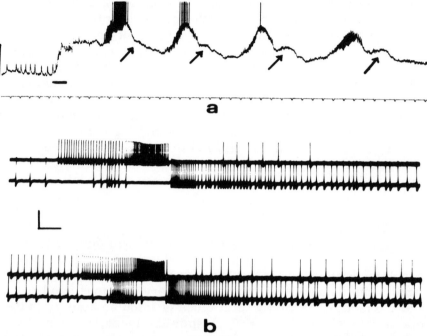

Fig. 3. (a) Effect of hyperpolarization during bursting in flexion neurone in intact animal preparation. During entire period of record, current was passed which maintained the neurone 20 mV hyperpolarized with respect to resting level in the absence of other stimulation. Compare with Fig. 1a (upper trace) or Fib. 2b(i). Although firing is greatly reduced particularly during the last 2 bursts, underlying PSP volleys are clearly enhanced. During interburst intervals, second depolarizing volleys (arrows) are revealed by this procedure. Marked depolarization early in record (bar) is caused by stimulation (salt solution placed on animal's skin) that elicits swimming response. Action potentials are truncated by recorder. (b) Effect of ouabain on flexion neurone bursting. Upper pair of traces is control response of ventral and dorsal flexion neurones exposed to normal sea water. After 5 min perfusion in 2×10^{-4} M ouabain in sea water, pattern and coordination of bursts are essentially unchanged. Calibration: (a) Marks - seconds; vertical bar - 40 mV. (b) 2 sec; 50 mV.

affected by this blocker of $Na^+ - K^+$ active transport (Fig. 3b). Bathing of the ganglion in fresh sea water reversed the mild effects of ouabain.

PLEURAL GANGLION, PARABOLIC BURSTER NEURONES

Three neurones, designated RP12, LP12 and LP13 located on the right and left pleural ganglia (Dorsett et al., 1973), regularly show recurring bursts of impulses over long periods under completely unstimulated conditions (Fig. 1b). These experiments were done using isolated ganglion preparations bathed in sea water in all cases, although there is evidence that similar bursting occurs in these same cells in the intact animal (T. Linder, unpublished observation).

The bursts in these neurones are characterized by trains of approximately 6-20 spikes on a depolarizing wave of many seconds duration. Following the last spike in the train, a depolarizing wave (3-10 sec duration) leads into a 5-15 mV hyperpolarization (the postburst hyperpolarization, PBH). The PBH lasts 10-200 sec, until the slowly building depolarizing phase carries the membrane potential to threshold and spiking begins again. The amplitude and duration of the PBH increases with the number of impulses in the preceding burst.

Altering the temperature of the solution bathing these neurones has well-defined and repeatable consequences. Bursting continues at temperatures from $10\text{-}12^\circ$ C which is normal for the animal in summer, up to at least 15° C. As temperature is lowered over a period of minutes, bursting is terminated abruptly at $8.0\text{-}8.5^\circ$ C. At and below 8.0° C, these neurones fire impulses continuously and regularly at 1-4/min with no tendency for grouping of impulses into bursts (Fig. 4a). As the temperature is raised again, bursting begins, initiated by a PBH. During abolition of bursting by low temperature, the membrane potential remains at approximately the level of the depolarized phase of the normal bursting cycle.

The pleural ganglion parabolic bursters were exposed to 150 mM Mg^{++} made by adding isotonic $MgCl_2$ to sea water in suitable proportions. This procedure has the effect of maintaining tonicity (940 milliosmols) but substitutes extra Mg^{++} for the ions normally present (principally Na^+). After 10-30 mins of perfusion, no substantial change in bursting activity was evident, nor was a change

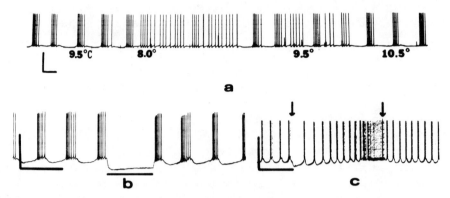

Fig. 4. (a) Bursting in LP12 terminated at 8.0°C. Neurone is
depolarized and fires continuously until temperature is raised
again to approximately 9.0°C, at which time bursting begins
again. (b) Hyperpolarization (bar) of LP13 reveals no underlying volley of PSPs nor a depolarizing wave at the time when
bursting should have occurred. Release from hyperpolarization
leads directly into a burst. Regularity of interburst interval
temporarily disrupted by period of hyperpolarization, with
first interval after release shorter than previous or following
average intervals. (c) Substitution of O K^+ sea water (between
arrows) abolishes bursting and causes depolarization with
regular firing until regular sea water perfusion resumed.
Calibration: (a), (b), 1 min; 50 mV, (c) 4 min; 50 mV.

produced when the high Mg^{++} solution was washed out again with
normal sea water.

Two affects of applied hyperpolarizing currents were noted.
First, over a range that did not block spiking entirely, maintained
hyperpolarizing currents produced an increase in the duration of
PBH. For instance, 5 nA injected into RP12 prolonged the average
interburst interval from 65 sec to 90 sec. Second, when hyperpolarization is increased until spikes are blocked, no underlying
volley of depolarizing synaptic potentials could be detected (Fig. 4b).

These same neurones were exposed to several agents supposed to
interfere with or block Na^+ - K^+ pumping. Solutions containing
lithium substituted for sodium, solutions containing zero potassium
(made up to isotonicity with extra Na^+), and solutions containing
2×10^{-5} g/ml ouabain or 3×10^{-4} M DNP (pH 6.7) all produced

substantially the same result. As is shown in Fig. 4c for a bathing solution containing 0 K^+, after 9 mins, bursting ceased altogether and instead the cell fired continuously from a resting level similar to the level during the depolarized phase of bursting. When this solution was replaced by normal artificial sea water containing 10 mM K^+, bursting commenced again within 2 min.

TRIGGER GROUP NEURONES

The trigger group neurones or TGNs, comprising a group of 30 neurones on each of the pleural ganglia, trigger escape swimming behaviour (Willows and Hoyle, 1969; Willows et al., 1973). Upon contact of the epithelium of the whole animal with the tube feet of starfish or with salt, the TGNs are excited by synchronous post-synaptic potentials which if sufficient in amplitude and duration cause accelerating bursts of spikes. These bursts are observed to occur synchronously throughout the population as a whole. In response to a constant depolarizing current injected into a single neurone, the population also can be made to fire accelerating bursts of spikes with a similar synchrony. Fig. 1c shows intracellular recordings from two TGNs. The two bursts on the left are spontaneously occurring. In response to a constant depolarizing current in one cell, these cells show four bursts (marked by bars) terminated by a prolonged hyperpolarization occurring after synchronous firing. The interburst interval is sometimes greater than 1 sec.

Bursting in the TGN system proved resistant to changes in temperature and to inhibitors of synaptic transmission and of electrogenic pumps. Bursting occurs in response to constant current at all temperatures from 5-15°C. In fact, the tendency to burst, and interburst intervals are enhanced at lower temperatures, Bathing the brain in sea water containing 2 x normal Mg ions (100mM) and 1/2 x normal Ca ions (2.5 mM) did not block bursting (Fig. 5). Both the depolarization underlying spike activity and the prolonged hyperpolarization at burst termination remain intact. Bathing the brain in Li^+ (substitited for Na^+) sea water which is supposed to block the sodium dependent electrogenic pump has no affect on the bursting in TGN cells.

Hyperpolarization of one cell in the TGN population causes a hyperpolarization of all the TGNs through the electrotonic junctions. As the hyperpolarization of a single TGN is increased the tendency to burst is decreased due to progressive hyperpolarization of all

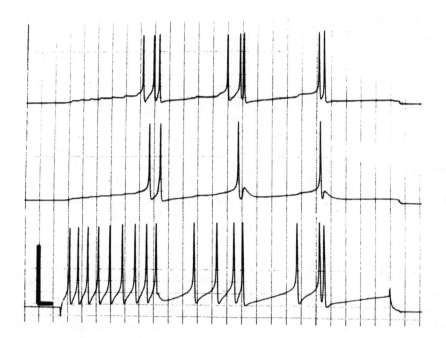

Fig. 5. Three TGNs simultaneously recorded. Ganglion bathed in 2 x normal Mg^{++} (100 mM) and 1/2 normal Ca^{++} (2.5 mM). Depolarization of neurone on bottom trace elicits normal bursting behaviour in this electrically coupled group. Electrical coupling evident from D.C. shift in upper two traces caused by current injection in neurone of lower trace. Compare with Fig. 1c. Calibration: 1 sec; 50 mV.

cells in the group. If sufficient, the hyperpolarization can prevent all cells except a   stimulated one from firing. In this case there is no burst formation but rather a smooth decline in spike frequency in the stimulated cell.

DISCUSSION

The results for this series of tests applied to three different bursting types, two having known functions in locomotion, are

summarized in Table 1. It is evident that the mechanisms underlying these bursting phenomena are distinctly separable one from
another. It is likely, for instance, that bursts in flexion neurones
are driven primarily by chemically mediated synaptic interactions
in agreement with earlier findings (Willows et al., 1973). The
reduction of burst rate at reduced temperatures is to be expected
in terms of a general rate reduction in all temperature dependent
processes that are chemically mediated. In particular, it is
expected and observed that action potential durations are greatly
prolonged, and peak burst frequencies are reduced. The underlying oscillations are not blocked, nor are the interactions that
lead to synergist-antagonist co-ordination. Similarly, the block
of the bursting mechanism and its underlying oscillations by high
Mg^{++} ion concentrations argues for a chemical synapse mediated
interaction. It would have been expected that endogenous driver
oscillations in the motor neurones (or electrical coupling to such
oscillations) would be unaffected even when chemical transmission
is blocked. The fact that no evidence whatever for membrane
potential oscillations was observed under these conditions argues
that endogenous pacemaker oscillations are not directly responsible for the flexion neurone bursts nor do they occur in neurones
that are electrically coupled to the motor neurones. It is possible
also that the failure of bursting to occur in high Mg^{++} may have
been caused by a blockage of the necessary inputs to initiate
bursting. Two possibilities remaining are that the bursts are
generated in pacemakers which are coupled to the motor neurones
by chemically mediated synapses or alternatively that the bursts
arise from chemically mediated synaptic interactions between the
motor neurones themselves. The former possibility is less likely
than the latter on the basis that the only endogenous pacemaker
bursting so far known in this nervous system is blocked (Fig. 3a)
at temperatures below 8.0°C whereas flexion neurone bursting is
not.

The effects of temperature, high magnesium exposure, hyperpolarization and Na^+ - K^+ pump blockers on bursting in RP12,
LP12 and LP13 are inconsistent with synaptic generating mechanisms. Instead, it is more likely that the cyclic bursting and the
underlying oscillations are generated endogenously. The most
direct evidence that the bursts are endogenous comes from the
observations that the oscillations continue unaffected by 150 mM
Mg^{++} in the bathing solution and that hyperpolarization blocks
bursting entirely, leaving no trace of underlying membrane potential waves. In addition, the fact that temperature reduction

	Temperature change	Exposure to high Mg^{++} concentration	Hyperpolarization	Exposure to agents that block Na^{+}-K^{+} pumping
Flexion Neurones	Burst rate slowed as temperature reduced. Co-ordination and pattern unaffected.	Blocked	Impulses blocked. Underlying PSP volleys enhanced but timing unaffected.	Unaffected (ouabain)
LP12, LP13, RP12	Bursting blocked at 8°C. During block neurone is depolarized and fires regularly.	Unaffected	Bursting and firing blocked. No underlying PSP volleys or waves observed during block.	During block, neurone is de-polarized and fires regularly. (O K^{+}, DNP, ouabain)
Trigger Group Neurones	Unaffected. Low temperatures produced slight enhancement of bursting tendency.	Unaffected	Bursting blocked in hyperpolarized neurone because firing inhibited. Bursting capability in other TGN's unaffected.	Unaffected. (Li^{+} substituted for Na^{+} in sea water.)

Table 1.   Effect of varied experimental conditions on bursting.

abruptly terminates bursting, suggests that the oscillations depend upon metabolic processes having a well-defined threshold. This is in contradistinction to both electrically and chemically mediated synaptic mechanisms which proceed essentially normally (although probably at a slowed pace) down to considerably lower temperatures. Finally, all the data obtained from experiments using agents that interfere with $Na^+ - K^+$ pumping are suggestive but not proof of the involvement of such pumps in producing the oscillations. Unfortunately, these tests (Li^+ substitution for Na^+, zero K^+, ouabain, DNP and temperature reduction) all interfere with maintenance of the normal resting potential, by blocking electrogenic pumping which in turn causes membrane depolarization. The depolarization in itself may cause the termination of bursting if the oscillatory mechanism depends upon membrane potential. Thus, the oscillatory mechanism might well be intact under all these conditions but merely incapable of normal expression owing to the depolarized condition of the membrane (D. Carpenter, personal communication). Thus, the available evidence does not permit a distinction to be made whether the LP12, LP13 and RP12 bursting depends upon cyclic activation of an electrogenic pump or upon recurring activation of a conductance change.

A neurone having similar bursting properties in Aplysia, R15, has been extensively studied and several endogenous mechanisms proposed (Strumwasser, 1968; Strumwasser and Kim, 1969; Wachtel and Wilson, 1973; Carpenter, 1973).

The TGN system proved virtually unaffected by all of the conditions applied to it except hyperpolarization, which blocked firing. The underlying mechanism apparently does not require either chemically mediated synaptic interactions, nor does it require electrogenic pumping. It has been shown (Willows and Hoyle, 1969; Willows et al., 1973; Getting and Willows, 1973) that these neurones are interconnected by electrically conducting junctions. The mechanisms we have proposed for burst formation (Getting and Willows, 1973) in this system involve: (i) regenerative build-up of excitation by positive feedback through the junctions and (ii) burst termination by two processes: development of a diphasic PSP with a large and prolonged hyperpolarizing phase when firing becomes nearly synchronous in many TGNs, and by the electrical "unloading" of TGNs when firing is absolutely synchronous, permitting the development of a larger and longer after-hyperpolarization following the last spike of each burst.

The findings reported here for the TGNs are consistent with the supposition that the interactions between TGNs that generate bursts are through electrical junctions.

The principle conclusion which can be drawn from the above is that there are distinct bursting mechanisms involved in different neurone groups in the central ganglia of this nudibranch mollusk. The most likely mechanisms include chemically mediated synaptic interactions (a detailed model for such interactions leading to bursting is provided in Willows et al., 1973), pacemaker oscillations endogenous to neurones and purely electrical interactions based upon close electrical coupling between a group of neurones. It is apparent also that no single bursting neurone type from this gastropod should be taken as a model for the study of generalized oscillatory or bursting phenomena since distinctly different processes are likely to be involved depending upon the neurone selected.

Acknowledgement: Research supported by N.S.F. Research Grant GB20351 to A.O.D. Willows, and P.H.S. Postdoctoral Fellowship to P.A. Getting.

REFERENCES

Bentley, D.R., 1969. Intracellular activity in cricket neurons during the generation of behaviour patterns. J. Insect Physiol. 15, 677-699.

Burrows, M., and Willows, A.O.D., 1969. Neuronal co-ordination of rhythmic maxilliped beating in brachyuran and Anomuran Crustacea. Comp. Biochem. Physiol. 31, 121-135.

Carpenter, D.O., 1973. Ionic mechanisms and models of endogenous discharge of Aplysia neurons. In Rhythms in Invertebrate Nervous Systems. (Ed. Salanki, J.) In press.

Davis, W.J., 1968. Lobster righting responses and their neural control. Proc. Roy. Soc. B, 70, 435-456.

Davis, W.J., 1969. The neural control of swimmeret beating in the lobster. J. Exp. Biol. 50, 99-117.

Davis, W.J., Siegler, M.V.S., and Mpitsos, G.J., 1973. Distributed neuronal oscillators and efference copy in the feeding system of Pleurobranchaea. J. Neurophysiol. 36, 258-274.

Dorsett, D.A., Willows, A.O.D., and Hoyle, G., 1969. Centrally generated nerve impulse sequences determining swimming behavior in Tritonia. Nature 224, 711-712.

Dorsett, D.A., Willows, A.O.D., and Hoyle, G., 1973. The neuronal basis of behavior in Tritonia IV. The central origin of a fixed action pattern demonstrated in the isolated brain. J. Neurobiol. 4, 287-300.

Elsner, N., 1969. Kommandofasern in Zentralnervensystem der Heuschrecke Gastrimargus africanus (Oedipodinae). Zool. Anz. 33, 465-471.

Getting, P.A., and Willows, A.O.D., 1973. Burst formation in electrically coupled neurons. Brain Res. In press.

Hoyle, G., 1970. Cellular mechanisms underlying behavior - neuroethology. In Advances in Insect Phys. (Eds. Trehern, J.E. and Beament, J.W.L.) Academic Press, Lond., pp. 349-444.

Kendig, J.J., 1968. Motor neurone coupling in locust flight. J. Exp. Biol. 48, 389-404.

Kennedy, D., Evoy, W.H., and Hanawalt, J.T., 1966. Release of coordinated behavior in crayfish by single central neurons. Science 154, 917-919.

Mendelson, M., 1971. Oscillator neurons in crustacean ganglia. Science 171, 1170-1173.

Miller, P.L., 1967. The derivation of the motor command to the spiracles of the locust. J. Exp. Biol. 46, 349-371.

Payton, B.W., Bennett, M.V.L., and Pappas, G.D., 1969. Temperature-dependence of resistance at an electrotonic synapse. Science 165, 594-597.

Strumwasser, F., 1968. Membrane and intracellular mechanisms governing endogenous activity in neurons. In Physiological and Biochem. Aspects of Nervous Integration (Ed. Carlson, F.D.) pp. 329-341.

Strumwasser, F., and Kim, M., 1969. Experimental studies of a neuron with an endogenous oscillator and a quantitative model of its mechanism. The Physiologist 12, 367.

Wachtel, H., and Wilson, W.A., 1973. Voltage clamp analysis of rhythmic slow wave generation in bursting neurons. In Rhythms in Invertebrate Nervous Systems. (Ed. Salanki, J.). In press.

Watanabe, A., 1958. The interaction of electrical activity among neurons of lobster cardiac ganglia. Jap. J. Physiol. 8, 305-318.

Wiersma, C.A.G., and Ikeda, K., 1964. Interneurons commanding swimmeret movements in the crayfish, Procambarus clarkii (Girard). Comp. Biochem. Physiol. 12, 509-525.

Wilson, D.M., 1966. Central nervous mechanisms for the generation of rhythmic behavior in arthropods. Symp. Soc. Exp. Biol. 20, 199-228.

Wilson, D.M., 1968. The nervous control of insect flight and related behavior. In Recent Advances in Insect Physiology. (Eds. Trehern, J.E. and Beament, J.W.L.) Academic Press, N.Y.

Willows, A.O.D., Dorsett, D.A., and Hoyle, G., 1973. The neuronal basis of behavior in Tritonia. III Neuronal mechanism of a fixed action pattern. J. Neurobiol. 4, 255-285.

Willows, A.O.D., and Hoyle, G., 1969. Neuronal network triggering a fixed action pattern. Science 166, 1549-1551.

Zucker, R.S., Kennedy, D., and Selverston, A.I., 1971. Neuronal circuit mediating escape responses in crayfish. Science 173, 645-650.

CRUSTACEAN WALKING

W. H. Evoy and C. R. Fourtner

Laboratory for Quantitative Biology, University of
Miami, Coral Gables, Florida and Department of
Physiology, University of Alberta, Edmonton, Canada

Recent approaches to a neuronal basis for crustacean locomotion have attempted to understand the interactions between
central patterning of motor output, systems for initiation of
movement and the interaction of proprioceptive signals with
these central factors. Analysis of locomotion has utilized
various techniques for measuring and comparing movements
of segmental appendages and their joints during walking and
swimming. In some cases, electrical recording of neuromuscular activity had aided these interpretations. Both intra-
and intersegmental co-ordinating mechanisms have been examined by observation of timing of movements of individual joints
or appendages with respect to the others.

The central motor score is thought to consist of central oscillatory systems for the generation of rhythmic motor outputs as
well as a separate network of neurones that co-ordinate the
activities of the motor oscillators. More direct evidence has
accumulated for 'command' or 'triggering' systems, mediated
by extrasegmental interneurones, that call out the general
modes of walking. Superimposed on the interacting neuronal
systems that make up this central score are a variety of sensory factors involving feedback from the movements themselves
as well as afferent influences such as vision and equilibrium.
Proprioceptive feedback has been approached by the study of
reflexes and by attempts to interfere with the sensory sources
by surgical ablation and by physical alterations of joint move-

ments. These procedures cause changes in otherwise regular aspects of locomotor co-ordination, indicating that joint movements, muscle tension and resistance to movement all modify the central score.

Because there is little direct evidence concerning the nature of the connections and activities of central neurones involved in walking, most of the hypotheses await neurophysiological and structural tests. Aspects of walking and swimming such as gaits or timing between limb movements may involve both intersegmental coupling and specific command systems. The interactions of all these factors have not, as yet, been exposed.

Walking in various organisms has been considered for many years to be a suitable phenomenon for the study of underlying neuronal mechanism, and crustaceans have received their due share of attention. Various approaches have been employed, but none of them, as yet, has resulted in a satisfactory picture of the way in which the central nervous system is organized to produce observed patterns of leg movements. Walking and some types of swimming in decapod crustacea involve the co-ordinated movements of from 2 to 5 pairs of legs (pereiopods), each of which has six or seven functional joints. Even the apparently straightforward task of accounting for all of these movements in time and in space is a complex and laborious one. Other modes of locomotion not covered in this paper involve the use of swimmerets, uropods and abdominal musculature.

A fairly extensive early literature during the past century has described behaviourally the use of the legs in walking and swimming crustaceans. Many of these early investigators employed surgical lesions or stimulation of ganglia and connectives in attempts to find control centres and pathways for activation and co-ordination of overt behaviour. This work has been extensively reviewed by Lochhead (1961) and by Bullock and Horridge (1965). This brief discussion will not review the material covered in these treatments but will instead concentrate primarily on efforts during the last 10 years that represent preliminary attempts to determine the mechanisms for co-ordination, control and initiation of walking and swimming as a result of interactions between activities of individual neurones.

Interpretations of crustacean walking and swimming have been influenced for many years by theories regarding the relative importances of central programming of movements and proprioceptive reflexes in the co-ordination of motor outputs. At one time, reflexes were thought to be responsible for much of the co-ordination of sequences of muscular contractions. More recently, it has been generally considered that such reflexes may modify motor programs, but the majority of workers are in agreement that most motor programs have a least a 'wired-in' basis in the organization of neurones in the central nervous system. However, there is as yet no definitive evidence for the existence of such a central program for the co-ordinated locomotory movements of the thoracic appendages of decapod crustacea.

Major questions regarding the neuronal basis of crustacean locomotion remain to be answered.

1. To what extent does a central motor score, genetically determined and laid down in the connections and activities of central neurones, exist as the basis for regular repeated contractions of the walking leg muscles? A few excellent examples of such hard-wired motor scores have been described in other systems, and a strong argument for their genetic basis was put forward by Wilson (1972).

2. What is the nature of the elements in a central motor score? Possibilities are single neuronal or network 'oscillators', 'command fibres', specific trigger systems, specific sensory inputs calling out motor patterns, reciprocity between neurones at the ganglionic level (perhaps preceding the motoneurones themselves), specific driver units in segmental ganglia, etc. While lines of direct evidence have been favourable to one or another of these viewpoints, in only a few motor systems has there been rigorous demonstration of central control of co-ordinated movements in the absence of any other factor.

3. How do sensory inputs modify the hypothetical motor score and under what conditions? How does this sensory modification relate to observed proprioceptive reflexes?

4. In all the observed modes of walking and swimming, the individual walking legs move in describable sequences. How is this relationship between outputs of segmental ganglia achieved? Some system of coupling between the final motor pathways to the individual legs appears to exist, but a neuronal basis has not been found.

SOME APPROACHES TO THE PROBLEMS

Gaits

Gaits have generally been categorized from observations of repeated identical sequences in the order of movements of the several walking legs. (In most Astacura and Brachyura the first pereiopod, the chela, does not always serve an obvious function in locomotion.) Many of the Decapoda have been observed to utilize two or more gaits, in some cases correlated with the speed of locomotion. In forward walking of crayfish, Procambarus blandgii and Orconectes virilis (Parrack, 1964), and in sideways walking of the fiddler crab, Uca pugnax (Barnes, in preparation), five or six such gaits have been recorded. Constancy of these gaits is low; the animals appear to shift rapidly from one sequence of leg movements to another, even during an otherwise constant bout of stepping.

Assignment of a sequence of stepping to one or another gait is generally based on observations of either lifting from or touching the substrate, the only discrete points in a step that can be used as a basis for comparison between legs. All degrees of overlap between steps may occur, and description of a gait does not account for variations in stroke duration between legs. Slight changes in the phase relations of leg movements cause a shift from one apparent gait to another when steps of one leg are in close coincidence with those of another. For this reason, gaits classified by order of leg use are most useful when steps of each leg are well separated from all others.

A commonly observed mode of locomotion in Crustacea appears to be a rough correspondence to movement of legs in alternating tetrapods, in which alternate legs of one side raise or touch at about the same time as legs of adjacent segments on the opposite side. This mode of locomotion would provide maximum stability for a slowly moving animal (Fig. 1A). In this and other gaits observed, the legs on a side of the animal tend to move in a more or less metachronal wave, one following the other. The several gaits can be achieved when varying degrees of overlap occur between beginnings and ends of the wave. Crayfish have been observed to develop a series of tripods when the waves overlap sufficiently (Parrack, 1964). While gaits have been useful for comparing stepping of different animals, they have not provided much insight

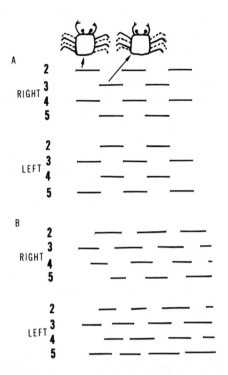

Fig. 1. Gaits in sideways walking of crabs. A. Theoretical
tetrapod gait, in which alternating legs on a side are in phase.
The raised legs are shown as dotted lines, those in contact
with the ground as solid lines. Bars represent the period of
time the dactylopodite is in contact with the ground. B. A
similar representation of measurements taken from films of
Cardisoma guanhumi during sideways walking. The two sides
show different apparent gaits and the left changes gait during
the record. Nevertheless, the metachrony of each side, although not perfect, is similar to that in the idealized tetrapod
situation.

into neuronal mechanisms that control stepping. The basic mode
of coupling between legs probably depends on neuronal systems
linking oscillatory activity that originates in segmental ganglia.
The efficacy of this coupling appears to be highly variable over
short periods of time and is very weak or perhaps nonexistent
in some animals.

In other studies where gaits have not been extensively analyzed, the qualitative descriptions of leg movements allow some comparison. Clarac and Coulmance (1971) show a few sequences of lateral walking at relatively low speeds in crabs; the gait appears to be metachronal. However, as walking speed increases, several gaits become apparent, and all roughly correspond to the alternating tetrapod. Cardisoma guanhumi shows a similar tendency to use an alternating tetrapod gait but shows rapid transitions from one mode of stepping to another as steps alter in duration and phase of movement with respect to others (Fig. 1B). In the ghost crab, Ocypode ceratophthalma, capable of speeds over 2 m/s, the alternating tetrapod situation appears to occur at lower speeds (Burrows and Hoyle, 1973). However, during very rapid running leg 5 or both legs 4 and 5 are held raised, and only legs 2 and 3 alternate on the trailing side of the animal. At the same time the legs on the leading side move only slightly and are held in a partially extended position with the outer surface of the dactyl occasionally skidding along the ground. The animals actually push off with the trailing legs, both of which may be off the ground simultaneously, so that the crab is leaping toward the leading side (op. cit. and Hafemann and Hubbard, 1969).

Swimming crabs also demonstrate highly variable co-ordination of leg movements. A dromid crab, Homola barbata, is capable of both lateral and forward swimming and uses a 4-3-2 sequence of walking leg movements for both; the chelae and fifth legs are not used (Hartnoll, 1970, 1971). The portunid crab, Callinectes sapidus, undergoes a complete transition from a walking gait involving legs 2, 3 and 4 when it taxis and takes off into sideways swimming (Spirito, 1972). As it taxis, the fifth legs begin to beat, and then the crab launches upward with trailing legs 1 through 4 extended horizontally. Legs 2, 3 and 4 on the leading side maintain an irregular beat similar to that during walking, and the two fifth legs now beat in phase to produce a propellor-like sculling motion.

In some instances it has been observed that the co-ordination or stepping rates of the two sides of the animal are different (Parrack, 1964; Clarac and Coulmance, 1971; Evoy and Fourtner, 1973), suggesting that the neuronal co-ordinating system may have strong ipsilateral connections but weak contralateral coupling.

Relative Timing of Leg Movements

A commonly applied method of investigating the timing of motor outputs that evoke movements in appendages has been to plot the occurrences of relative points in time of an identifiable stage of the movement as a relative phase histogram. The several Crustacea examined in this way show different degrees of coupling between the different walking legs although in no case does coupling seem as constant as in some other systems such as the abdominal swimmerets or some insect walking legs.

The general pattern during sideways walking in crabs is that relative phase histograms of adjacent legs show peaks near 0.5; those of alternate ipsilateral legs show peaks near 0.0 or 1.0; those of segmental leg pairs 0.5 (Barnes, in preparation; Evoy and Fourtner, 1973). The co-ordination of crayfish legs during forward walking is somewhat less regular. Phase relations between legs 2, 3 and 4 on the same side are not as precise as in crabs but show a tendency toward the same sort of co-ordination (Fig. 2A1). Changes in relative phase are seen with each step, but there does not seem to be any tendency to maintain one phase relation for several steps and then shift to another relationship (Fig. 2A2). Phase relations between the fifth leg and any other ipsilateral leg are extremely variable in crayfish, and the fifth leg tends to step at a higher frequency than the others (Fig. 2B). Thus, coupling between the last walking leg and other legs seems to be weaker or more variable than coupling between the rest of the legs.

Even more complex phase relations are seen in the strokes of legs in swimming crabs. Homola barbata, when swimming forward, has mean relative phases of about 0.3 between adjacent and between alternate ipsilateral legs (Hartnoll, 1970). Phase relations between the beats of ipsilateral legs 2, 3 and 4 during sideways swimming in Callinectes sapidus are similar to those seen during walking in this and other crabs (Spirito, 1972). There are no significant constant phase relations between the fifth and other ipsilateral walking legs during the sculling motion. However, the last legs are quite tightly coupled; there is a latency of about 35 msec between the beats of the leading and trailing sides.

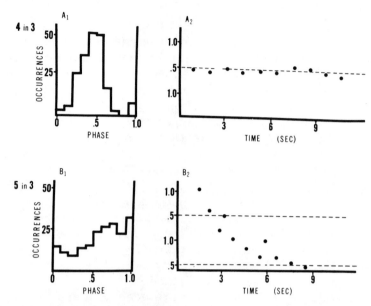

Fig. 2. Relative phase relations between walking legs in Procambarus clarkii. A1. Relative phase histogram of steps of the fourth leg in relation to those of the third ipsilateral leg. A2. Instantaneous phase plot of a portion of the data used in plotting the histogram in A1. In this presentation, relative phase is shown for each step during the sequence of walking. B1. Relative phase histogram of steps of the fifth leg in relation to the third ipsilateral leg. B2. Instantaneous phase plot of a portion of the data shown in B1. The fifth leg stepped somewhat more rapidly than the others. Mean interval between steps in msec: Leg 2, 1.13; leg 3, 1.21; leg 4, 1.13; leg 5, 0.98.

Motor Co-ordination of Walking Leg Muscles

Electrical recording of nerve and neuromuscular activity from the legs of walking animals has revealed several features of neuromuscular co-ordination in individual legs. The general rule is that antagonistic muscles are driven by reciprocal excitatory bursts during the stepping cycle. The clearest reciprocity is seen between muscles driving joints that participate in the major return- and powerstrokes of locomotion. In crabs, walking sideways, clear reciprocity is generally seen between the levator and depressor of the coxopodite-basipodite (C-B) joint as well as between flexor and extensor of the meropodite-carpopodite (M-C) joint, which is responsible for most of the excursion of the legs in this mode of walking (Atwood and Walcott, 1965; Clarac and Coulmance, 1971). In Ocypode ceratophthalma, this reciprocity is seen on both sides of the animal at slower walking speeds but during running occurs only on the trailing side; the meropodite muscles on the leading side discharge nearly tonically as the animal skids on the dactyls (Burrows and Hoyle, 1973).

Other walking leg muscles of crabs show some cyclical activity during walking, but reciprocity is not as clear. The closer muscle of the propodite-dactylopodite (P-D) joint tends to fire in phase with the M-C flexor and the P-D opener with the M-C extensor, but these muscles rarely show completely silent periods (Atwood and Walcott, 1965; Barnes et al., 1972; Burrows and Hoyle, 1973). Some cyclical activity is also seen in the stretcher and bender muscles of the carpopodite-propodite (C-P) joint but again is less clearly defined than in the muscles of the M-C joint. Thus, the distal joints appear to provide leverage and fine adjustment but to contribute little to movement during the step.

Precise timing occurs between the more proximal joints that participate in posture of the leg during walking and the muscles of the M-C joint. In Carcinus sp., the C-B levator is active in synchrony with the M-C flexor and is silent during activity of the M-C extensor on the trailing side of the animal. However, on the leading side, the relationships are reversed, that is, the C-B levator and the M-C extensor fire in synchrony and are silent during flexion (Clarac and Coulmance, 1971). In Ocypode ceratophthalma, the relationship between discharges in M-C and C-B muscles was similar to that in Carcinus sp. except that the M-C muscles were activated slightly ahead of the C-B muscles (Burrows and Hoyle, 1973). During forward walking in crayfish the depressor of the fifth walking leg discharges in almost perfect synchrony with the M-C extensor (Grote, 1973). Comparison of myograms from the depressor area is difficult because there are three or four distinct heads of the muscle system, which may operate independently to cause different directions of movement.

The presence of specific inhibitors to P-D opener and C-P stretcher muscles in brachyurans raised the possibility that some

control over these muscles, both activated by a single excitatory
axon, might be achieved by selective activation of these inhibitors.
Atwood and Walcott (1965) noted suppressed amplitudes of potentials recorded from these muscles at the beginnings of the bursts
and attributed the suppression to inhibition. Recordings with a
suction electrode of the efferent fibres to these muscles in
Cardisoma guanhumi walking on a treadmill showed overlap
between the bursts of the opener and stretcher inhibitors and
the bursts of the shared excitatory axon (Barnes et al., 1972).
However, both the comparison of the bursts of the inhibitory axons
during walking to the bursts evoked by passive joint movements
and the phase relations between inhibitory and excitatory impulses indicate that the inhibitors are not used to effectively
separate contractions of the two muscles (Spirito et al., 1972;
Bush, 1962, 1965).

EVIDENCE REGARDING A CENTRAL PROGRAM
FOR WALKING

Atwood and Wiersma (1967) evoked rhythmic movements of
walking legs in crayfish upon stimulation of fibres in the circumoesophageal connectives. However, the legs of these animals
were not touching the surface, and it was noted that the movements did not appear identical with those of walking. Similar
command fibre stimulation of crayfish on a circular treadmill
has evoked discrete aspects of walking (Bowerman and Larimer,
1972, 1974b). Five command fibres have been identified in the
circumoesophageal connectives that, when stimulated at 50-
100/sec, evoked forward walking; another 4-5 fibres evoke
backward walking. Walking leg movements are generally metachronous and show the same sort of variable coupling noted in
studies of freely walking animals. Walking generally continued
only as long as the stimulation was maintained and could not be
evoked if legs were not in contact with the moveable treadmill.
The latter observation is suggestive of considerable interaction
of proprioceptive influences with a central score to be discussed
in the next section. Other fibres were found that caused various
postural changes; at least one of these may also be involved in
control of walking (Bowerman and Larimer, 1974a). This class
of command fibres caused a turning posture to the right or left
and could operate in concert with locomotor commands to bring
about changes in direction. The necessity of activation of central
pathways along with a situation in which normal walking move-

ments occurred (contact with and free movement in relation to the substrate) indicate that both central commands and appropriate proprioceptive signals are necessary to maintain co-ordinated locomotor activity.

Other investigations dealing with observations of motor patterns have suggested a central motor program. The differences between the patterns of motor output to the distal walking leg muscles during walking and those in resistance reflexes in Cardisoma guanhumi indicate that these reflexes are inappropriate to the normal patterns of locomotor co-ordination (Barnes et al., 1972). Marked differences between outputs to legs on the two sides of the animal during swimming in Callinectes sapidus and rapid running in Ocypode ceratophthalma have been cited as evidence for an overriding central motor score (Spirito, 1972; Burrows and Hoyle, 1973). The beat of maxillipeds in the gill chambers of several crabs shows a good correlation with the direction of sideways walking; these appendages generally beat only on the trailing side of the body (Burrows and Willows, 1969). The authors speculate that, because both trailing legs and maxillipeds utilize extensor muscles for the power stroke, identical central control may influence the excitability of both sets of appendages. The relatively constant duration of motor bursts to the levator muscle as well as clean reciprocity between antagonistic muscles have led Clarac and Coulmance (1971) to propose a model for central control of walking in Carcinus sp. This model suggests that a central 'command system' activates the levator motoneurones and that their activity is further modified by afferent input from proprioceptors located for the most part at the M-C joints.

It seems likely that the several distinct modes of locomotion seen in Crustacea indicate the presence of a multiplicity of motor scores that organize different relationships of activity within the same populations of motoneurones. This selective activation probably involves the activity of command interneurones that may in turn trigger ganglionic co-ordinating cells and are themselves triggered in specific ways upon appropriate integration of a variety of inputs. Initiation and modulation of stepping in crayfish by visual stimulation from a moving stripe pattern indicate that movement detection is an important factor in calling out or maintaining walking (Davis and Ayers, 1972). Tactile stimulation is certainly a factor and clearly provides a directional stimulus for walking as can be readily seen by tapping any crustacean from the side, front, or rear.

Intersegmental co-ordination of the movements of the individual walking legs is a complicated and difficult problem. The comparative evidence indicates considerable variation in tightness of coupling between segmental outputs. This is particularly obvious in the case of crayfish forward walking in which movements of fifth legs are poorly coupled, if at all, with those of the more anterior legs. Rapid transition from one apparent gait to another may be due to slight changes in phasic coupling between segmental motor outputs.

Until we have information on the neuronal makeup of the motor outputs and connections between them, both ipsilaterally and contralaterally, it will not be possible to tell whether apparent gaits are due to separately commanded motor scores or to variations in the coupling influence between segmental motor systems. Evaluations of studies of leg movements suggest a possible system of coupling in which there is inhibitory coupling between hemisegmental oscillator systems ipsilaterally, with perhaps a similar but weaker coupling between contralateral hemisegmental systems (Spirito, 1973; Evoy and Fourtner, 1973). However, excitatory coupling cannot be ruled out completely in any of these very general models. Another difficulty lies in the hypothesized oscillators. This term has been used rather loosely in connection with Crustacean walking and is based on the cyclic nature of muscle contraction and relaxation. Demonstrations of non-spiking oscillators, apparently driving or at least co-ordinating repeating motor outputs makes this hypothesis very attractive (Mendelson, 1971). Coupling between such segmental oscillatory motor drives could involve a system of interneurones, similar to that suggested by Graham (1972) for insect walking, that could be triggered either by the segmental oscillatory activity or by proprioceptive inputs or by both. The considerable variability of intersegmental coupling would seem to favour such an interneuronal system, rather than a repertory of commands calling out specific stepping sequences. All such speculation regarding generation and co-ordination of motor activity must await testing by direct neurophysiological exploration of the central nervous system.

PROPRIOCEPTIVE MODIFICATIONS OF WALKING

Only a few of the possible sensory modifications of walking leg movements have been explored. Upon immobilization of the M-C or other joints of a walking leg, there are detectable changes in

the output to that leg as well as to other legs, but stepping continues
as long as the tip of the dactylopodite of the bound leg can contact
the surface (Clarac and Beaubaton, 1969; Clarac and Coulmance,
1971; Barnes et al., 1972). Binding the M-C joint of a crayfish
fifth walking leg at a 90° angle results in a latency shift between
the M-C extensor and the C-B depressor so that the extensor
burst leads that of the depressor by as much as 100 msec (Grote,
1973, and in preparation). In crayfish, co-ordination between
walking leg joints may involve reflex interactions initiated by
receptors of different joints (Moody, 1970). However, when a
leg of Cardisoma guanhumi was tied so that the M-C, C-P and
P-D joints were free to move but could not touch the ground,
movements of that leg became irregular and reduced in amplitude
(Evoy and Fourtner, 1973). At the same time, a definite change
in the relative phase of movements between the remaining legs
was noticed similar to the results of autotomy on Uca pugnax
(Barnes, in preparation). In crayfish, a leg amputated at the
meropodite moved erratically and weakly, but when an artificial
extension was attached so that it could contact the ground, normal
movements were restored (Grote, 1973). These results suggest
the presence of receptors in the proximal leg segments specialized
for detecting stresses occurring during the step. Input from these
receptors may interact with the central oscillatory and coupling
system. These receptors could be either those described by Wales
et al. (1971), Clarac et al. (1971), or those of Ripley et al. (1968)
and Roberts and Bush (1971).

A few attempts have been made to selectively ablate portions of
the sensory system in otherwise intact crabs. Clarac and Coulmance
(1971) altered movements of the C-B joint in a leg with its M-C
joint blocked by crushing the musculature of the meropodite and
thereby apparently unlinking the sensory inputs. Removal or
interruption of the mechanical linkage of a muscle receptor system
in the meropodites of several legs resulted in excessive flexion of
that joint during walking in Cardisoma guanhumi (Fourtner and
Evoy, 1973). However, a similar procedure in Cancer magister
resulted in interference with postural adjustment in a stationary
animal but did not appear to alter walking (Evoy and Cohen, 1971).

Resistance reflexes were evoked during walking in Cardisoma
guanhumi by applying joint movements to a walking leg at different
phases of the step cycle (Barnes et al., 1972). Resulting discharge
patterns of efferent fibres to distal leg muscles were similar to
those evoked by passive joint movements in a quiescent animal

(Bush, 1963, 1965; Spirito et al., 1972). Thus, the resistance reflexes can break into the ongoing motor patterns of walking and are presumed to act as a modifying influence to adjust for irregularities in movement.

Walking crabs respond to increased load, imposed by walking up steep grades or by applying a brake to a treadmill, by either extending the powerstroke duration, thereby generating increased building of tension (Evoy and Fourtner, 1973), or by increasing the motor output frequency to the powerstroke muscles (Fourtner and Evoy, 1973). The sensory source for this timing is unknown but could involve either proprioceptive signalling of the end of the step or tension-monitoring systems described by MacMillan and Dando (1972). It is likely that these tension receptors associated with the tendons of walking leg muscles modify motor output during walking. Clarac and Dando (1973) stimulated the afferent nerves of these receptors in the meropodite of Cancer pagurus and found that, at low stimulus intensities, motor discharge to the muscle of origin was suppressed, but that at higher stimulation intensities, excitation of both the muscle of origin and its antagonist occurred. Although these reflexes can modify spontaneous efferent activity and activity resulting from passive joint movement, it remains to be seen how they interact with walking. When the animal walks up a grade, restoration of movements in a leg tied in levation indicates that the load response is distributed intersegmentally. This response could be due to direct proprioceptive influences or could be ascribed to interaction of the proprioceptive signal with an intersegmental coupling system (Evoy and Fourtner, 1973).

There are undoubtedly a host of other sensory interactions that influence either the co-ordination or the excitability of the motor outputs. Some of these are likely to involve proprioceptive feedback from leg joint and muscle activity. There are also regulatory influences on stepping from sources other than direct proprioceptive feedback, such as the statocysts (Roye, 1972). One major task at hand, if neuronal control of Crustacean walking is to be developed as a useful system for the exploration of a relatively sophisticated motor system, is to account for the interactions of the sensory modification with motor score. It may well be that this problem will be inseparable from an elucidation of the nature of the central systems for initiation and co-ordination of movements.

Acknowledgement: Supported in part by NSF Grant GB 30605, NIH Training Grant HD 00187 and NIH Postdoctoral Fellowship F02 NS 54893.

REFERENCES

Atwood, H.L., and Walcott, B., 1965. Recording of electrical
  activity and movement from legs of walking crabs. Can. J.
  Zool. 43, 657-665.
Atwood, H.L., and Wiersma, C.A.G., 1967. Command interneurons
  in the crayfish central nervous system. J. Exp. Biol. 46,
  249-261.
Barnes, W.J.P., Spirito, C.P., and Evoy, W.H., 1972. Nervous
  control of walking in the crab, Cardisoma guanhumi. II. Role
  of resistance reflexes in walking. Z. Vergl. Physiol. 76,
  16-31.
Bowerman, R.F., and Larimer, J.L., 1972. Command fibers in the
  circumoesophageal connectives of crayfish. Amer. Zool. 12,
  692.
Bowerman, R.F., and Larimer, J.L., 1974a. Command fibers in the
  circumoesophageal connectives of crayfish. I. Tonic fibers.
  J. Exp. Biol. In press.
Bowerman, R.F., and Larimer, J.L., 1974b. Command fibers in the
  circumoesophageal connectives of crayfish. II. Phasic fibers.
  J. Exp. Biol. In press.
Bullock, T.H., and Horridge, G.A., 1965. Structure and Function
  in the Nervous Systems of Invertebrates. W.H. Freeman and Co.,
  San Francisco.
Burrows, M., and Hoyle, G., 1973. The mechanism of rapid running
  in the ghost crab, Ocypode ceratophthalma. J. Exp. Biol. 58,
  327-349.
Burrows, M., and Willows, A.O.D., 1969. Neuronal coordination of
  rhythmic maxilliped beating in Brachyuran and Anomuran Crustacea.
  Comp. Biochem. Physiol. 31, 121-135.
Bush, B.M.H., 1962. Proprioceptive reflexes in the legs of
  Carcinus maenas L. J. Exp. Biol. 39, 89-105.
Bush, B.M.H., 1963. A comparative study of certain limb reflexes
  in decapod crustaceans. Comp. Biochem. Physiol. 10, 273-290.
Bush, B.M.H., 1965. Leg reflexes from chordotonal organs in the
  crab, Carcinus maenas. Comp. Biochem. Physiol. 15, 567-587.
Clarac, F., and Beaubaton, D., 1969. Perturbations réversibles des
  programmes locomoteurs induites par blocage articulaire chez le
  crabe Carcinus. Compt. Rend. Soc. Biol. 163, 2646-2649.
Clarac, F., and Coulmance, M., 1971. Le marche latérale du crabe
  (Carcinus): Coordination des mouvements articulaires et regulation
  proprioceptive. Z. Vergl. Physiol. 73, 408-438.
Clarac, F., and Dando, M.R., 1973. Tension receptor reflexes in
  the walking legs of the crab, Cancer pagurus. Nature 243, 94-95.
Clarac, F., Wales, W., and Laverack, M.S., 1971. Stress detection
  at the autotomy plane in the decapod Crustacea. II. The function
  of the receptors associated with the cuticle of the basi-
  ischiopodite. Z. Vergl. Physiol. 73, 383-407.

Davis, W.J., and Ayers, J.L. Jr., 1972. Locomotion: control by positive feedback optokinetic responses. Science 177, 183-185.

Evoy, W.H., and Cohen, M.J., 1971. Central and peripheral control of arthropod movements. In Advances in Comparative Physiology and Biochemistry, Vol. 4. (Ed. Loewenstein, O.) Academic Press, N.Y., pp. 225-266.

Evoy, W.H., and Fourtner, C.R., 1973. Nervous control of walking in the crab, Cardisoma guanhumi. III. Proprioceptive influences on intra- and intersegmental coordination. J. Comp. Physiol. 83, 303-318.

Fourtner, C.R., and Evoy, W.H., 1973. Nervous control of walking in the crab, Cardisoma guanhumi. IV. Effects of myochordotonal organ ablation. J. Comp. Physiol. 83, 319-329.

Graham, D., 1972. A behavioural analysis of the temporal organisation of walking movements in the first instar and adult stick insect (Carausius morosus). J. Comp. Physiol. 81, 23-52.

Grote, J.R., 1973. Sensory and Motor Control of Stepping in the 5th Leg of the Crayfish, Procambarus clarkii. M.S. Thesis, Univ. of Miami.

Hafemann, D.R., and Hubbard, J.I., 1969. On the rapid running of ghost crabs, Ocypode ceratophthalma. J. Exp. Zool. 170, 25-32.

Hartnoll, R.G., 1970. Swimming in the Dromiid crab, Homola barbata. Anim. Behav. 18, 588-591.

Hartnoll, R.G., 1971. The occurrence, methods and significance of swimming in the Brachyura. Anim. Behav. 19, 34-50.

Lochhead, J.N., 1961. Locomotion. In Physiology of Crustacea. Vol. II, (Ed. Waterman,T.H.) Academic Press, N.Y., pp. 313-364.

MacMillan, D.L.,and Dando, M.R., 1972. Tension receptors on the apodemes of muscles in the walking legs of the crab, Cancer magister. Mar. Behav. Physiol. 1, 185-208.

Mendelson, M., 1971. Oscillator neurons in crustacean ganglia. Science 171, 1170-1173.

Moody, C.J., 1970. A proximally directed intersegmental reflex in a walking leg of the crayfish. Amer. Zool. 10, 501.

Parrack, D.W., 1964. Stepping Sequences in the Crayfish. Ph.D. Thesis, Univ. of Illinois.

Ripley, S.H., Bush, B.M.H., and Roberts, A., 1968. Crab muscle receptor which responds without impulses. Nature 218, 1170-1171.

Roberts, A., and Bush, B.M.H., 1971. Coxal muscle receptors in the crab: the receptor current and some properties of the receptor nerve fibers. J. Exp. Biol. 54, 515-524.

Roye, D.B., 1972. Evoked activity in the nervous system of Callinectes sapidus following phasic stimulation of the statocysts. Experientia 28, 1307-1309.

Spirito, C.P., 1972. An anlysis of swimming behavior in the portunid crab, Callinectes sapidus. Mar. Behav. Physiol. 1, 261-276.

Spirito, C.P., Evoy, W.H., and Barnes, W.J.P., 1972. Nervous control of walking in the crab, Cardisoma guanhumi. I. Characteristics of resistance reflexes. Z. Vergl. Physiol. 76, 1-15.

Wales, W., Clarac, F., and Laverack, M.S., 1971. Stress detection at the autotomy plane in the decapod Crustacea. I. Comparative anatomy of the receptors of the basi-ischiopodite region. Z. Vergl. Physiol. 73, 357-382.

Wilson, D.M., 1972. Genetic and sensory mechanisms for locomotion and orientation in animals. Amer. Sci. 60, 358-365.

NERVOUS CONTROL OF WALKING IN THE COCKROACH

K. G. Pearson, C. R. Fourtner and R. K. Wong

Department of Physiology, University of Alberta
Edmonton, Canada

Over the past few years there have been significant
advances in our knowledge of the nervous events underlying
the leg movements of walking insects. These include (1)
the precise description of the discharge patterns of identified motoneurones and the correlation of electrophysiological
and behavioural data, (2) the demonstration of central
rhythm generators for producing the basic rhythmicity of
leg movements, (3) the recording of intracellular events in
motoneurones and interneurones during rhythmic leg movements, and (4) the effects on motor output of changes in
feedback from leg receptors. The most intensively studied
animal has been the cockroach. For this animal it is clear
that central mechanisms determine the basic rhythmicity
and reciprocity in the activity supplying the muscles producing the alternate flexion and extension movements of the
femur. Preliminary studies indicate that non-spiking interneurones are involved in the central patterning of motor
output.

Reflexes from two groups of leg receptors also play an
important part in patterning the motor output during walking
in the cockroach. (1) The afferents from the campaniform
sensilla of the trochanter strongly excite extensor motoneurones and are maximally active during the extension
phase of leg movement. This reflex therefore functions to
reinforce the centrally generated extensor burst and provides

a mechanism to compensate for any variations in load. The input from the campaniform sensilla also depresses the rate of rhythmic leg movements by prolonging the duration of the extensor bursts. This inhibitory influence is important in regulating the rate of stepping and in co-ordinating the stepping movements of different legs. (2) The receptors of the hair plate on the trochanter are excited during the flexion movements and their removal leads to more intense and pro- longed flexor burst during stepping (resulting in an exagger- ated stepping movement). The reflexes from this group of receptors appear to be organized so as to limit the magnitude and duration of flexor bursts and to facilitate the initiation of extensor activity.

It is now quite clear in both invertebrates and vertebrates that the basic rhythmicity in the motoneuronal activity underlying rhythmic movements is generated in systems of neurones located entirely within the central nervous system (DeLong, 1971; Kater et al., 1973). Furthermore, it is clear that for most systems the centrally generated motor output can be modified by input from various groups of peripheral sensory receptors. The degree to which sensory input can influence the motor output appears to be related to the extent that there can be unpredictable variations in external conditions. Rather surprisingly, we have very little knowledge of either the cellular basis for the central generation of rhythmic burst activity in motoneurones or the precise function of feedback from peripheral receptors.

There is no doubt that sensory feedback from a variety of leg receptors is very important in regulating the motor output during walking in cats (Lundberg, 1969; Grillner, 1973, this Symposium), crabs (Clarac and Coulmance, 1971; Evoy and Fourtner, 1973, this Symposium) and insects (Usherwood and Runion, 1970; Pearson, 1972; Pearson and Iles, 1973). However, the precise conditions under which the input from any group of leg receptors is utilized is not clear for any of these animals although numerous suggestions have been made (Lundberg, 1969; Grillner, 1973, this Symposium; Evoy and Fourtner, 1973; Pringle, 1961; Pearson, 1972; Pearson and Iles, 1973). A feature of the leg movements in walking animals is the large degree of variability even when the animal is walking on a flat surface (Stuart et al., this Symposium; Evoy and Fourtner, 1973; Burns, 1973; Graham, 1972). Although no measurements have been made, it seems reasonable to suppose

that this variability increases when the animals walk over uneven
surfaces. A particularly challenging problem is to determine the
extent to which variations in proprioceptive signals can account
for the variable leg movements, and whether these signals function
to adjust automatically the motor output to compensate for unexpected changes in external conditions.

Our knowledge of the nervous control of insect walking has
increased enormously over the past few years. The system controlling leg movements in the walking cockroach is the best
understood, but many features of this system are common with
those in other insect species. The aim of this article is to review
briefly the recently published and unpublished work on the nervous
mechanisms controlling walking in the cockroach, with an emphasis
on those features which appear common in the nervous control of
rhythmic movements in other animals.

NORMAL LEG MOVEMENTS

The movements of individual legs and the co-ordination of
stepping movements in different legs during normal walking have
recently been analyzed in considerable detail for the cockroach
(Delcomyn, 1971a), locust (Burns, 1973) and stick insect (Graham,
1972). The most common stepping pattern in the cockroach and
locust is the tripod gait in which the stepping of the fore and hind
leg on one side and the middle leg on the opposite side alternates
with the stepping of the other three legs. For the cockroach,
Periplaneta americana, the rate of leg movements can be as
high as 24 steps/sec, and the tripod gait is used whenever the
animals walk at rates higher than about 2 steps/sec. First
instar stick insects most commonly use a tripod gait but at times
use the adult gait in which the lag between the stepping of the
hind and fore legs is significantly less than the total step period.

Another common feature of the movements of individual legs
in insects is that with changes in walking speed the change in
duration of the swing phase (protraction) is considerably smaller
than the change in duration of the stance phase (retraction). Thus,
an increase in the rate of stepping results primarily from a
decrease in the duration of retraction. This feature is also seen
in the leg movements of other animals (Miller and van der Burg,
this Symposium; Szekely et al., 1969). For the insect species
studied so far the time of protraction is typically between 50 and 150

msec and the ratio of the protraction time to the retraction time
varies from 0.2 to 1.0 in slowly walking and rapidly running
animals respectively.

In the cockroach there are two phases of movement of the
middle and hind legs in each stepping cycle, and four phases for
the fore legs (Fig. 1). These phases can be seen by noticing the

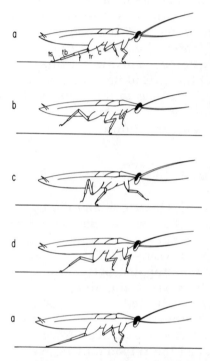

Fig. 1. Schematic diagram showing the various phases of
movement in the three ipsilateral legs of a walking cockroach.
Protraction of the hind and fore legs alternates with protraction
of the middle leg. In the hind and middle legs there are two
phases of movement of the femur in each stepping cycle:
flexion during protraction and extension during retraction. For
the forelimbs there are four phases of movement of the femur:
flexion during the first part of protraction and the first part of
retraction (b and d), and extension during the latter parts of
protraction and retraction (c and a). Abbreviations: c - coxa;
tr - trochanter; f - femur; tb - tibia; ts - tarsus.

movements of the femur relative to the coxa. During protraction
of the fore legs there is initially a flexion movement which is
followed by extension. This latter movement results in the leg
being extended at the beginning of retraction. During retraction
an initial flexion movement of the femur is followed by extension.
In the other two pairs of legs the flexion and extension movements
of the femur occur only during protraction and retraction respectively. These differences between the movements of the fore legs
and the movements of the middle and hind legs increases the complexity of this system and adds to the difficulty of determining the
nervous mechanisms controlling the leg movements in the different
segments. A comparable situation exists in the system controlling
walking in mammals where there are two phases of hip movement
and four phases of knee and ankle movements in each stepping
cycle (Engberg and Lundberg, 1969).

ACTIVITY IN MOTONEURONES DURING WALKING

The activity in various leg motoneurones has been recorded
during walking in locusts and cockroaches (Hoyle, 1964; Runion
and Usherwood, 1968; Usherwood et al., 1968; Usherwood and
Runion, 1970; Burns, 1972; Pearson, 1972; Pearson and Iles,
1973). In the cockroach the rhythmic flexion and extension movements of the femur are produced by bursts of activity in motoneurones supplying the coxal levator and depressor muscles respectively (Pearson, 1972). Fig. 2 shows the activity recorded
from these muscles in a cockroach walking in a straight line on a
horizontal surface. At walking speeds between 2 and 10 steps/sec
two excitatory motoneurones are active during the flexion movements; extension movements are produced by activity in a single
slow motoneurone. For walking speeds less than 2 steps/sec only
the smaller of the two levator motor units is active while above
10 steps/sec large fast motor units are recruited to both the
levator and depressor muscles. The orderly recruitment of
larger motor axons as the walking speed increases is another
example of the size principle (Henneman et al., 1965; Davis,
1971; Stein and Milner-Brown, this Symposium). As the walking
speed increases the durations of both the flexor and extensor
bursts decrease, and for any walking speed these durations
correspond closely to the behavioural measurements of protraction
and retraction times respectively (Pearson, 1972).

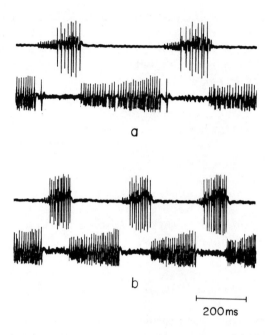

a

b

|—————————|
200 ms

Fig. 2. Reciprocal burst activity recorded from the coxal
levator (top) and depressor (bottom) muscles in the hind leg
of a freely walking cockroach. The alternate contractions
of these muscles produce the flexion and extension movements of the femur respectively. For stepping rates between
2 and 10 steps/sec two slow motor axons are active during
femur flexion, while only a single motoneurone is active
during femur extension (from Pearson, 1972).

At all walking speeds in the cockroach the reciprocity of
activity in motoneurones supplying the coxal levator and depressor
muscles is maintained. There have been reports of co-activation
of motoneurones innervating antagonistic muscles in walking
locusts (Hoyle, 1964) and cockroaches (Ewing and Manning, 1966).
There is some doubt, however, whether this phenomenon actually
occurs. The lack of clarity in the early records from the cockroach prevents any confident assertion of its existence, while in
the locust a clear reciprocity is seen in the records made from
the flexor and extensor tibiae muscles by Usherwood et al. (1968)
when the animals were walking at speeds where Hoyle (1964)

reported co-activation of the same muscles. In more recent studies Burns (personal communication) has also failed to observe any co-activation of antagonistic motoneurones in the locust hind leg. However, in the fore and middle legs the slow extensor tibiae motoneurone is not inactive during flexor bursts whereas the fast extensor tibiae motoneurone always discharges reciprocally with the flexor motoneurones.

A close correlation exists between the timing of the bursts in motoneurones to the coxal levator muscles in the three ipsilateral legs of the cockroach and the stepping pattern in these three legs. Fig. 3 shows bursts of activity recorded from the coxal levator

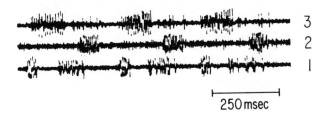

250 msec

Fig. 3. Burst activity recorded from the coxal levator muscles of the hind (3), middle (2) and fore (1) legs of a freely walking cockroach. Contractions in these muscles produce flexion movements of the femur. The bursts in the hind and middle legs alternate and their occurrence corresponds to the stepping movement in each of these limbs. Two fore leg bursts are seen for each hind leg burst. The more intense and shorter in duration begins just prior to the hind leg burst. This burst of activity is responsible for producing the flexion movement of the femur during the first part of protraction. The other fore leg burst produces femur flexion during the initial part of retraction.

muscles in the hind, middle and fore legs of a cockroach walking in a straight line on a horizontal surface. The phase of the middle leg burst in the hind leg cycle is approximately 0.5 for all but the slowest walking speeds. There are two fore leg bursts for each burst in the middle and hind legs. These two fore leg bursts occur during the two flexion phases of the femur. One burst

begins just before the hind leg burst, and its phase within the hind
leg cycle is usually slightly less than 1.0 except at very slow
walking speeds. This fore leg burst is shorter in duration and
more intense than the other fore leg burst and is responsible for
producing the flexion movement of the femur during the initial
part of fore leg protraction. The magnitude of the phase values
mentioned above and their lack of variation with walking speed
corresponds to the behavioural observation that a tripod gait is
used over a wide range of walking speeds. The difference in the
motor output to the forelimbs compared to that to the middle and
hind legs is particularly intriguing, for the problem immediately
arises of how two flexor bursts are generated during each stepping
cycle. Do central mechanisms operate to produce both bursts, or
is the oscillator basically similar to that postulated for the middle
and hind legs (see below) with the additional burst generated
reflexly? At present we cannot even attempt to answer this
question.

CENTRAL PATTERNING OF ACTIVITY IN MOTONEURONES

There has been considerable discussion in the past about the
extent to which the motoneuronal activity is patterned centrally
and the importance of sensory feedback in determining the motor
output (Hoyle, 1964; Wilson, 1966). This discussion is far from
over, but recent work has led to a number of specific proposals
(Pearson and Iles, 1970, 1973; Pearson, 1972). Although central
patterning probably occurs in the walking systems of all insects,
only in the cockroach and milk-weed bug have we any direct evidence
for its occurrence (Pearson, 1972; Hoy and Wilson, 1969). In both
these animals rhythmic motor output persists after removal of all
sensory input from leg receptors. Significantly the patterns of
activity in these deafferented preparations are similar in some
aspects to those seen in rhythmically moving intact legs. For
example, the reciprocal relationship between the two levator and
single depressor motoneurones seen in walking cockroaches (Fig. 2)
is also seen in the same three motoneurones of the middle and hind
legs of deafferented preparations. There is rarely any overlap of
activity in antagonistic motoneurones in both deafferented preparations and walking animals. In addition, the durations of the
levator bursts are relatively constant and similar in magnitude to
the durations observed in walking animals (Pearson and Iles, 1970;
Pearson, 1972). These similarities indicate that the rhythmic
motor output seen after deafferentation is related to walking, and

constitute strong evidence that a central rhythm generator produces the levator bursts. Moreover, they also indicate that central connections ensure the strict reciprocity in the activity of antagonistic motoneurones. However, not all features of the motor output are similar in walking and deafferented preparations. In the latter there is no obvious relationship between the durations of the levator bursts and the frequency at which the bursts occur, nor is the discharge rate of either the levator or depressor motoneurones within a burst clearly related to burst frequency. These differences could be due either to the lack of direct segmental proprioceptive effects on the system producing the rhythmic reciprocal motor output, or to differences in the activity of central command neurones controlling the central rhythm generator, or to a combination of both. At present we do not know which of these possibilities accounts for the differences in motor output.

After removal of all sensory input from leg receptors the levator bursts in the middle and hind legs rarely overlap; the hind leg burst tending to occur immediately after the middle leg burst, or vice versa. This negative correlation indicates some form of central inhibitory coupling between the two segments. Within the connectives joining the middle and hind segments there exist interneurones which discharge in phase with the levator bursts in either the hind segment or the middle segment (Pearson and Iles, 1973). These interneurones could mediate mutual inhibitory coupling between the levator burst generating systems in the two segments, but whether they do has not yet been determined. Nevertheless, we can conclude that central inhibitory pathways exist between the adjacent rhythm generating systems and that these pathways probably ensure that the two adjacent legs do not step at the same time. Again, as for the motor output for a single segment, there are differences in the temporal relationships of the middle and hind leg levator bursts in deafferented preparations and walking animals. An attempt has been made to explain these differences by the lack of segmental proprioceptive influences in the deafferented preparations (Pearson and Iles, 1973).

At present virtually nothing is known about the cellular basis of the rhythmic burst generation in vertebrate and invertebrate locomotory systems (Grillner, this Symposium; Willows et al., this Symposium). For the cockroach walking system it has been postulated that the reciprocal levator and depressor bursts are produced by activity in a bursting interneurone, or a system of bursting interneurones, which periodically excites the levator

motoneurones and inhibits the ongoing activity in the depressor
motoneurone (Pearson and Iles, 1970; Pearson, 1972). It appears
reasonable to suppose that the patterning of the motor output
depends on activity in an interneuronal network rather than on
coupling between motoneurones, for antidromic stimulation of
either set of motoneurones has no effect on activity in antagonists
(Pearson and Iles, 1970). In the locust too there is no evidence
for positive coupling between agonist or inhibitory coupling
between antagonist motoneurones active during rhythmic leg
movements (Hoyle and Burrows, 1973).

In an attempt to determine the cellular basis for the central
rhythm generator in the cockroach we have recorded intracellularly
from motoneurones and interneurones in the third thoracic ganglion
during rhythmic leg movements. We have found nothing to support
the earlier proposal that a bursting pacemaker or bursting system
of interneurones drives the levator motoneurones. Explorations
in most regions of the ganglion failed to reveal any cell which in
addition to discharging spikes in-phase with the levator bursts
also produced activity in the levator motoneurones when a depolarizing current was applied to evoke spike activity. On the other
hand, we regularly penetrated two distinct types of non-spiking
interneurones which when depolarized had a profound effect on the
activity of levator motoneurones. In both types there were
rhythmic membrane potential depolarizations which were either
in-phase, Type I (Fig. 4a), or out-of-phase, Type II (Fig. 4b),
with the bursts of activity in the levator motoneurones. Intracellularly applied depolarizing currents to Type I interneurones
readily elicited activity in the levator motoneurones (Fig. 5).
Significantly only those motoneurones active during walking movements were excited, and the order of recruitment with increasing
stimulus strengths was identical to that which occurs in a
walking animal. Thus it appears probable that this type of interneuron is associated with the system of neurones producing
the burst activity in the levator motoneurones during walking.
Applied depolarizing current to Type II interneurones inhibited
any ongoing activity in levator motoneurones, the larger motoneurones being silenced first.

A critical question is whether or not these non-spiking interneurones are part of the rhythm generating system, or simply
interneurones intercalated between this system and the motoneurones. We have no data to decide between these possibilities,

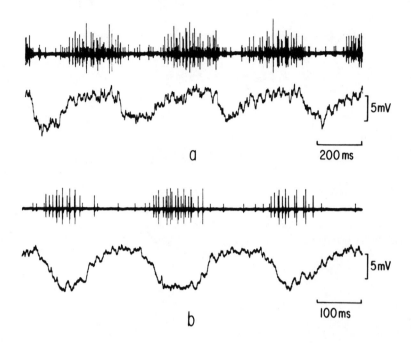

5mV

200 ms

a

5mV

100ms

b

Fig. 4. Oscillatory activity recorded intracellularly from two
types of non-spiking interneurones in the third thoracic ganglion
of the cockroach during rhythmic leg movements. Top traces -
activity recorded from motor axons innervating the coxal
levator muscles; bottom traces - intracellular records.
(a) In this neurone (Type I) the depolarizations occur at the
same time as the bursts of activity recorded from motor
axons supplying the coxal levator muscles. (b) In this neurone
(Type II) the depolarizations occur during the periods between
the levator bursts. Applied depolarization of Type I interneurones strongly excites the levator motoneurones (Fig. 5)
whereas a depolarization of Type II interneurones inhibits
the ongoing activity in levator motoneurones.

for we have not yet observed the effects on the rhythm of short
applied current pulses to these neurones. However, there seems
no doubt that they are associated with the system of neurones
producing rhythmic leg movements. In addition to the rhythmic
membrane oscillations and the specific effects of applied stimulation, these interneurones are located in a region of the ganglion
which when damaged by slight probing with microelectrodes

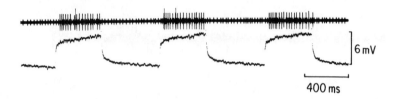

Fig. 5. Excitation of three motoneurones innervating the coxal
levator muscles upon depolarization of a Type I non-spiking
interneurone. Top trace - record from nerve to coxal levator
muscles; bottom trace - change in membrane potential in
Type I interneurone. (The depolarizing currents were applied
through the recording electrode using a balanced bridge circuit.)
The action potentials with the two largest amplitudes in the top
record are from the two slow motor axons active during stepping
(Fig. 2), while the small amplitude action potential is from the
branch of a common inhibitory motoneurone. Note that all three
motoneurones are excited without any spike activity in the interneurone.

results in the abolition of rhythmic leg movements. Other regions
of the ganglion can be repeatedly probed without the abolition of
these movements.

Another important question is whether the basic rhythmicity
depends entirely upon the oscillations in a single pacemaker cell,
or whether oscillations are generated by the interaction of a number
of neurones. Our present data are insufficient to answer this
question, although the finding of more than one type of non-spiking
interneurone favours the latter possibility. Mendelson (1971) has
proposed that a single non-spiking interneurone is responsible
for generating the respiratory rhythm in crustaceans. However,
there is nothing in his results which excludes the possibility that
the non-spiking cells he recorded from were individuals in a
system of non-spiking neurones.

REFLEX REGULATION OF MOTOR OUTPUT

In walking insects it is quite apparent that sensory input from leg receptors is important in determining the motor output. One indication is the difference between the motor output in walking animals and deafferented preparations (see Central Patterning Activity in Motoneurones). The most direct indication, however, is that removal of certain groups of receptors, or alteration of the sensory input by a change in loading, can markedly change the motor output. Although these changes have been observed in a number of studies, in some cases it is unclear how the sensory input is utilized in patterning the motor output. For example, in the locust removal of tarsal receptors or the femoral chordotonal organ in a metathoracic leg causes a decrease in the intensity of output in the slow and inhibitory motoneurones to the extensor tibiae muscles, as well as a slowing of the stepping movements (Usherwood and Runion, 1970). Our lack of knowledge of the reflex effects from these receptors, and the role of central patterning in the locust, prevents any concise explanation for this changed motor output following receptor ablation.

Two groups of sensory receptors, the campaniform sensilla and hair-plates of the trochanter, have been found to be important in regulating the motor output of the coxal levator and depressor motoneurones in the hind leg of a walking cockroach. The campaniform sensilla of the trochanter are located in the cuticle and respond to cuticular distortions which presumably occur during the leg retraction phase of walking (Pringle, 1938; 1961). On the other hand, the receptors of the hair-plate are excited during flexion movements of the femur and are thus presumably active during leg protraction. Removal of the hair-plate leads to a more intense and prolonged burst in the levator motoneurones and consequently to an exaggerated protraction movement. An exaggerated stepping movement also occurs in the legs of stick insects following the removal of the coxal hair-plates (Wendler, 1966). We have discovered three reflex effects elicited by activity in the hair-plate receptors: (1) monosynaptic excitation of the slow coxal depressor motoneurone; (2) a short latency inhibition of the coxal levator motoneurones; and (3) a depression of the rate of bursting in the levator motoneurones. The inhibitory pathways to the rhythm generator and levator motoneurones very likely function to limit the intensity and duration of the levator bursts during walking, while the excitatory pathway to the depressor motoneurone could facilitate the initiation of the bursts of activity in this motoneurone.

It is probable that this latter pathway also functions to stabilize
leg posture during standing. Any imposed flexion movement will
excite the hair receptors and therefore reflexly increase the level
of activity in the depressor motoneurone. This will increase the
force in the depressor muscle, and hence the flexion movement
will be resisted.

There are at least two reflex effects elicited by activity in the
campaniform sensilla: (1) a strong excitation of the slow coxal
depressor motoneurone (Pringle, 1961; Pearson, 1972); and (2)
a strong inhibition of the system producing the levator bursts
(Pearson and Iles, 1973). Since these receptors are probably
excited during leg retraction, their excitatory effect will facilitate
the activity in the depressor motoneurone (which is active during
retraction). This reinforcing effect of the feedback from the
campaniform sensilla provides a mechanism for load compensation.
For example, if the animal begins to walk up an incline, there
will be a greater resistance to leg extension, an increased activity
in the campaniform sensilla and consequently an increased
contractile force in the depressor muscle to give a stronger
extension movement. The positive feedback effect from the
campaniform sensilla to the depressor motoneurone is limited
by two mechanisms. Firstly, as the femur extends there will
be a decrease in the degree of distortion of the trochanter due to
a decrease in the bending moment at the coxa-trochanter joint,
and secondly, as the animal moves forward more of the load
carried by the extending leg will be carried by the other legs
thus decreasing the stresses in the cuticle of the trochanter
(Pringle, 1961). Thus, these two limiting effects ensure that the
positive feedback pathway does not irreversibly turn on the
depressor motoneurone.

When the resistance to the retraction movement of the leg is
increased (for example when the animals drag a small weight or
walk up an inclined surface) the rate of stepping decreases. The
obvious explanation for this effect is that it results from increased
activity in the inhibitory reflex pathway from the campaniform
sensilla to the rhythm generating system. The functional importance of this reflex pathway does not become apparent until we
consider how the stepping movements in the different legs are
co-ordinated. Earlier we mentioned that the rhythm generating
systems in adjacent ipsilateral segments are centrally coupled
by one or more inhibitory pathways, thus ensuring that no two
adjacent ipsilateral legs step at the same time. If the animal

only ever walked on flat horizontal surfaces then this central
connection could be sufficient for ensuring the correct sequence
of leg movements. However, it is quite clear that cockroaches
can walk with remarkable dexterity over uneven surfaces which,
a priori, suggests a high degree of reflex control of intersegmental co-ordination during this behaviour. The inhibitory
reflex pathway from the campaniform sensilla to the rhythm
generating systems provides an ingenious mechanism for this
reflex control. If the activity in the inhibitory afferent pathway
is above a certain level then the rhythm generating system will
be inactivated and no stepping movement produced. Thus, when
the load carried by a leg is high that leg will not step. As the
load is reduced the inhibitory input to the rhythm generating
system will become insufficient to prevent this system from
producing another burst in the levator motoneurones and the leg
will step. Therefore, as the animal moves over a rough and
unpredictable terrain, the load in some legs will be sufficient to
prevent them from stepping while the load in the other legs will
be insufficient to prevent a stepping movement. Put another way,
stepping movements only occur in those legs carrying the least
load. Once the stepping leg finds a solid support this leg will
begin to carry some of the animal's weight and thus result in a
decrease in load carried by one or more of the other legs. This
may be sufficient to allow stepping in the unloaded leg, or legs.
Subject to the condition that no two adjacent ipsilateral legs step at
the same time, there may not necessarily be any precise and predictable temporal relationship between the stepping movements
of the different legs when the animal walks over very rough surfaces.

Here we have only discussed what we know of the function of
the reflexes arising from the hair-plate and campaniform sensilla
of the trochanter. Undoubtedly, sensory input from other groups
of leg receptors is important in regulating the motor output,
perhaps different groups being utilized under different conditions.
For example, the sensory regulation could be quite different
when the animal walks upside down beneath a horizontal surface
compared to that when it walks upright on a flat surface. At
present we do not know the functional significance of the input
from any other groups of leg receptors in the cockroach.

CONCLUSIONS

Despite fairly intensive efforts over the past few years, we are still a long way from fully understanding the nervous control of insect walking. Nevertheless, there have been some significant advances which include: (1) the precise description of the motor output and the correlation of behavioural and electrophysiological data (Burns, 1972, 1973; Pearson, 1972; Pearson and Iles, 1973); (2) the demonstration of central rhythm generators in the cockroach and milk-weed bug (Pearson, 1972; Hoy and Wilson, 1969) and central inhibitory coupling between these generators in the second and third thoracic segments of the cockroach (Pearson and Iles, 1973); (3) the existence of non-spiking interneurones in the third thoracic ganglion of the cockroach which either excite or inhibit those levator motoneurones active during walking (see Central Patterning Activity in Motoneurones); and (4) the determination of the function of certain reflex pathways in regulating the motor output in the cockroach (see Reflex Regulation of Motor Output). At present all models of the walking systems in insects are extremely qualitative (Wilson, 1967; Delcomyn, 1971b; Graham, 1972; Pearson, 1972; Pearson and Iles, 1973) and only those proposed for the cockroach make any prediction about the cellular events occurring in motoneurones and interneurones. Apart from their usefulness in suggesting additional experiments, these models provide a convenient means for summarizing our current knowledge. Such a summary is shown in Fig. 6 for the organization of the system controlling rhythmic movements of the femur in hind legs of the cockroach. The two central elements of this system consist of (1) a rhythm generator which periodically excites the flexor motoneurones and inhibits the ongoing activity in the extensor motoneurones, and (2) a central command input which produces activity in the rhythm generator and drives the extensor motoneurone. At present little is known about either of these elements although recent work indicates that the central rhythmicity could be generated in a system of non-spiking interneurones (see Central Patterning Activity in Motoneurones). Superimposed on these central elements are two reflex systems. The first from the hair-plate of the trochanter functions during femur flexion, and the other from the campaniform sensilla of the trochanter functions during femur extension. The behavioural significance of these two reflex systems has been discussed in Reflex Regulation of Motor Output).

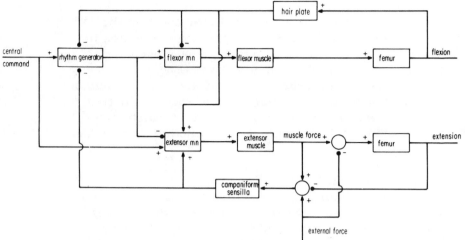

Fig. 6. Block diagram showing some of the known and postulated organization of the system controlling rhythmic movements of the femur in the hind legs of a walking cockroach.
The central elements in this system are discussed in the
section on Central Patterning Activity in Motoneurones, and
the functional properties of the reflex pathways from the
campaniform sensilla and hair-plate are discussed in the
section on Reflex Regulation of Motor Output.

There are two features of general interest in the function of
these two reflex systems. The first is the reinforcing effect on
the activity in the extensor motoneurone by the feedback from
the campaniform sensilla. A functionally similar reinforcing
effect has been described for a number of other motor systems
in vertebrates and invertebrates (Lundberg, 1969; Euler, 1966;
Davis, 1969; Paul, 1971; Kater and Rowell, 1973). Significantly,
these reflexes have only been found to reinforce the activity in
motoneurones controlling muscles in which there can be unpredictable variations in load during contraction. It seems reasonable to conclude, therefore, that reinforcing reflexes in all
animals provide a simple mechanism for at least partially
compensating for unpredictable changes in external conditions.

The second interesting feature of the reflex organization
shown in Fig. 6 is that the feedback from the hair-plate receptors
functions to limit femur flexion and facilitates the initiation of
femur extension. A functionally similar reflex system has been
described in the swimmeret system of the lobster (Davis, 1969)

and the masticatory system of the snail (Kater and Rowell, 1973),
while there is a possibility that in the cat reflexes function to
facilitate the termination of the flexion phase of movement at
the knee and initiate the first extension phase (Engberg and
Lundberg, 1969; Lundberg, 1969). Thus, it appears in a number
of systems that reflexes function to facilitate the termination
of activity in motoneurones supplying muscles in which the
load is unlikely to change from one cycle to another, or during
a single contraction.

     Research on insect walking will probably develop along three
main lines in the near future: (1) in determining more precisely
the function of sensory feedback from different groups of leg
receptors and how the sensory input interacts with the central
elements to produce functionally significant changes in motor
output; (2) in determining the cellular basis for the central generation of rhythmic motor output; and (3) in identifying and determining the properties of central command interneurones. There
are many challenging problems in all three of these areas.
Anticipating future developments is extremely exciting for even
our present rudimentary knowledge leaves us with a sense of
wonder at the intricacy, subtlety and unity of the mechanisms
controlling and co-ordinating rhythmic leg movements in insects.

REFERENCES

Burns, M.D., 1972. The control of walking in Orthoptera. Ph.D.
   Thesis, Univ. Glasgow.
Burns, M.D., 1973. The control of walking in Orthoptera. I. Leg
   movements in normal walking. J. Exp. Biol. 58, 45-58.
Clarac, F., and Coulmance, M., 1971. La marche latérale du crabe
   (Carcinus); coordination des mouvements articularies et régulation
   proprioceptive. Z. vergl. Physiol. 73, 408-438.
Davis, W.J., 1969. Reflex organization in the swimmeret system of
   the lobster. I. Intrasegmental reflexes. J. Exp. Biol. 51,
   547-563.
Davis, W.J., 1971. Functional significance of motoneuron size and
   soma position in swimmeret system of the lobster. J. Neurophysiol.
   34, 274-288.
Delcomyn, F., 1971a. The locomotion of the cockroach, Periplaneta
   americana. J. Exp. Biol. 54, 443-452.
Delcomyn, F., 1971b. The effect of limb amputation on locomotion in
   the cockroach, Periplaneta americana. J. Exp. Biol. 54, 453-469.
DeLong, M., 1971. Central Patterning of movement. Neurosci. Res.
   Prog. Bull. 9, 10-30.
Engberg, I., and Lundberg, A., 1969. An electromyographic analysis
   of muscular activity in the hindlimb of the cat during unrestrained
   locomotion. Acta Physiol. Scand. 75, 614-630.

Euler, C.V., 1966. The control of respiratory movement. In Breathlessness (Ed. Howell, J.B.L., and Campbell, E.J.M.). pp. 19-32.

Evoy, W.H., and Fourtner, C.R., 1973. Nervous control of walking in the crab, Cardisoma guanhumi. III. Proprioceptive influences on intra- and intersegmental coordination. J. Comp. Physiol. 83, 303-318.

Ewing, A.W., and Manning, A., 1966. Some aspects of the efferent control of walking in three cockroach species. J. Ins. Physiol. 12, 1115-1118.

Graham, D., 1972. A behavioural analysis of the temporal organization of walking movements in the first instar and adult stick insect (Carausius morosus). J. Comp. Physiol. 81, 23-52.

Grillner, S., 1973. On the spinal generation of locomotion. In Sensory Organization of Movements (Ed. Batuev, A.S.) In Press.

Henneman, E., Somjen, G., and Carpenter, D.O., 1965. Functional significance of cell size in spinal motoneurons. J. Neurophysiol. 28, 560-580.

Hoy, R.R., and Wilson, D.M., 1969. Rhythmic motor output in leg motor neurons of the milkweed bug, Oncopeltus. Fed. Proc. 28, 588.

Hoyle, G., 1964. Exploration of neuronal mechanisms underlying behaviour in insects. In Neural Theory and Modelling. (Ed. Reiss, R.). Stanford Univ. Press, pp. 346-376.

Hoyle, G., and Burrows, M., 1973. Neural mechanisms underlying behavior in the locust, Schistocerca gregaria. I. Physiology of identified neurons in the metathoracic ganglion. J. Neurobiol. 4, 3-41.

Kater, S.B., Heyer, C., and Kaneko, C.R.S., 1973. Identifiable neurons and invertebrate behavior. In Neurophysiology (Physiology Series). MTP Int. Rev. Sci. (Ed. Hunt, C.) In Press.

Kater, S.B., and Rowell, C.H.F., 1973. Integration of sensory and centrally programmed components in generation of cyclical feeding activity in Helisoma trivolvis. J. Neurophysiol. 36, 142-155.

Lundberg, A., 1969. Reflex control of stepping. Nansen Memorial Lecture to Norwegian Academy of Sciences and Letters.

Mendelson, M., 1971. Oscillator neurons in crustacean ganglia. Science 171, 1170-1173.

Paul, D.H., 1971. Swimming behavior of the sand crab, Emerita analoga (Crustacea, Anomura). III. Neuronal organization of uropod beating. Z. vergl. Physiol. 75, 286-304.

Pearson, K.G., 1972. Central programming and reflex control of walking in the cockroach. J. Exp. Biol. 56, 173-193.

Pearson, K.G., and Iles, J.F., 1970. Discharge patterns of coxal levator and depressor motoneurones of the cockroach, Periplaneta americana. J. Exp. Biol. 52, 139-165.

Pearson, K.G., and Iles, J.F., 1973. Nervous mechanisms underlying intersegmental co-ordination of leg movements during walking in the cockroach. J. Exp. Biol. 58, 725-744.

Pringle, J.W.S., 1938. Proprioception in insects. II. The action
    of the campaniform sensilla on the legs. J. Exp. Biol. 15,
    114-131.
Pringle, J.W.S., 1961. Proprioception in arthropods. In The Cell
    and the Organism. (Ed. Ramsay, J.A. and Wigglesworth, V.B.).
Runion, H.I., and Usherwood, P.N.R., 1968. Tarsal receptors and
    leg reflexes in the locust. J. Exp. Biol. 49, 421-436.
Szekely, G., Czeh, G., and Voros, G., 1969. The activity pattern
    of limb muscles in freely moving normal and de-afferented newts.
    Exp. Brain Res. 9, 53-62.
Usherwood, P.N.R., and Runion, H.I., 1970. Analysis of the mechani-
    cal responses of metathoracic extensor tibiae muscles of free-
    walking locusts. J. Exp. Biol. 52, 39-58.
Usherwood, P.N.R., Runion, H.I., and Campbell, J.I., 1968. Structure
    and physiology of a chordatonal organ in the locust leg. J. Exp.
    Biol. 48, 305-323.
Wendler, G., 1966. The co-ordination of walking movements in arthro-
    pods. Symp. Soc. Exp. Biol., No. 20. Nervous and Hormonal
    Mechanisms of Integration, pp. 229-250.
Wilson, D.M., 1966. Insect walking. Ann. Rev. Entomol. 11, 103-122.
Wilson, D.M., 1967. An approach to the problem of control of
    rhythmic behavior. In Invertebrate Nervous Systems. (Ed. Wiersma,
    C.A.G.). Univ. Chicago Press, pp. 219-230.

LOCOMOTION IN THE SPINAL CAT

S. Grillner

Department of Physiology, University of Göteborg
Göteborg, Sweden

The locomotion of the hindlimbs in the low spinal cat (Th 12) is described as well as some common features in the spinal neuronal circuitry in the spinal and the decerebrate preparations in which locomotion can be elicited. Three different spinal preparations are considered: chronic spinal cats in which the spinal cord was transected 7-14 days after birth, acute spinal cats in which the noradrenergic precursor DOPA or the noradrenergic receptor stimulator Clonidine was injected i. v. These preparations can utilize their hindlimbs to walk on a treadmill with a speed dependent on the belt speed. The duration of the stance phase shortens as the speed increases while the swing phase is much less influenced as under intact conditions. The EMG activity of the prime movers in hip, knee and ankle is similar to that of the intact cat and the extensor activity starts before the foot touches the ground; the muscle force is adequate for support. At lower speeds the two hindlimbs alternate as in walk or trot but at higher speeds the activity of the two hindlimbs is almost synchronous as in the cat's gallop.

In these three spinal walking preparations and in the mesencephalic walking preparation a particular type of discharge with a long central latency and a long duration can be evoked after a short train of stimuli to a peripheral nerve. Another common feature seems to be a depression of reflex effects evoked with short latency from cutaneous and high threshold

515

muscle afferents. These effects are considered in relation to
the central generation of locomotion and possible reflex interactions. The possible contribution of the noradrenergic descending system in releasing the spinal interneuronal network
responsible for the generation of locomotion is discussed.

The nervous generation of locomotion in vertebrates can essentially be regarded as due to an intraspinal interneuronal network,
which generates the sequential activation of the different muscles
in the step cycle of the individual limb (Brown, 1911, 1914; Taub
and Berman, 1968; Szekely et al., 1969; for a review of the arguments see Grillner, 1973). The nature of this central interneuronal
network or generator is at present unknown; two main alternatives
have been discussed: (1) An oscillator arrangement with two reciprocally organized interneuronal "half centres" (Brown, 1911,
1914; Jankowska et al., 1967b; Wilson, 1964; Wilson and Waldron,
1968), one half centre controlling one muscle group and the other
the antagonist muscles. When the first half centre is active, it
will block the activity of the other centre, but the interneurones
of the first centre will cease being active due to accumulated re-
fractoriness and thereby release the activity of the second half
centre. In this way a rhythmic reciprocal activity of the two half
centres could arise. (2) An arrangement in which the responsible
interneurones are connected in a closed chain, i.e. a circular
arrangement. The different interneurones in the chain are connected with different muscle groups and thus continuous activity
in this chain would result in alternating activity in the different
muscle groups (Szekely, 1968; Gurfinkel et al., 1973).

It is also not clear if there is one master generator for each
limb which interacts with the generators of the other limbs to
produce the interlimb coordination or if the individual muscles
or muscle groups in one limb are controlled by functionally
separate generators whose activity can be coupled to each other.
However, from the results on locomotion in spinal cats discussed
below, this central generator network appears to be influenced and
regulated from the periphery. Normally there is an interaction
between the periphery and the central generator and presumably
the former is of great importance although the basic structure of
the cycle is laid down centrally.

If locomotion is essentially generated on a spinal level, we can
consider to what extent the locomotion of the spinal animal resem-

bles that of the intact cat and what changes occur in the spinal
cord when it becomes capable of generating locomotion. The
present paper will discuss locomotion and the spinal circuitry in
the chronic spinal cat, and the acute spinal cat after the injection
of DOPA or Clonidine i.v., and compare these results with the
findings on the high decerebrate cat that walks after a stimulation
of a certain region in the brain stem (Shik et al., 1966) and the
intact cat.

CHRONIC SPINAL CATS

Locomotion

Cats spinalized at lower thoracic or upper lumbar level can
after some period show the features of the chronic spinal preparation. If the cat is held such that the hips are extended it will
very often show the alternating flexion and extension movements
of the hindlimbs which has been called "spinal stepping" (Freusberg, 1874; Sherrington, 1910). If kittens are spinalized in such
a way, they can "learn" to use their hindquarters for walking and
standing (Phillippson,1905; Shurrager and Dykman, 1951; Kozak
and Westerman, 1966).

In a series of 8 kittens spinalized between 7-16 days after birth
(Forssberg, Grillner and Sjöström, unpublished), all could walk
on a treadmill with a speed dependent on the treadmill and with a
muscle force adequate to support the animal (cf. below). Of these
cats, one walked and galloped with ease, three cats used their
hindlimbs regularly during walking but always had some difficulty,
the remainder (4) did not regularly use their hindlimbs but dragged
themselves along with their forelimbs. If the hindquarters were
prevented from falling over they could, however, walk and support
themselves with their limbs.

Already 1-2 days after spinalization the hindlimbs showed the
activity typical of locomotion if they were held over a treadmill
with their hindlimbs touching the moving band. This could be at
a stage when the eyes had not yet opened and when the limbs had
not yet developed the necessary force to support the animal either
in the operated or the normal kittens. Already at this stage the
hindlimbs could show either the typical alternating activity of the
two hindlimbs in walking or a virtually simultaneous flexion and

extension of the hindlimbs as normally occurs in the cat's gallop.
At higher belt speeds the pattern typical of gallop occurred more
often. If a 49-day-old kitten, which could use its hindlimbs for
walking and standing on open ground, was put on a treadmill, its
first step would be walking (alternating) if the treadmill was
started at a speed of 0.25 m/sec in 78% of the trials. Otherwise,
the first step would be as in a gallop but then it would change to
a walk in the second or third step. On the other hand, if the speed
was 0.45 m/sec the first step was as in a gallop in 90% of the
trials. In the remainder the alternating pattern of walking was
seen but it would then change over to a gallop in the second or
third step. The difference between the two groups was significant
(P < 0.001). This was true independent of whether the kitten was
standing with the two limbs at the same frontal level (as it normally
does) or if the limbs were put in a diagonal fashion before starting
the treadmill. Similar findings have been obtained in all cats and
hence it can be concluded that the lumbosacral spinal cord itself
can generate either the alternating activity of the hindlimbs typical
of walk or trot or the virtually simultaneous activity typical of
gallop. The type of gait that the chronic spinal cats "choose"
seems to depend on the speed with which the limbs are brought
backwards (and for the first step possibly also the acceleration),
i.e. movements particularly in the hip joints.

   The step cycle can be divided into two parts (Fig. 1 replotted
from data from Engberg and Lundberg, 1969, and Kulagin and Shik,
1970), the period during which the foot is in contact with ground
(stance phase) and the period during which it is brought forward
and placed on the ground (swing phase). The duration of the stance
and the swing phase was analyzed in these preparations by having
a small silver plate on the foot pad of one limb which makes contact
with the conducting belt each time the foot touches the belt. Fig. 2A
shows the relation between the speed of the belt and the duration of
swing and stance phase. It is apparent that particularly the stance
phase shortens as the speed increases. If the stance phase is
plotted in a log-log fashion (Fig. 2B) the relation appears straight
and hence the relation between the speed and stance duration
appears to be a power function. The relation found here is very
similar to the one found for mesencephalic (Kulagin and Shik, 1970)
and intact cats (Goslow and Stuart, 1973). The latter authors also
found that a power function fitted their data well.

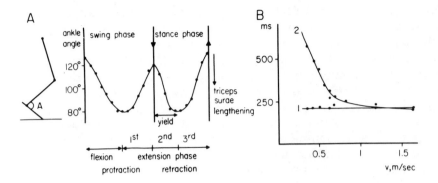

Fig. 1. Joint angles and the relative duration of swing and stance phase during locomotion at different speeds. A shows the joint angles in the ankle (< A) during one step cycle in a cat's gallop (replotted from Engberg and Lundberg, 1969). The different terms used for the different parts of the cycle are indicated in the graph. B shows the duration of the stance phase (2) and the swing phase (1) during locomotion at different speeds in a mesencephalic cat (replotted from Kulagin and Shik, 1970).

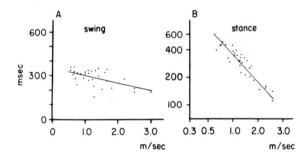

Fig. 2. Duration of stance and swing phase during locomotion at different speeds in a chronic spinal cat. 3.5 month old cat spinalized at L1 at an age of 9 days. The duration of the stance phase was revealed by means of a small silver plate on the foot pad of the left hindlimb, which made contact with the conducting treadmill belt each time the foot was placed on the belt. In A the duration of the swing phase is plotted versus the speed of locomotion on a linear scale; to the right (B) is the corresponding graph for the stance phase plotted on a log-log scale. Note the straight relationship in B indicating a power function.

This graph (Fig. 2B) reflects simply that the cat traverses the same distance during each stance phase independently of the speed, i. e. the leg (mainly the hip joint) appears to traverse the same number of degrees during all speeds. This is quite interesting in relation to the turning points in the step cycle. This seems for the intact cat to hold true mainly for trot and walk. In the intact cat's gallop when the lower spine takes an active part (Goslow and Stuart, 1973) the distance which the cat traverses during each stance phase increases as can be deduced from the records presented by Stuart et al. (this Symposium) and also by Kulagin and Shik (1970). This increase does not seem to involve an increase in the number of degrees traversed in the hip joint (see Engberg and Lundberg, 1969; Goslow and Stuart, 1973).

In the intact cat the extensor activity usually starts some 30-60 msec before the foot touches the ground. Similar results are shown for chronic spinal cats in Fig. 3. Two thin wires were introduced into the muscle recorded from and the stance phase was recorded by a silver plate on the foot pad. The extensor activity started consistently prior to placing the foot. The interval was somewhat more variable than in the intact preparation which might be expected since the position of the hindquarters varies more in the spinal than in the intact walking cat. It is also shown that the duration of the extensor EMG decreases as the speed of locomotion increases as does the duration of the stance phase. For flexor muscles the pattern is more variable; in some cases a biphasic activity occurs with a peak in the period between stance and swing and another in the end of the swing phase, while in others a more continuous flexor activity occurs. For the muscles investigated, i. e. the prime movers of the knee and the ankle, the EMG pattern is very similar to that of the walking intact cat (Engberg and Lundberg, 1969).

Adjustments in the Chronic Spinal Preparation

During standing in the chronic spinal cat usually the hindlimbs adjust themselves so that they stand at the same level and carry the same weight. If the left hindlimb carries more weight than the other, e.g. due to a movement of the front part (Fig. 4A), the whole "left" limb will be lifted up and abducted (Fig. 4B) and placed again in a more adequate position (Fig. 4C). This can be readily shown also if the hindquarters are pushed as indicated by the arrow. As the result of the movement of the left limb in B or

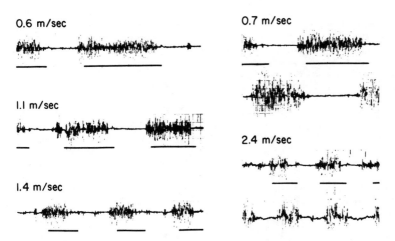

Fig. 3. Extensor activity during locomotion at different speeds
in a chronic spinal cat. The recordings are from a 3.5 month
old cat spinalized 9 days after birth at L1. The cat was
standing with its forelimbs on a platform while the hindlimbs
were on a treadmill belt, which could be moved at different
speeds. The recordings to the left and the upper recordings
in right series are from the left vastus lateralis (knee extensor)
while the lower recordings are from the right vastus lateralis.
The EMG was recorded with two thin wires (insulated except
for the tip) that were introduced in each of the muscles (see
Forssberg and Grillner, 1973). The bars below indicate the
period during which the foot was in contact with the treadmill
belt (see text). Time calibration, distance between each thick
vertical line corresponds to 50 msec. The speed of the belt is
indicated above each series. Note in the left series that the
stance phase shortens as the speed increases, while the swing
phase is more constant. The two recordings to the right show
walk at 0.7 m/sec and a gallop at 2.4 m/sec. Note the different
phase relationship in walk and gallop and that the left limb
leads the right limb somewhat in the latter case (Forssberg,
Grillner and Sjöström, unpublished).

due to other circumstances the right limb might be placed in a
too abducted position. If so, an adjustment by lifting the limb will
often occur combined with an adduction followed by placing the
limb in a more proper position. When the front part of the cat turns

spinal cat from behind

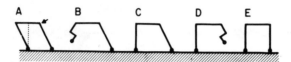

Fig. 4.   Adjustments of the hindlimbs in the chronic spinal
cat.   Each figurine is meant to represent a chronic spinal cat
from behind.   In A the hindlimbs are in an awkward position
with the left limb carrying most of the weight.   B shows the
adjusting movement occurring, i. e. lifting up the left limb -
adducting and placing it again in a proper position (C).   In C
the right limb is still not properly placed and an adjustment
takes place by a corresponding procedure as in D except for
adduction in the hip.   In E the adjustment is completed.

the hindquarters follow by such adjustments.   If the foot during
such a postural adjustment or during walking does not get proper
contact with the surface the limb is lifted up and placed again;
this can go on repeatedly until the foot gets proper contact.

Already 2-3 days after the kittens were spinalized "tactile
placing reactions" occurred.   Thus, if the cats were held with the
hips somewhat extended, touch to the dorsum of the foot with a
brush resulted in a lifting up of the hindlimb followed by a
re-extension of the limb and a prompt placing of the foot in a
more "rostral" position.   Touching either the medial or the lateral
side could result in sideways placing in the proper direction.
These placing reactions appear similar to the ones usually described
as cortical reflexes (Amassian et al., 1973), although Amassian
(1972) recently described that they occur also after decortication
in kittens.   No attempt has as yet been made to record the latencies
of the placing reactions observed in chronic spinal kittens in
order to show an identity, but a very similar type of integrated
reflex can be due to a true spinal circuitry.   These placing
reactions are probably of importance at least during "spinal
locomotion", e.g. if the hindlimbs meet with an obstacle touching
the dorsum of the foot.

LOCOMOTION IN SPINAL CATS AFTER DOPA
OR CLONIDINE I. V.

In the acute spinal cat only phasic reflexes can be evoked but
neither tonic stretch reflexes nor spinal stepping. After an
injection of DOPA i.v., both can be evoked (Grillner, 1969a, b),
and, if such a cat is put on a treadmill (Budakova, 1971 and
unpublished), it can walk with a speed related to the speed of the
treadmill belt. Strong evidence supports the hypothesis that the
effect of the noradrenaline precursor DOPA, when injected i.v.
in an acute spinal cat is to release NA from the terminals of
descending reticulospinal NA-fibres (Andén et al., 1966b). All
monoaminergic terminals in the cord belong to descending NA- or
5-HT fibres (Carlsson et al., 1964). Hence the effect of DOPA
can with reasonable certainty be regarded as that of a selective
activation of the noradrenergic reticulospinal system. If so, the
effect of DOPA should largely be mimicked if a pure noradrenergic
receptor stimulator like Clonidine (Andén et al., 1970) was
injected i.v. into a spinal cat. Indeed, locomotion on the treadmill
occurs also after this drug with a speed dependent on the treadmill
speed (Fig. 5) and with an EMG activity that for at least the prime
movers of the limb corresponds well to that of walking intact cat
(Forssberg and Grillner, 1973). The extensor EMG activity also
begins prior to the foot contacting the ground (Forssberg and
Grillner, unpublished) and the muscle force is adequate to
support the animal. When the treadmill is stopped the EMG
activity commences in the extensors and the animal remains
standing for some period of time and even adjusts the position
of the two limbs. As for the chronic spinal preparation, the gait
of the two hindlimbs can shift between the alternate gait as in
trot and walk and a more or less synchronous activation as in
gallop.

WHAT HAPPENS IN THE SPINAL CORD?

What changes occur in the spinal circuitry when the spinal cord
changes from being inactive in the acute spinal state to being
capable of generating co-ordinated locomotion after (1) an i.v.
injection of DOPA or Clonidine, or (2) the plastic changes
occurring in the development of the chronic spinal state, or (3)
the effects exerted on the spinal cord from the mesencephalic
"locomotor region" in the high decerebrate cat. The effects of
DOPA in the spinal cat on reflex transmission to alpha motoneurones

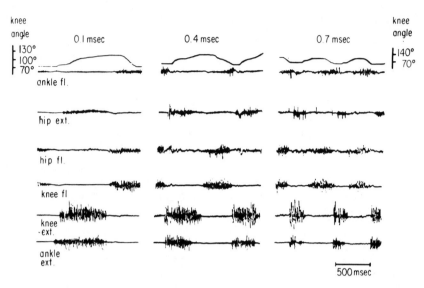

Fig. 5. Locomotion in the acute spinal cat injected with
Clonidine i. v. Decerebrate, acute spinal (Th 12) cat without
anaesthesia injected with Clonidine i. v. (200 µg/kg). The cat
had its hindlimbs on a treadmill belt which was moved with a
speed of 0. 1, 0. 4 or 0. 7 m/sec. The EMG activity was
recorded with two thin enamelled wires insulated except for
the tip which were introduced into each muscle. The prime
movers of one hindlimb were recorded simultaneously, i. e.
an ankle flexor (anterior tibial), a hip extensor (adductor
magnus), a hip flexor (iliopsoas), a knee flexor (semitendinosus),
a knee extensor (vastus lateralis) and ankle extensor (lateral
gastrocnemius). The knee joint angle was recorded in the
uppermost trace. Note that the extensor activity shortens with
increasing speed (from Forssberg and Grillner, 1973).

(Andén et al., 1966a; Jankowska et al., 1967a), gamma motoneurones (Bergmans and Grillner, 1969; Grillner, 1969b), interneurones (Jankowska et al., 1967b) and primary afferents (Andén
et al., 1966c) have been analyzed in some detail. For the other
walking preparations some of these data have been obtained.

The reflex transmission in the short latency reflex paths from
cutaneous and high threshold muscle afferents (gr. II and III) to
alpha motoneurones (i. e. mainly excitation of flexors and inhibition
of extensors) is depressed after DOPA i. v. (Andén et al., 1966a).

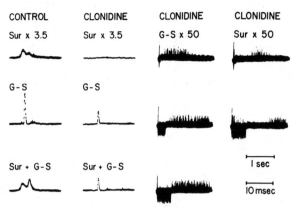

Fig. 6. Reflex transmission in an acute spinal cat injected
with Clonidine i.v. The cat was decerebrated, without anaesthesia,
and spinalized at Th 12 and afterwards curarized and given
Clonidine (200 μg/kg i.v.). The recordings in the two left
columns are from the L7 ventral root and each represents 8
averaged responses. The left series shows the response to
stimulation of the sural nerve at 3.5 times threshold and a
monosynaptic test reflex from gastrocnemius-soleus (G-S).
When the test response is conditioned by stimulation of the
sural nerve the test response is abolished. After Clonidine
the sural nerve gives no response with identical stimulation
parameters. The test (stimulation parameters were changed)
on the other hand, is unchanged when conditioned by the sural
nerve. Hence, it can be concluded that the short latency transmission from the sural nerve to gastrocnemius-soleus motoneurones is depressed after Clonidine. Note also that the response to stimulation of the sural nerve itself is also depressed.
The response to a train (interval 3.3 msec) of pulses to the G-S
(50 times threshold) and the sural nerves (50 times threshold)
is shown to the right in a L7 ventral root filament. The lower
records are with progressively increasing train duration. Note
that the late discharges are delayed as the train increases.
Time calibration 1 sec for the right two columns and 10 msec
for the two left columns.

Correspondingly short latency transmission to extensors has been
found to be depressed after Clonidine i.v. (Fig. 6; Grillner,
unpublished) and also during stimulation of the mesencephalic
locomotor region (Grillner and Shik, 1973; Fig. 7) in the high
decerebrate cat. Whether this is so also for the chronic spinal cat

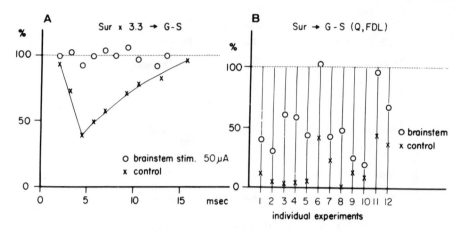

Fig. 7. Depression of short latency transmission from the
sural nerve to an extensor during stimulation of the "mesencephalic locomotor region". The recordings are from a pre-
collicular post mammillary decerebrate cat without anaesthesia
The "mesencephalic locomotor region" is stimulated with
50 μA at 60 Hz which prior to the curarization gave rise to
locomotion on the treadmill. Conventional test conditioning
technique (see Fig. 6). In A is shown (crosses) the time course
of the depression of the monosynaptic test reflex when it is
preceded by a volley to the sural nerve. During mesencephalic
stimulation (open circles) the inhibition of the test response is
abolished. In B is shown the depression of the test reflex for
different experiments before (crosses) and during (open circles)
brainstem stimulation (from Grillner and Shik, 1973).

is difficult to know since a comparison cannot be made in the
same preparation.

Although the short latency effects from these afferents are
depressed after DOPA strong effects with much longer latency
and a duration of half a second or more can, nevertheless, be
evoked from the same afferents (Andén et al., 1966a; Jankowska
et al., 1967a). Such "late discharges" involve activation of both
alpha-, dynamic and static gamma-motoneurones (Grillner, 1969a).
Both extensor and flexor muscles can be activated but their
discharges are then reciprocally organized. After Clonidine
similar "late discharges" can be evoked (Fig. 6) and with the
same particular feature as for DOPA regarding the effect of

repetitive stimulation, i. e. the discharge starts only after the
end of stimulation and if the stimulus train is prolonged the onset
of the discharge is delayed until the stimulation is ended. The
same type of reflex discharge can be obtained also in the chronic
and spinal preparation (Fig. 8; Forssberg, Grillner and Sjöström,
unpublished; similar observations were made also by Lundberg

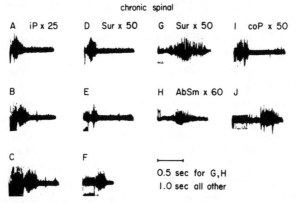

Fig. 8. "Late discharges" in a chronic spinal cat. The cat
was 6 months old and spinalized at an age of 8 days. The cat
was decerebrated, without anaesthesia and curarized. The
recordings are from a filament to semitendinosus. In A-C
the ipsilateral peroneal nerve was stimulated with a train of
pulses (interval 3. 3 msec) at increasing duration of the train
(strength 25 times threshold). D-F show the corresponding
records for the sural nerve (50 times threshold) and I-J for
the contralateral peroneal nerve. G shows the record in D
with a faster time base. H shows the response to stimulation
of the nerve to anterior biceps semitendinosus. Note that the
"late discharge" is delayed as the train duration increases.

and Vyklicky, unpublished). In the fourth preparation used
experimentally for locomotion, i. e. in the high decerebrate cat,
the stimulation of the mesencephalic locomotor region also
facilitates the appearance of such late discharges.

Hence, the present rather limited data indicate that the occurrence of "late reflex discharges" is a common feature in the
different preparations in which locomotion can be evoked; another
common feature seems to be a depression of the short latency
transmission.

It was suggested earlier (Jankowska et al., 1967a, b; Lundberg, 1969) that the central circuitry generating the locomotor pattern should be identical with that of the interneuronal system responsible for the reciprocally organized "late discharges" in flexors and extensors occurring after DOPA. This suggestion has since received indirect support by the finding that locomotion can be elicited after DOPA (Grillner, 1969a; Budakova, 1971) and that similar "late discharges" as well as locomotion occur both in the spinal cat after Clonidine (Forssberg and Grillner, 1973; Grillner, unpublished) in the chronic spinal state (see above; Forssberg, Grillner and Sjöström, unpublished), and also during stimulation of the mesencephalic locomotor region (Grillner and Shik, 1973). It is therefore possible that the different spinal interneurones recorded by Jankowska et al. (1967b) during "late discharges" in the DOPA preparation could represent part of the generator itself (cf. above) but they might also be interneurones intercalated between the generator and the motoneurones or other target neurones. Orlovsky and Feldman (1972) have recorded neurones in the spinal cord which are active in phase with the locomotion also in deafferented preparations. As discussed in the first part of this paper, even the principal arrangement of this generator is as yet unknown.

How is the interneuronal network generating the "late discharges" released? The possibility that continuous activity in the short latency pathway blocks the "late discharges" has been discussed and, as a consequence, a blockage of the short latency pathways should (as e.g. after DOPA), automatically cause a release of the late reflex system (Jankowska et al., 1967a). This possibility is attractive but it should be noted (see also Engberg et al., 1968) that a depression of the short latency reflex transmission can occur without a release of the late "reflex system" as in the decerebrate cat. Which descending systems cause the release of the interneuronal generator responsible for locomotion? Is it identical with the "late discharge system" or not? Since both the noradrenergic receptor stimulator Clonidine and the noradrenergic precursor DOPA give rise to locomotion, it would suggest that reticulospinal noradrenergic fibres would be responsible, particularly since stimulation of the "mesencephalic locomotor region" in many aspects mimics the effect of DOPA on the spinal cord (Grillner and Shik, 1973). These similarities are rather striking as is evident from Table 1 which compares the different effects known for the mesencephalic and the three spinal walking preparations. The possible involvement

	Mesencephalic preparation locom. reg. stim.	Spinal Preparations		
		DOPA	Clonidine	Chronic
Walk on treadmill	+[1]	+[2]	+[3]	+[4]
Tonic effects a) depression of short latency effects from FRA	+[5]	+[6]	+[7]	?
b) effect on alpha-motoneurone excitability	~0[5]	~0[6]	~0[7]	?
c) effect on discharge rate of gamma	+[8]	+[9]	?	?
Phasic alternate activity in flexor and extensor a) alpha moto-neurones	+[10]	+[11]	+[7]	+[4]
b) static gamma	+[8]	+[9]	?	?
c) dynamic gamma	+[12]	+[9]	?	?
d) depression of Renshaw inhibition during phasic activity	+[13]	+[14]	?	?

Table 1. Comparison between the "mesencephalic walking cat" and the low spinal cat (Th 12) injected with DOPA i.v. The different statements in the table are based on the following papers: 1) Shik et al. (1966), 2) Grillner (1969a), Budakova (1971), Forssberg and Grillner (1973), 3) Forssberg and Grillner (1973), 4) Grillner, Forssberg and Sjöström (unpublished), 5) Grillner and Shik (1973), 6) Anden et al. (1966a), 7) Grillner (unpublished), 8) Severin et al. (1967a), Severin (1970), 9) Grillner (1969a, b), Bergmans and Grillner (1969), 10) Severin et al. (1967b), 11) Anden et al. (1966a), Jankowska et al. (1967a), 12) In the decorticate preparation, dynamic gamma activity appears to take part (Perret and Buser, 1972), whereas it is unknown for the mesencephalic preparation), 13) Severin et al. (1968), 14) Bergmans et al. (1969). The phasic activity in 9 and 11 refers to the reciprocal late reflex discharges in flexors and extensors.

of the noradrenergic system has received further support by
experiments with the noradrenergic alpha-receptor-blocker
phenoxybenzamine (blocking e.g. the effect of DOPA on the
spinal cord). If this drug is given to a mesencephalic cat,
stimulation of the locomotor region at a strength that prior to
the injection gave rise to locomotion has no effect, even if the
stimulation strength is very much increased (Grillner and Riman,
unpublished). Preliminary experiments suggest that also the
effect on short latency transmission to alpha motoneurones
(Grillner and Shik, 1973) is blocked after phenoxybenzamine
(Grillner and Riman, unpublished). Thus, the evidence for the
involvement of the noradrenergic system seens compelling.
However, such an important circuit as these generator interneurones may well be controlled not only by one but by several
descending systems.

The findings in the cats in which the spinal cord was transected
at an early age and in which all descending fibres have degenerated
can of course not be explained by an involvement of noradrenergic
fibres but must be due to a release of the "interneuronal stepping
generator" due to plastic changes in the cord itself.

If we consider the generator a spinal black box of unknown
design, it is clear from the results discussed above for example
in chronic spinal preparations that this generator is not auto-
nomous but can be influenced by peripheral events; the duration
of the stance phase changes with the speed of locomotion as well
as the interlimb co-ordination (walk or trot versus gallop).
Various evidence indicates that movements particularly in the
hip have an important role for the regulation of this generator
(see Grillner, 1973). In this respect a new observation (Grillner,
unpublished) may be relevant. Changes of the position in the hip
joint can cause a reversal of late reflex effects to antagonist
muscles (Fig. 9; Clonidine preparation, for details see legend).
It should be noted that with hip extension the reflex effects result
in flexion which would be the subsequent phase in the step. With
hip flexion, on the other hand, extensor activation occurs which
would correspond to the onset of the extension phase. Somewhat
similar results were obtained by Magnus (1924) in chronic spinal
dogs using a knee tap as stimulus.

Fig. 10 shows a speculative diagram for the control of locomotion. The NA-system (and possibly others) releases the inter-

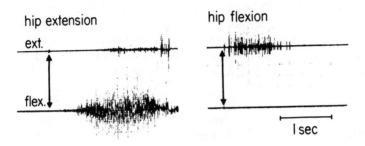

hip extension   hip flexion

ext.

flex.

I sec

Fig. 9. Reflex reversal by changes in the hip joint position.
From an acute spinal cat injected with 250 µg/kg Clonidine.
The EMG recordings (as in Fig. 4) are from left vastus
lateralis (knee extensor), and left semitendinosus (knee
flexor). The left common peroneal nerve was stimulated
(arrows) with a short train (6 pulses at an interval of 3.3
msec) at a strength of 20 times threshold. When the hip was
extended the stimulus caused strong flexor activity whereas
with the hip flexed the same stimulus did not influence the
flexor at all but gave a marked extensor activation (see text)
(Grillner, unpublished).

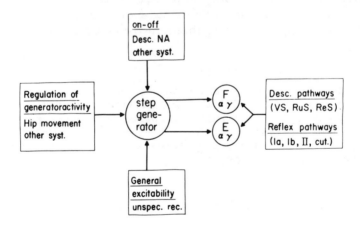

Fig. 10. Speculative diagram of the circuitry involved in the
generation of locomotion (see text).

neuronal step generator and allows its operation; its general excitability is also influenced by unspecific peripheral bilateral input (cf. Wilson, 1964; Shik et al., 1966; Forssberg and Grillner, 1973; Grillner, 1973). The actual phasic activity of the generator can be influenced by the hip movement and other peripheral sources. These factors thus control the basic cir-cuitry responsible for the main features of locomotion.

Superimposed on this activity, the motoneurones will receive signals from muscle spindles and other receptors and also from the descending systems that are known to be phasically active in locomotion, such as the vestibulo-, rubro- and reticulospinal pathways (Orlovsky, 1970, 1972a, b). Such control signals can act to continuously adjust each step cycle optimally with the help of for example the cerebellum. Also directly superimposed on the motoneuronal activity could be signals concerning activation of particular groups of muscles as needed when changing direction of locomotion or for the proper placing of the limb, etc.

The various results discussed in this paper emphasize the large capacity of the spinal cord in generating much more complex motor acts than for example the flexor reflex and the stretch re-flex. Perhaps it is useful to consider the possibility that during evolution the neuronal substrate for standard motor acts like locomotion and various adjusting reflexes has been located at the lowest possible level and that the higher centres do not generate these movements themselves but can initiate them and also act in continuously modifying these movements to best suit the actual external conditions.

Acknowledgement: This work was supported by the Swedish Medical Research Council proj. no. 14X-3026. The skillful assistance of Mrs. Margreth Svanberg is greatfully acknowledged as well as the participation in the different series of experiments by Mr. H. Forssberg, Dr. E. Riman and Mr. A. Sjöström and the constructive remarks on the manuscript by Dr. T. Hongo.

REFERENCES

Amassian, V.E., Weiner, H., and Rosenblum, M., 1972. Neural systems subserving the tactile placing reaction: A model for the study of higher level control of movement. Brain Res. 40, 171-178.

Amassian, V.E., and Ross, R., 1973. Development in the kitten of
   control of contact placing by sensorimotor cortex. J. Physiol.
   230, 55-56 P.
Andén, N.-E., Jukes, M.G.M., Lundberg, A., and Vyklický, L.,
   1966a. The effect of DOPA on the spinal cord. 1. Influence
   on transmission from primary afferents. Acta Physiol. Scand.
   67, 373-386.
Andén, N.-E., Jukes, M.G.M., and Lundberg, A., 1966b. The effect
   of DOPA on the spinal cord. 2. A pharmacological analysis.
   Acta Physiol. Scand. 67, 387-397.
Andén, N.-E., Jukes, M.G.M., Lundberg, A., and Vyklický, L. 1966c.
   The effect of DOPA on the spinal cord. 3. Depolarization
   evoked in the central terminals of ipsilateral Ia afferents by
   volleys in the flexor reflex afferents. Acta Physiol. Scand.
   68, 322-336.
Andén, N.-E., Corrodi, H., Fuxe, K., Hökfelt, B., Hökfelt, T.,
   Rydin, C., and Svensson, T., 1970. Evidence for a central
   noradrenaline receptor stimulation by Clonidine. Life Sci. 9,
   513-523.
Bergmans, J., and Grillner, S., 1969. Reciprocal control of
   spontaneous activity and reflex effects in static and dynamic
   γ-motoneurones revealed by an injection of DOPA. Acta Physiol.
   Scand. 77, 106-124.
Bergmans, J., Burke, R., and Lundberg, A., 1969. Inhibition of
   transmission in the recurrent inhibitory pathway to motoneurones. Brain Res. 13, 600-602.
Brown, T.G., 1911. The intrinsic factors in the act of progression in the mammal. Proc. Roy. Soc. 84, 308-319.
Brown, T.G., 1914. On the nature of the fundamental activity of
   the nervous centres; together with an analysis of the condition-
   ing of rhythmic activity in progression, and a theory of the
   evolution of function in the nervous system. J. Physiol.
   48, 18-46.
Budakova, N.N., 1971. Stepping movements evoked by a rhythmic
   stimulation of a dorsal root in mesencephalic cat. Fiziol. Zh.
   (Mosk.). 57, 1632-1640. (In Russian).
Carlsson, A., Falck, B., Fuxe, K., and Hillarp, N.-Å., 1964.
   Cellular localization of monoamines in the spinal cord. Acta
   Physiol. Scand. 60, 112-119.
Engberg, I., and Lundberg, A., 1969. An electromyographic
   analysis of muscular activity in the hindlimb of the cat during
   unrestrained locomotion. Acta Physiol. Scand. 75, 614-630.
Engberg, I., Lundberg, A., and Ryall, R.W., 1968. Reticulospinal
   inhibition of transmission in reflex pathways. J. Physiol.
   194, 201-223.
Forssberg, H., and Grillner, S., 1973. The locomotion of the
   acute spinal cat injected with Clonidine i.v. Brain. Res. 50,
   184-186.

Freusberg, A., 1874. Reflexbewegungen beim Hunde. Pflügers Arch. Physiol. 9, 358-391.

Goslow, G.E., Jr., and Stuart, D.G., 1973. The cat step cycle. 1. Joint angles and muscle lengths during unrestrained locomotion. J. Morphology. In press .

Grillner, S., 1969a. Supraspinal and segmental control of static and dynamic γ-motoneurones in the cat. Acta Physiol. Scand. 327, 1-34.

Grillner, S., 1969b. The influence of DOPA on the static and the dynamic fusimotor activity to the triceps surae of the spinal cat. Acta Physiol. Scand. 77, 490-509.

Grillner, S., 1973. On the spinal generation of locomotion. In Sensory Organization of Movements. (Ed. Batuev, S.) Leningrad.

Grillner, S., and Shik, M.L., 1973. On the descending control of the lumbosacral spinal cord from the "mesencephalic locomotor region". Acta Physiol. Scand. 87, 320-333.

Gurfinkel, V.S., Kostyuk, P.G., and Shik, M.L., 1973. On some possible modes of descending control of the spinal cord activity in connection with the problem of motor control. In Proceedings of Symposium Papers, Fourth International Biophysics Congress.

Jankowska, E., Jukes, M.G.M., Lund, S., and Lundberg, A., 1967a. The effect of DOPA on the spinal cord. 5. Reciprocal organization of pathways transmitting excitatory action to alpha motoneurones of flexors and extensors. Acta Physiol. Scand. 70, 369-388.

Jankowska, E., Jukes, M.G.M., Lund, S., and Lundberg, A., 1967b. The effect of DOPA on the spinal cord. 6. Half-centre organization of interneurones transmitting effects from the flexor reflex afferents. Acta Physiol. Scand. 70, 389-402.

Kozak, W., and Westerman, R., 1966. Basic patterns of plastic change in the mammalian nervous system. In Nervous and Hormonal Mechanisms of Integration. Soc. Exp. Biol. Symp. 20, 509-544.

Kulagin, A.S., and Shik, M.L., 1970. Interaction of symmetrical limbs during controlled locomotion. Biofizika. 15, 171-178. (Eng. transl.).

Lundberg, A., 1969. Reflex control of stepping. The Nansen Memorial Lecture V. Universitetsforlaget, Oslo. 1-42.

Magnus, R., 1924. In Körperstellung. Springer, Berlin.

Orlovsky, G.N., 1970. Influence of the cerebellum on the reticulospinal neurones during locomotion. Biofizika. 15, 928-936. (Eng. transl.).

Orlovsky, G.N., 1972a. Activity of vestibulospinal neurons during locomotion. Brain. Res. 46, 85-98.

Orlovsky, G.N., 1972b. Activity of rubrospinal neurons during locomotion. Brain Res. 46, 99-112.

Orlovsky, G.N., and Feldman, A.G., 1972. Classification of lumbosacral neurons according to their discharge patterns during evoked locomotion. Nejrofiziologija. 4, 410-417. (In Russian).

Perret, C., and Buser, P., 1972. Static and dynamic fusimotor activity during locomotor movements in the cat. Brain Res. 40, 165-169.

Phillippson,M., 1905. L'autonomie et la centralisation dans le système nerveux des animaux. Trav. Lab. Physiol. Inst. Solvay Bruxelles . 7, 1-208.

Severin, F.V., 1970. The role of the gamma motor system in the activation of the extensor alpha motor neurones during controlled locomotion. Biophysics. 15, 1138-1145 (Eng. transl.).

Severin, F.V., Orlovsky, G.N., and Shik, M.L., 1967a. Work of the muscle receptors during controlled locomotion. Biophysics. 12, 575-586.

Severin, F.V., Shik, M.L., and Orlovsky, G.N., 1967b. Work of the muscles and single motoneurones during controlled locomotion. Biofizika. 12, 762-772. (Eng. transl.).

Severin, F.V., Orlovsky, G.N., and Shik, M.L., 1968. Recurrent inhibitory effects on single motoneurones during an electrically evoked locomotion. Bull. Exp. Biol. Med. 66, 3-9. (In Russian).

Sherrington, C.S., 1910. Flexion-reflex of the limb, crossed extension reflex, and reflex stepping and standing. J. Physiol. 40, 28-121.

Shik, M.L., Severin, F.V., and Orlovsky, G.N., 1966. Control of walking and running by means of electrical stimulation of the mid-brain. Biofizika. 11, 756-765. (Eng. transl.).

Shurrager, P.S., and Dykman, R.A., 1951. Walking spinal carnivores. J. Comp. Physiol. Psychol. 44, 252-262.

Székely, G., 1968. Development of limb movements: Embryological, physiological and model studies. In Ciba Foundation Symposium on Growth of the Nervous System. (Ed. Wolstenholme, G.E.W. and O'Connor, M.) J. & A. Churchill Ltd., Lond., pp. 77-93.

Székely, G., Czéh, G., and Vörös, G., 1969. The activity pattern of limb muscles in freely moving normal and deafferented newts. Exp. Brain Res. 9, 53-62.

Taub, E., and Berman, A.J., 1968. Movements and learning in the absence of sensory feedback. In The Neurophysiology of Spatially Oriented Behaviour. (Ed. Freedman, S.J.) Dorsey Press. pp. 173-192.

Wilson, D.M., 1964. The origin of the flight-motor command in grasshoppers. In Neuronal Theory and Modeling. (Ed. Reiss, R.F.) Stanford Univ. Press. pp. 331-345.

Wilson, D.M., and Waldron, I., 1968. Models for the generation of the motor output pattern in flying locust. Proc. I.E.E.E. 56, 1058-1064.

TIME CONSTRAINTS FOR INTER-LIMB CO-ORDINATION IN THE CAT DURING UNRESTRAINED LOCOMOTION

D. G. Stuart, T. P. Withey, M. C. Wetzel and
G. E. Goslow, Jr.

Departments of Physiology and Psychology, University
of Arizona, Tucson, Arizona, and Department of
Biological Sciences, Northern Arizona University,
Flagstaff, Arizona

Unrestrained walking, trotting and galloping by adult cats is
analyzed cinematographically. Classical models, which have
previously characterized quadrupedal gait by "idealized" footfall formulas and support durations, can be revised from the
present data to specifically describe cat locomotion. The
number of limbs supporting the body weight and the sequence
in which they are placed on the ground are largely a function of
forward speed. Even within one gait and at a given speed,
however, the same cat can be observed to vary its support
pattern markedly in different strides, such as a
transition in mid-flight from a rotatory to a transverse gallop.
On the basis of these findings we then propose that, since locomotion can thrive under a variety of conditions both across and
within gaits, the locomotor control program has <u>facultative</u>
capability.

In spite of the facultative capability, normalized gait patterns
have proved valuable for analysis of the temporal constraints
within which proprioceptive, propriospinal, and vestibulo
(otolith)-spinal traffic must operate if they are to assist in the
control of stepping. Although adequate time is available for
autogenetic and interlimb load compensatory reflexes to occur

at most forward speeds, there is indication that interactions
between proprioceptive input and the locomotor program might
change on the transition from gait to gait. Our measurements
to date have not suggested a potential role for long propriospinal
pathways in normal stepping. Precise relations exist between
near-sinusoidal variations in vertical head acceleration and
footfall patterns in walking, trotting and galloping. The amplitude of excursions appears sufficient to activate the otolith
apparatus in every gait. Our approach to the study of locomotion
has not produced a completed neural control synthesis at this
stage, but rather it strongly emphasizes events and times with
which the nervous system must contend in order to provide
four-legged stepping.

INTRODUCTION

The substantial literature on the properties and connections of
muscle afferents, spinal neurones, and brainstem neurones has
contributed little to date to our understanding of the neural control
of locomotion. This is partly because of a shortage of requisite
information about the nature of the stepping acts themselves. It
is particularly unfortunate that the most severe shortage exists
for the cat, whose central and peripheral neural pathways have
been studied so intensively. Philippson's (1905) step cycle provided an early model for cinematographic analysis of the mechanics
of a single limb's step sequence (Fig. 1), and was subsequently
valuable to Engberg and Lundberg (1969), Gambarjan et al. (1971)
and Grillner (1972) in their examination of natural stepping movements. We have recently showed how a further cinematographic
analysis of the hindlimb stepping movements of unrestrained cats
during low and high speed locomotion can contribute to understanding the demands made by locomotor movements on muscle
performance and proprioceptor response (Goslow et al., 1973a, b,
c). The present report shows how the same cinematographic
records can be used to assess the four-legged stepping sequence.
Several models have been used previously to systematically present idealized interlimb sequences in various animals (cf Muybridge,
1899; Howell, 1944; Hildebrand, 1966; Roberts, 1967; Gray, 1968).
These models are considered in relation to our own data on the gaits
employed by domestic cats. The report will show how the gait descriptions can then be used to evaluate the time constraints within which
proprioceptive input, propriospinal traffic, and vestibulospinal

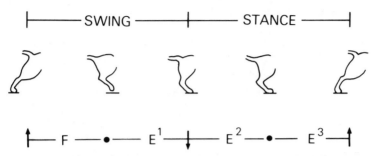

Fig. 1. A schematic representation of the step cycle of a
single limb. This simple sketch for the LH limb has been
used in our previous introductions to stepping (Goslow et al.,
1973a, b, c; Stuart et al., 1972). The four phases of the step
cycle as originally defined by Philippson have been given equal
allotments of time. The flexion (F) phase begins as the foot is
thrust off the ground, at which time there is beginning flexion
at hip, knee and ankle joints. This phase ends as extension
(E^1) begins in knee and ankle. These movements of limb
flexion and early extension comprise the swing (transfer)
phase of the step. The stance (support) phase involves progressive extension of the hip. During the second extension
phase (E^2) the knee, ankle and metatarsophalageal joints
yield (i.e. flex) with the weight of the body while in the third
extension phase (E^3) there is extension at all joints of the
hindlimb.

traffic must operate to be of value in the control of stepping.

METHODS

The locomotion of 11 adult cats weighing 2-3 Kg was photographed
with a 16 mm camera at 64 frames/sec. For walking and trotting
sequences the cats were trained to move parallel to an 18 ft background (ruled with a grid of 10 cm squares and bowed into a semicircle with a radius of 21 ft). Walking and trotting were tracked
and filmed from the centre of the semicircle. For the gallop, the
cats ran along a straightaway (40 ft long) covered with indoor-
outdoor carpeting. A stationary camera was positioned perpendicular to and 10-25 ft from a background grid mounted on the far
side of the straightaway. The camera did not track the gallop, and
to reduce parallax the only stride analyzed was the one with the

centre-most position relative to the framed sequence.

Single frame analysis permitted measurement of: (1) the duration of time each leg was on and off the ground (the swing and stance phases for all four legs); (2) vertical displacements of the head (ground to eye); and, (3) angular displacements of the head (angle between the horizontal and a line connecting the nose and eye). Step cycles with unusual head movements were excluded. As described elsewhere in detail (Goslow et al., 1973a), a sequence of India ink marks on the shaved hindlimb, lower back and pelvis permitted measurement of hip, knee and ankle joint angles of the left hindlimb such that this limb's step cycle could be divided into its F, E^1, E^2, and E^3 epochs (Fig. 1). All times derived from film analysis were entered onto standard paper tape which was then processed with a digital computer (DEC Lab 8/e).

RESULTS AND COMMENTS

Gaits Employed by Cats

An early classification scheme (cf Muybridge, 1899) divided quadrupedal gaits into symmetrical (e.g. walk, trot and pace) and asymmetrical (e.g. canter, gallop and half-bound). The distinction is based on the spacing of strike times for the four feet. In symmetrical gaits the two fore feet strike the ground successively at intervals that are of constant duration, and the same is true of the two hind feet. In asymmetrical gaits the times of footfall are not evenly spaced in this manner. In a gallop, for example, the right hind foot may strike the ground 30 msec after the left hind foot, but more than 300 msec may then intervene before the left hind foot touches the ground again.

Another widely used classification scheme described the support pattern of various gaits (Muybridge, 1899; Howell, 1944). All gaits were considered to have eight epochs, one for each of the four footfalls and one for each period that a foot is suspended. A "footfall formula" then noted the number of feet supporting the body in the successive epochs. It was adopted widely (cf Gray, 1968; Roberts, 1967), although Hildebrand (1966) has pointed out a major limitation in that it does not represent durations of support.

The "gait diagram" of Hildebrand (1959; 1962, 1966) includes

these durations, as well as all of the information of previous
schematics. For this reason it serves as a useful model which
we follow in our own study of the cat. The diagram appears in
Figs. 2-5. Horizontal lines are assigned, from top to bottom,
to the left hind (LH), left fore (LF), right fore (RF) and right
hind (RH) limbs. Continuous thick horizontal lines indicate the
duration of each limb's stance phase (foot on ground), and open
spaces indicate the swing phase (foot off ground). The sequence
(stride) is begun and ended with LH limb placement, as the cat
moves from left to right. It should be noted that by this method
a "stride" (one complete cycle of motion) and a "stride interval"
(its duration) are both defined in terms of the movement of the LH
limb, rather than the more cumbersome plotting of the completed
successive step cycles of all four limbs.

The cat employs the fast walk, trot and gallop to far greater
extent than other gaits. There is sufficient individual variation
in both the usage and nature of these preferred gaits, however,
that it is necessary to evaluate individual strides and also employ
a normalization procedure that permits presentation of represen-
tational data for neurophysiological analysis.

Walking

Usual descriptions of the walk add several characteristics to
the paramount requirement of symmetrical footfalls. Howell
(1944), noting that in the walk there is always at least one foot on
the ground, described several idealized support patterns that depend on speed. In slow walking, epochs in which three limbs are
on the ground are interspersed with periods in which all four
limbs support the body weight (pattern 4, 3, 4, 3, 4, 3, 4, 3),
while in fast walking, the pattern becomes 3, 2, 3, 2, 3, 2, 3, 2.
The two-legged epochs alternate between contralateral fore- and
hindlimbs (diagonal support) and ipsilateral fore- and hindlimbs
(lateral support). With further increase of speed, the support
pattern was said to be 3, 2, 1, 2, 3, 2, 1, 2 and eventually 2, 1,
2, 1, 2, 1, 2, 1 in the running walk (amble). Later workers
(Gray, 1968; Roberts, 1967) have implied that all eight phases
are of equal duration, and both emphasized that in the walk the
order of footfalls is LH, LF, RH, RF (if the sequence begins with
LH). Finally, Hildebrand (1966) added that in a walk each foot's
contact time with the ground is longer than 50% of the total stride
interval, a further arbitrary criterion which we have adopted for

the present.

None of the criteria described above addresses the issue of variability or exceptions to the idealized patterns, although the rigidity of linkages in time is obviously important to any neurophysiological analysis of stepping. Fig. 2 illustrates five individual walk

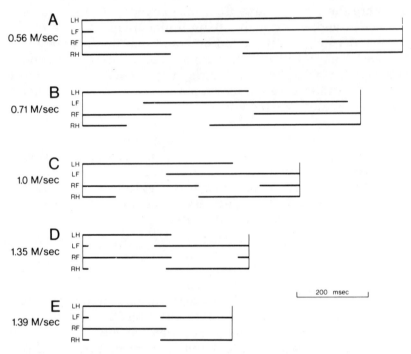

Fig. 2. Different patterns of walking. Gaits are represented by use of Hildebrand's (1959) "gait diagram". (For explanation see text.) The forward speeds at which these single stride measurements were made are shown in M/sec. The A, B, C and D gaits were used by a single 3.0 Kg cat. The E gait is from another cat, weighing 2.9 Kg. Abbreviations in this and subsequent figures: LH, left hindlimb; LF, left forelimb; RF, right forelimb; and RH, right hindlimb.

patterns, parts A-D being for a single cat. An overall orderly change of support pattern accompanied increase of forward speed to the extent that periods of diagonal support became more synchronized, and the periods of lateral or three-legged support became shorter. Note also that A approximates the idealized slow

4, 3, 4, 3, 4, 3, 4, 3 pattern of support and B possesses the 3, 2, 3, 2, 3, 2, 3, 2 pattern of a moderate walk. The strike order is also invariant at LH, LF, RH, RF until the fastest speed, E. Moreover, successive footfalls at each girdle were approximately evenly spaced, as is required in a symmetrical gait.

There were some marked discrepancies, nevertheless, from previous descriptions of the walk. Some support patterns were quite atypical, such as C-E in which there were no periods of lateral support. Neither D (4, 2, 3, 4, 2, 3) nor E (4, 2, 4, 2) corresponds to an idealized support pattern at high speed walking. Although both of the latter gaits are walks by the 50% criterion, the cats appear to be trotting (see Fig. 3). Another discrepancy is

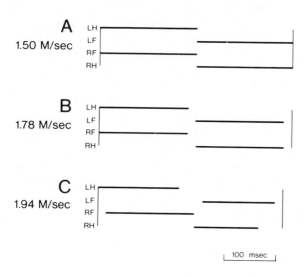

Fig. 3. Different patterns of trotting. These three patterns (single strides) are taken from two different cats (A and B from a 2.3 Kg cat, and C from a 2.9 Kg cat). The A and B gaits were seen to far lesser extent than the C gait.

that the five support patterns shown were not completely related to forward speed. In the same or different cats, A occurred at speeds from 0.53-0.70 M/sec, B from 0.60-0.80 M/sec, C from 0.70-1.1 M/sec, D from 1.3-1.5 M/sec, and E from 1.34-1.5 M/sec. Perhaps the most striking departure from classical gait models, apart from the overlapping speeds at which discrete patterns could occur, was that in none of the five strides represented in Fig. 2

did the various support epochs even approach a constant duration.
Even in the B stride with its 3, 2, .3, 2, 3, 2, 3, 2 pattern, the
support epoch durations varied over a ten-fold range (30-300 msec).

Trotting

By conventional definition (Howell, 1944; Gray, 1968) the trot
is attained when periods of two-legged diagonal support are alternated with periods in which all four limbs are off the ground, with
the support pattern 2, 0, 2, 0 in a completely synchronized trot
(the diagonal step cycles perfectly time-locked). Data (on horses)
of Marey (1879) that were cited as if general by Gray (1968) imply
that the periods of diagonal support are twice as long as the periods
of no support. In an incompletely synchronized trot, which is more
typical, either the fore- or hindlimb of a diagonal pair strikes first.
Gray (1968) described an idealized pattern of eight phases (2, 1, 0,
1, 2, 1, 0, 1), with the duration of periods when a diagonal pair is
on the ground being three times as long as when only one or no
limbs are supporting the body. For both synchronized and asynchronized trots the walking sequence of LH, LF, RH, RF changes
to LH-RF, RH-LF. Since, however, a given limb may strike
slightly earlier or later in one or both diagonal pairs, a large
number of theoretical support diagrams could be drawn (cf
Hildebrand, 1966). It is evident that this way to represent the
trotting stride would only obscure its principal feature, the long
periods of diagonal support.

The cats in this study trotted at speeds from 1.5-2 M/sec, although trotting speeds up to at least 3.7 M/sec have been observed
on a treadmill (unpublished data). Fig. 3 shows that as with the
walk, several distinct patterns were seen within the same range of
speeds, yet the support sequences depended somewhat on forward
speed. At relatively slow speeds (1.5-1.8 M/sec for A and 1.56-
1.9 M/sec for B) synchronized trots were sometimes observed,
although A has no unsupported phase, while the B pattern is the
idealized 2, 0, 2, 0. Note that contrary to what previous literature
suggests, the duration of zero support in B is far less than the
diagonal epochs. C shows an asynchronous trot, which was common
over the same range and at slightly higher speeds (i.e. 1.74-2 M/sec).
Howell contended (1944) that in the fast trot the forefoot always
leaves the ground before the contralateral hindfoot, but this was
not true for our fast trot, C.

Galloping and Half-bounding

At high speeds (above 2.6 M/sec in the present study), the cat may employ one of three asymmetrical gaits: the transverse gallop (fore- and hindfeet strike in the same order), the rotatory gallop (fore- and hindfeet strike in opposite order), or the half-bound (hindfeet strike simultaneously and forefeet alternately). Contact intervals of left and right feet of a pair tend to be equal, but fore contact intervals may differ from hind contact intervals (cf Hildebrand, 1962). Roberts (1967), following Muybridge's (1899) early statement that the cat prefers the transverse gallop, has claimed that the idealized pattern for the cat is 2, 1, 0, 0, 1, 2, 1, 2. The period of zero support follows the thrust off of the hindlimbs.

Fig. 4 shows the three patterns for a single cat moving at substantial speed. Stride rates are equal, although stride length (not shown), and hence forward velocity, vary. In A the cat is using a rotatory gallop at a forward

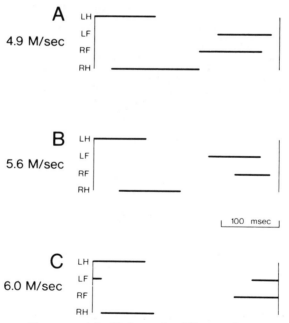

Fig. 4. The gallops and half-bound. These three gaits (single strides) were used by a single 2.5 Kg cat at the indicated speeds. A is a rotatory gallop, B a transverse gallop, and C a near half-bound.

speed of 4.9 M/sec. Note that the single period of zero support occurs after fore- (rather than hind-) limb thrust off, and that the support pattern is 1, 2, 1, 1, 2, 1, 0. B shows the transverse gallop at 5.6 M/sec, with two periods of zero support (1, 2, 1, 0, 1, 2, 1, 0). In other instances (not shown) it was clearly evident for both gallops that a period of zero support could follow thrust-off of the forelimbs or the hind, or both. C shows a slightly asynchronized half-bound with a characteristically long period of zero support. These strides are all of identical duration and near-identical swing-stance epochs, yet the four-legged rhythms differ substantially. The three patterns are used by the cat at all galloping speeds, and we have records of cats changing from one pattern to another in midflight while moving over both stationary terrain (present data) and while running on a treadmill (Wetzel et al., this Symposium). In both this study and on the treadmill, however, the rotatory gallop is the preferred gait.

Normalization Procedures

Fig. 5 shows representative gait diagrams for the preferred gaits, as taken from 4 cats. The walking gait included several step cycles from each cat: 4, 3, 7 and 4 respectively. Cycles were not necessarily successive but rather were selected on the basis of their relatively similar durations (530-703 msec) and relatively similar forward speeds (0.6-0.95 M/sec). For each step cycle a + (on ground) or 0 (off ground) value was assigned to each foot for each cinematographic frame (taken at intervals of 15.6 msec). A modified Fourier transform was then used to convert all the step cycles into an equal number of data points. With the aid of a computer (DEC Lab 8/e) the corresponding points in each step cycle were summed and divided by the number of step cycles used. The average values varied between 0 and +1 and were rounded to one of these two numbers. Similar transforms were made for head movements and for the F, E^1, E^2, and E^3 epochs of the LH cycle. The same normalizing procedures were used for trotting cycles of the same 4 cats (6-8 step cycles for each, with durations of 343-468 msec and forward speeds from 1.5-2.0 M/sec). Our data on galloping were limited to 2 cats and included but one step cycle each of rotatory (296 and 358 msec durations at 4.54 and 4.72 M/sec) and transverse (280 and 343 msec at 5.64 and 6.0 M/sec) type.

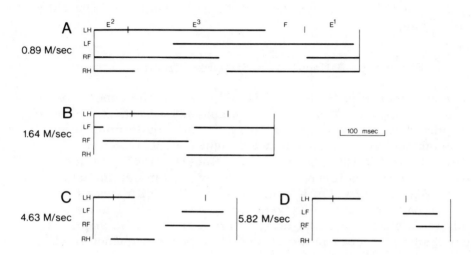

Fig. 5. Normalized gaits. A shows a normalized walking gait (see text for technique) based on 18 step cycles from 4 cats. Short vertical lines transect the LH step cycle and divide it into its E^2, E^3, F and E^1 epochs. B shows a trotting gait based on 27 step cycles from the same 4 cats. C shows a rotatory gallop based on single steps from 2 of the 4 cats. D shows a transverse gallop which is also based on single step cycles from the same 2 cats.

The representative walk in Fig. 5A is at relatively fast speed (0.89 M/sec) and contains the idealized eight support epochs (3, 2, 3, 2, 3, 2, 3, 2). The durations of three-legged support epochs (ranging from 87.4-106 msec), are similar to epochs of diagonal support (88 and 94.2 msec), but epochs of ipsilateral support are far shorter (13.1 and 17.5 msec). This normalized gait closely resembles gaits B and C of Fig. 2. The representative trot, as would be expected from real but minor variations in footfall timings from stride to stride, is not completely synchronized, but the periods of two-legged diagonal support consume most of the cycle (LH-RF 190.3 msec and RH-LF 181 msec). None of the other support epochs exceeds 20.6 msec. The gallops are quite conventional, like those in Fig. 4. It is not implied, in summary, that these normalized gait diagrams are invariant for all cats in this weight range at the indicated speeds. We would rather

emphasize that the main elements of the gaits can be brought out
by the technique.

Summary: A Facultative Stepping Rhythm

In accordance with Hildebrand (1966), we find the concept of an
eight phase support pattern that was emphasized by the early workers to be of limited usefulness. It is, in fact, quite misleading
when combined with the view that the eight epochs are of equal
duration (Roberts, 1967; Gray, 1968). Roberts (1967) has described the footfall patterns for a variety of mammals, including
the cat. His survey led him to propose that "the differences between the patterns of limb movements in various gaits arise
mainly from differences in timing within a single basic sequence,
rather than differences in the organization of the sequence itself".
Surprisingly, he does not define the basic sequence. Our
present data do not refute that the progression from walking to
trotting is very likely characterized by continuously changing interlimb phase differences, with increasing synchronization of diagonal
limbs. The conversion to galloping, however, appears to be discontinuous. Nor are the subtle changes easily explainable that
occur within the ranges of walking, trotting and galloping speeds.
On the basis of these findings we then propose that both across
and within gaits locomotion can thrive under more than one set of
conditions. In other words, the stepping generator is <u>facultative</u>
in nature.

TIME CONSTRAINTS IN STEPPING

Fig. 5 lends itself to consideration of the time constraints within
which certain types of proprioceptive, propriospinal and vestibulo-
spinal traffic must operate if they are to assist in the control of
stepping. The data in no way prove that a given reflex or transmission along a specific pathway is involved in stepping, but rather
emphasize whether or not the times are compatible with such
potential events.

Proprioceptive Reflexes

Consideration is here limited to load compensatory reflexes
whose afferent signals are initiated in the E^2 phase of each limb's
step cycle when the foot strikes the ground. Load reception is
presumably a function for both spindles and tendon organs in

extensors, with reflex changes in tension being evoked in both the same and other limbs. Grillner (1972) has recently shown that the shortest latency from receptor activation (as, for example, for the foot strikes) to onset of an autogenetic reflex change in tension (increase or decrease) in ankle extensors is about 30 msec. Considerably longer, up to 100 msec, might be required to balance tension among individual motor units to attain a new steady tension. Other latencies important for compensation are far smaller. Differences in the sum of afferent and efferent transmission times from hip as opposed to ankle muscles are about 4 msec for reflexes of group I origin and 8 msec for group II; differences in central segmental delay between Ia, Ib and group II reflexes are about 1-5 msec; differences between ipsilateral and contralateral reflexes are about 2-5 msec; and even the difference between lumbosacral and brachial reflex times of hip (or knee) extensor origin is only of the order of about 8-18 msec (Miller et al., 1973a). Apparent input times will decrease as forward speed increases and the E^2 activated input verges on synchronous volleys (Goslow et al., 1973b). Taking all of these differences into account, however, would allow a conservative prediction for proprioceptive reflexes in even distal muscles of approximately 50 msec for reflexes in the same girdle (e.g. LH to LH or RH) and 60 msec for reflexes to the other girdle (e.g. LH to LF or RF).

In Fig. 5 the duration of E^2 is 77 msec for the LH cycle of the walk, 86 msec for the trot, and 46 msec for the rotatory gallop. In only two of 29 measurements of E^2 time for the walk was its duration greater than 100 msec. The shortest E^2 time encountered was 31 msec in fast rotatory gallops. Durations as short as these have prompted both Grillner (1972, 1973a, b) and Stuart and Goslow (1972) to comment that reflex effects evoked at the beginning of E^2 in the ankle extensors cannot become manifest until the subsequent E^3 phase and in truly high speed locomotion perhaps even appear during subsequent cycles. It is then obvious that much of the load compensation is attributable to the visco-elastic properties of the extensor muscles themselves, already active before each foot strikes the ground (for full review of this important point, see Grillner, 1972).

Since so many of the segmental reflexes and synaptic connections between muscle afferents and motoneurones appear to have evolved as if to assist in the control of stepping (cf. Easton, 1972; Engberg and Lundberg, 1969; Lundberg, 1969), however, it is probably safer not to assume that reflex load compensation is excluded. Elsewhere we have argued that while it is valuable to separate E^2

from E^3 in a descriptive definition of the step cycle, the extensor muscles are actually undergoing a single mechanical event: an active stretch-shorten cycle for knee and ankle extensors and an isometric contraction-shortening cycle for hip extensors (Goslow and Stuart, 1972; Goslow et al., 1973a). Viewed in this light, the entire stance phase is the functionally significant epoch for load compensation achieved by both the affected limb and the other support limbs. In Fig. 5 this duration for LH is 500 msec in the walk, 200 msec in the trot and 92 msec in the rotatory gallop. The shortest stance duration we have observed to date is 62-78 msec in rotatory gallops at forward speeds between 6.8 and 7.3 M/sec.

Table 1 illustrates the limbs that are available for load compensatory reflexes (meaning that the foot is supported) and the epoch of the cycle in which the compensaticn could occur (based on 50 msec latency from strike time of the reference limb to the target limb(s) in the same girdle, and a 60 msec latency if the target limb(s) is in the other girdle). In the normalized walk of Fig. 5 there is time available for compensation by three of the four limbs, the homonymous limbs being affected in late E^2 and throughout E^3. The other two limbs are potentially available for reflex effects in the E^3 epoch of a step cycle that was initiated before that of the reference limb. In the trot and gallop load compensation would be limited to two limbs (diagonals in trotting and pairs in galloping). It is perhaps significant for the walk and trot that compensation is possible for any foot which is contacting the ground. The situation is somewhat different for a gallop, where the interlimb effects are more restricted. In particular, for the paired forelimbs, a proprioceptive reflex initiated by the strike of the lead (most advanced of a pair) foot (LF) would have its effect so late in E^3 of the following foot (RF) that it would probably be ineffective. The same relationship holds for the leading (RH) and following (LH) hindfeet. Nevertheless, there is a potential interaction in the gallop which would be of great functional use. In each girdle, the reflex effect of the trailing foot would coincide with the initiation of E^2 in the lead foot. Any enhancement here would be particularly valuable because the body mass has just been thrust toward this leading limb, and it must now provide sufficient force to counteract the markedly increased load as well as to complete its own thrust-off. In the forelimbs, in fact, such a reinforcement might be especially important since the forelimbs always support a greater percentage of the body weight than do the hindlimbs during walking (Manter, 1938), and presumably during trotting and galloping also. Note further that

Gait	Reference Limb[a]	Step Cycle Epoch Available for Reflex Compensation			
		LH	LF	RH	RF
Walk 0.89 M/sec	LH	E^2-E^3[b]	---[c]	E^3	E^3
	LF	E^3	E^2-E^3	---	E^3
	RH	E^3	E^3	E^2-E^3	---
	RF	---	E^3	E^3	E^2-E^3
Trot 1.64 M/sec	LH	E^2-E^3	---	---	E^2-E^3
	RF	E^2-E^3	---	---	E^2-E^3
	RH	---	E^2-E^3	E^2-E^3	---
	LF	---	E^2-E^3	E^2-E^3	---
Rotatory Gallop 4.63 M/sec	LH	E^3	---	E^2-E^3	---
	RH	E^3	---	E^3	---
	RF	---	E^2-E^3	---	E^3
	LF	---	E^3	---	E^3

a - Perturbed as foot strikes ground at onset of E^2. Limbs are listed in the order of their strike sequence as shown in Fig. 5.

b - Implying that a compensatory effect could come in E^2 and continue into E^3.

c - Foot unsupported

Table 1. Epochs of each limb's step cycle in which a potential load compensatory reflex could occur (based on values of Fig. 5, with predicted times of 50 msec if a response was initiated in the same girdle and 60 msec if it was initiated in another girdle).

the forelimbs always strike alternately at high speed while the
hindlimbs may strike simultaneously as in the half-bound.

Propriospinal Pathways

Long ascending and descending propriospinal pathways would
seem well suited for rapid linkage of hind- and forelimb step
cycles (for review see Jane et al., 1964; Miller et al., 1973a).
The latency of early discharges in shoulder flexor motoneurones
after hindlimb nerve stimulation is only about 8-18 msec (Miller
et al., 1973a) and around 10 msec for the descending system (cf.
Lloyd, 1942). There are also long latency effects in both enlargements that are unmasked by L-DOPA (35-80 msec in the brachial
cord, Bergmans et al., 1973; 50-200 msec in the lumbar cord,
Jankowska et al., 1967a, b). It is not known whether or not such
long latencies are operative during natural locomotion. If, however,
such a potentially long time span is involved, it is difficult for us
to suggest for the present data meaningful interlimb linkages that
are derived from the temporal characteristics of the two primary
stride variables, strike time and contact duration. No successive
strike times for the four limbs in the walk are less than 118 msec
(normalized walk, Fig. 5A), and the strike times between ipsilateral fore- and hindlimbs in the trot (Fig. 5B) and the gallop
(Fig. 5C) are even greater. The strike time difference between
diagonal limbs in the trot is 20-22 msec. These limbs may also
strike in perfect synchrony (Fig. 3). Strike time intervals
between paired forelimbs or hindlimbs in the gallop are about
40 msec, and the footfall pattern varies facultatively from a
half-bound to a rotatory or transverse gallop. Contact durations
(stance intervals) do not lend themselves to serving as indices
of propriospinal activity, since they all exceed 100 msec, and
epochs during which 1, 2, 3 or 4 limbs support the body are
quite variable.

The thoughtful work of Miller and his colleagues (1973a, b)
has outlined a somewhat different and potentially promising
approach to relating locomotor movements to propriospinal
activity. They have stated that long ascending propriospinal pathways may take part in the normal elaboration of stepping and contribute facilitation to the flexors of the forelimb once the ipsilateral
hindlimb has begun its first extension phase leading to its placement on the ground. Contralateral effects are weaker but also
may act to facilitate flexion. For cats trained to move on a

treadmill they observed in walking and trotting above a forward speed of 1 M/sec a consistent time-locking of 40 msec between the onset of E^1 in the hindlimb and the onset of F in the ipsilateral forelimb. A significant time-locking of EMGs of appropriate hindlimb and forelimb muscles was also found at an interval of 30-50 msec; an interval that was significantly less variable than the total step period. It was also suggested that the long descending system might reciprocally facilitate extension of the hindlimb, while the forelimb is carried forward in flexion (Miller et al., 1973a and this Symposium).

We did not observe a 40 msec time-locking but rather the time interval between the F-E^1 junction for LH and the onset of F in LF (see Footnote 1) was 109 msec for the normalized walk and 125 msec for the trot (Fig. 5). For both gaits any facilitation of ipsilateral forelimb motoneurones that followed the onset of E^1 in a hindlimb by 40 msec would occur during E^3 of the forelimb rather than the F phase. It is possible, of course, that facilitation could coincide with the onset of flexor EMG activity which occurs prior to lift-off (Engberg and Lundberg, 1969). In the gallop this potential coupling could not be evaluated since it would differ so markedly between the transverse and rotatory modes.

Our data on variability (computed from the data of Fig. 5) were in accord with the findings of the Miller group (1973a, b) only to the extent that the standard deviations for the "$F \cdot E_{1LH}$-F_{LF}" interval (33 msec for the walk and 23 msec for the trot) were smaller than the standard deviations of the total stride duration (71 msec and 32 msec for the walk and trot, respectively). A different interpretation would be implied if relative magnitudes of means and standard deviations were compared. For the walk, the mean stride interval of the LH foot was 603 msec and the coefficient of variation (s.d./mean x 100) was 12, whereas the mean "$F \cdot E_{1LH}$-F_{LF}" time was 109 msec and the coefficient of variation was 30. In fact, the value of 30 for the coefficient of variation exceeded all measured values for various subcomponents of the stride duration (stance, swing, F and E_1). Similarly, in the trot (27 strides) the coefficient of variation for the "$F \cdot E^1_{LH}$-F_{LF}" time was 19 (exceeding that of almost every sub-duration of the stride), while for the stride duration it was only 8. It is well to remember that these measures of variance are limited in their accuracy by the film frame interval of 15 msec.

The complexity of both propriospinal transmission (which may
subserve any or all of generalized excitation to the central program, load compensation, and the supply of corrective signals
via the rapidly conducting component) and the stepping sequence
itself (its facultative nature) suggest that the discovery of rigid
time linkages may be elusive. Our treadmill data also differ from
those of the Miller group (Wetzel et al., this Symposium). These
comments in no way should detract from the value of the Miller
group's approach, with its rigorous specifications of synaptic
connections that are made by long ascending propriospinal
neurones to motoneurones destined for the forelimb musculature.

Vestibulo-Spinal Considerations

When humans (Melvill Jones, 1971; Melvill Jones and Watt,
1971a, b) or cats (Melvill Jones and Watt, personnal communication)
are dropped from a height, a vestibulo- (otolith) spinal reflex
contributes to the onset of extensor EMG activity in the limb
before it strikes the ground. An otolith-spinal reflex might also
periodically reinforce stepping provided there is: (1) sufficient
change in linear vertical acceleration during locomotion to activate
the otolith organs; (2) appropriate time delays between such activation and the onset of EMG activity in the extensors; and (3) an
"open" reflex pathway. Our present data cannot help with the third
consideration but do show substantial vertical displacements of
the cat's head during stepping that are precisely related to the
four-legged sequence.

Fig. 6 shows the time relations between the four-legged
stepping sequence in the normalized walk, trot and gallop and
normalized vertical displacements of the head (eye to ground).
Note that there are two near-sinusoidal perturbations of the head
(upper curve in each diagram) per stride for the walk and trot and
one for the gallops (and half-bound also). In the walk and trot this
near-sinusoidal displacement curve is as smooth as the head
reaches its highest point as at the lowest point. In the rotatory
and transverse gallops the displacement profile is sharper around
the lowest head height, but recall that the two gallop diagrams are
based on but two strides each. Note that there are no periods of
non-support in the walk and trot, and that in the gallops the two
periods of non-support do not correspond to times when the head
is either at its highest or lowest point, but rather when it is
rising or falling. Fig. 6 also shows vertical head acceleration

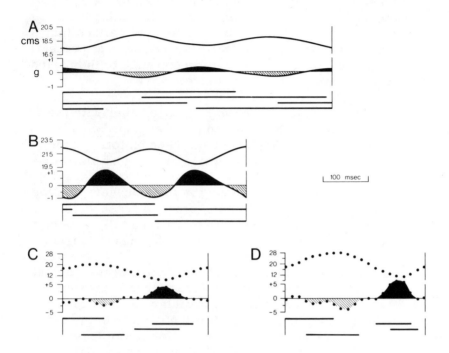

Fig. 6. Vertical head displacements in relation to the four-legged stepping sequence. The gait diagrams (lower records in each part) are those shown in Fig. 5. Also shown are the vertical displacements of the head throughout these stepping cycles (distance in cm from eye to ground) and the changes in vertical acceleration (1 g = 980 cm/sec^{-2}). Areas encased by zero g (defined in text) and positive g values are shaded in black while those for negative g are cross-hatched.

curves (middle tracing in each diagram). Since the displacement curves are assumed to be periodic, the effects of random fluctuations, due to measurement errors, were suppressed by using Fourier-transform methods (see Footnote 2) to restrict the frequency range of the information used in estimating the acceleration (second derivative of displacement) curves. Acceleration is expressed in g units relative to the point (labelled zero) at which the velocity of head displacement is constant. By this convention positive g values are located above the zero line (black areas), and the maximum value corresponds to the lowest

position of the head. Negative g values are located below zero
(hatched areas), and the minimum corresponds to the highest
position of the head. A limitation of the normalized gallops (parts
C and D) is that too few data are included (or available at present)
to show if the extended zero g periods corresponding to the periods
of non-support are true breaks in the curve.

The peak absolute g values shown in Fig. 6 together with their
rise time from zero (and for the walk and trot an approximate
frequency of near-sinusoidal displacement based on total stride
duration) included: for the walk + 0.4 g in 67 msec (3.5 Hz); for
the trot + 1.1 g in 42 msec (5 Hz); for the rotatory gallop + 3.7 g
in 59 msec and - 2.6 g in 56 msec; and, for the transverse gallop
+ 6 g in 55 msec and - 4.2 g in 92 msec. Some of these values
exceed the limit of a 1 g change that exists for free fall, and they
correspond to periods of two-legged support. A constant angle
was maintained (within a measurement error of + 7°) between the
ground and a line joining the eye and nose. It appears that the cat
keeps its head erect by·active muscle contraction that presumably
is controlled in part by reflexes of semicircular canal origin.
It has recently been shown that many otolith afferents in the cat
respond to changes in vertical head acceleration of far less magnitude than 0.1 g (Melvill Jones, personnal communication). Such
a low-threshold suggests that otolith afferents are strongly activated by the sinusoidal vertical head accelerations that occur in
every gait.

In addition to a feasible g threshold for a vestibulo-spinal response, its latency must be appropriate for stepping. Watt and
Melvill Jones (personnal communication) have found a mean
latency for the otolith-spinal reflex of 55 msec (s.d. = 32.4 msec)
between initiation of the fall and the first peak of extensor EMG
activity. While different otolith afferents have recently been
shown to fire at all phases of a sinusoidal variation in vertical
acceleration (Melvill Jones, personnal communication), we would
suggest that net input becomes progressively more intense as
vertical head acceleration proceeds from zero g to a peak of
negativity or positivity. In Fig. 6, in the walk, such an epoch
begins at least 59 msec before placement of each limb. Given the
high variance of the 55 msec otolith-spinal response, and
assuming extensors display an abrupt increase in the EMG activity
at least 20 msec before each limb strikes the ground (Engberg
and Lundberg, 1969), there is probably time for an otolith-spinal
response. In the trot the epochs of building negativity begin from

53 to 82 msec before placement of diagonal pairs of limbs. In the gallops fore- and hindlimb placements are related quite precisely in time to prior peaks of both positive and negative g. The positive peaks precede LH placement by 97 msec in the rotatory gallop and 56 msec in the transverse gallop. The negative peaks precede the first forelimb footfall by 70 msec in the rotatory gallop and 69 msec in the transverse gallop.

Although suggestive regularities of timing exist for all gaits, further discussion must await the availability of more data on the nature of otolith-spinal activity during locomotor type changes in vertical head acceleration. If an otolith-spinal reflex is to operate it must contend, however, with kinesiological constraints very similar to those presented in Fig. 6.

IMPLICATIONS FOR FUTURE WORK ON THE
NEURAL CONTROL OF STEPPING

This report has surveyed the boundaries of our current insight into the time constraints that are important for locomotion in the cat. Many technical barriers stand between past (and present) systems of gait analysis and the rigorous specification of different patterns of stepping. The overall theoretical problem is even more challenging. Our own mission is to work toward a general model that can encompass the true facultative nature of the neural control program as it operates within and between gaits. In the context of afferentation, we showed that while some appropriate load com-Pensatory reflexes may be postulated reasonably for every gait, their organization must differ between gaits. Similarly, any hypothesis of an effective proprio-spinal linkage between hind- and forelimbs cannot in its present form incorporate data for all gaits. Finally, current knowledge of the vestibulo-spinal apparatus is insufficient to account for either the orderliness of successive points on the vertical acceleration curve of the head, or the seductively close relationship between some of its points and the successive strike times of the feet. Any general model must eventually be valid over all these domains, from the hidden properties of the central program, through the mechanical and neural events during a single limb's step cycle, to the extra-ordinary external manifestation of rhythmic four-legged stepping.

Footnote 1:   The Miller group measures this interval from the peak of LH knee flexion to the onset of LF elbow flexion. Our measurement is from the peak of the LH ankle flexion to LF lift-off. While conceding the need for a standard method for making these measurements, careful consideration of our data on unrestrained cats on open terrain (Goslow et al., 1973a) indicates that our measurement of the coupling interval cannot differ appreciably from a value derived from knee-to-elbow measurement.

Footnote 2:   The acceleration curves were obtained from the eye position data through use of fast Fourier transform methods (cf. Cooley et al., 1969). Each position curve is assumed to be periodic, with period P. For each nominal eye position curve X, described by N points, a discrete Fourier transform was performed, to obtain an estimate of the spectrum of the position $F_X (n\Delta\omega)$, n = 0, 1, 2, ..., N., where $\Delta\omega$ is the fundamental frequency, $\Delta\omega = 2\pi/P$. The acceleration waveform will also be periodic with the same period, and the acceleration spectrum may be found as $F_A(n\Delta\omega)$ $= -(n\Delta\omega)^2 F_X(n\Delta\omega)$; here we used only the first four harmonics, i.e. n = 1, 2, 3, and 4. This was done to suppress the rather high measurement noise inherent in the type of visual film interpretation used. The acceleration curves were then estimated from $F_A(n\Delta\omega)$ by taking the inverse discrete Fourier transform.

Acknowledgements: Supported in part by USPHS grant NS 07888 and General Research Support Funds of the University of Arizona and its College of Medicine (USPHS grants FR 07002 and FR 05675). T.P.W. held summer fellowships from the Fan Kane Foundation (1972) and the Muscular Dystrophy Associations of America, Inc. (1973). Mr. Jolyon Barker from Oxford University, England, assisted in the data analysis and was supported by a summer fellowship (1972) from the Fan Kane Foundation. Gratefully acknowledged are Dr. J.V. Wait's assistance with part of the computer analysis, and the criticisms of Dr. Milton Hildebrand and our fellow participants Drs. Sten Grillner, Geoffrey Melvill Jones and Simon Miller.

REFERENCES

Bergmans, J.S., Miller, S. and Reitsma, D.J., 1973. Influence of L-DOPA on transmission in long ascending pathways in the cat. Brain Res., in press.
Cooley, J.W., Lewis, P.A.W. and Welch, P.D., 1969. The fast Fourier transform and its applications. Trans. on Education, I.E.E.E. 12, pp. 27-34.

Easton, T.A., 1972. On the normal use of reflexes. Amer. Sci. 60, 591-599.

Engberg, I. and Lundberg, A., 1969. An electromyographic analysis of muscular activity in the hind limb of the cat during unrestrained locomotion. Acta Physiol. Scand. 75, 614-630.

Gambarjan, P.P., Orlovskii, G.N., Protopopova, T.Y., Severin, F.V. and Shik, M.L., 1971. The activity of muscles during different gaits and adaptive changes of moving organs in Family Felidiae. Trudy Zool. Inst. Akad. Nauk USSR 48, 220-239 (In Russian).

Goslow, G.E., Jr., and Stuart, D.G., 1972. Neural control of the cat step cycle: Nature and role of lengthening contractions. Abstr. Soc. Neurosci., p. 189.

Goslow, G.E., Jr., Reinking, R.M. and Stuart, D.G., 1973a. The cat step cycle: I. Hind limb joint angles and muscle lengths during unrestrained locomotion. J. Morphol., 141, 1-41.

Goslow, G.E., Jr., Stauffer, E.K., Nemeth, W.C. and Stuart, D.G., 1973b. The cat step cycle. Responses of muscle spindles and tendon organs to passive stretch within the locomotor range. Brain Res. 60, 35-54.

Goslow, G.E., Jr., Reinking, R.M. and Stuart, D.G., 1973c. Physiological extent, range and rate of muscle stretch for soleus, medial gastrocnemius and tibialis anticus in the cat. Pflüg. Arch. 341, 77-86.

Gray, J., 1968. Animal Locomotion. Norton, N.Y., pp. 265-282.

Grillner, S., 1972. The role of muscle stiffness in meeting the changing postural and locomotor requirements for force development by the ankle extensors. Acta Physiol. Scand. 86, 92-108.

Grillner, S., 1973a. Muscle stiffness and motor control - forces in the ankle during locomotion and standing. In Proceedings of the Second International Symposium on Motor Control. Plenum Press, N.Y. In press.

Grillner, S., 1973b. On the spinal generation of locomotion. In Sensory Organization of Movements, Leningrad. In press.

Hildebrand, M., 1959. Motions of the running cheetah and horse. J. Mammal. 40, 481-495.

Hildebrand, M., 1962. Walking, running and jumping. Amer. Zool. 2, 151-155.

Hildebrand, M., 1966. Analysis of symmetrical gaits of tetrapods. Folio Biotheor. 6, 1-22.

Howell, A.B., 1944. Speed in Animals. Hafner, N.Y., pp. 217-247.

Jane, J.A., Evans, J.P. and Fisher, L.E., 1964. An investigation concerning the restitution of motor function following surgery to the spinal cord. J. Neurosurg. 21, 167-171.

Jankowska, E., Jukes, M.G.M., Lund, S. and Lundberg, A., 1967a. The effect of DOPA on the spinal cord. 5. Reciprocal organization of pathways transmitting excitatory action to alpha motoneurones of flexors and extensors. Acta Physiol. Scand. 70, 369-388.

Jankowska, E., Jukes, M.G.M., Lund, S. and Lundberg, A., 1967b.
    The effect of DOPA on the spinal cord. 6. Half-centre organ-
    ization of interneurones transmitting effects from flexor
    reflex afferents. Acta Physiol. Scand. 70, 389-402.
Lloyd, D.P.C., 1942. Mediation of descending long spinal reflex
    activity. J. Neurophysiol. 5, 435-458.
Lundberg, A., 1969. Reflex control of stepping. Nansen Memorial
    Lecture to Norwegian Academy of Sciences. Universitetsforlaget,
    Oslo, pp. 7-40.
Manter, J.T., 1938. The dynamics of quadrupedal walking. J. Exp.
    Biol. 15, 522-540.
Marey, E.J., 1879. Animal mechanism: a treatise on terrestrial
    and aerial locomotion. International Science Series. Appleton,
    N.Y., 283 pp.
Melvill Jones, G., 1971. Is there a vestibulo-spinal reflex
    contribution to running? Barany Society Meeting; Toronto Univ.
Melvill Jones, G. and Watt, D., 1971a. Observations on the control
    of stepping and hopping movements in man. J. Physiol. 219,
    709-727.
Melvill Jones, G. and Watt, D., 1971b. Muscular control on landing
    from unexpected falls in man. J. Physiol. 219, 729-737.
Miller, S., Reitsma, D.J. and van der Meché, R.G.A., 1973a.
    Functional organization of long ascending propriospinal pathways
    linking lumbo-sacral and cervical segments in the cat. Brain
    Res. In press.
Miller, S., van Berkum, R., van der Burg, J. and van der Meché,
    F.G.A., 1973b. Interlimb coordination in stepping in the cat.
    J. Physiol. 228, 30-31P.
Muybridge, E., 1899. Animals in Motion. Dover, N.Y. pp. 19-72.
Philippson, M., 1905. L'autonomie et al centralisation dans le
    systems nerveux des animaux. Trav. Lab. Physiol. Inst. Solvay
    (Bruxelles) 7, 1-208.
Roberts, T.D.M., 1967. Neurophysiology of postural mechanisms.
    Plenum Press, N.Y. pp. 153-175.
Stuart, D.G. and Goslow, G.E. Jr., 1972. Neural control of the
    cat step cycle: Nature and role of proprioceptive inputs.
    Abstr. Soc. Neurosci., p. 212.
Stuart, D.G., Mosher, C.G. and Gerlach, R.L., 1972. Properties and
    central connections of Golgi tendon organs with special refer-
    ence to locomotion. In Research Concepts on Muscle Development
    and the Muscle Spindle. Excerpta Medica, Amsterdam, pp. 139-166.
Wetzel, M.C., Atwater, A.E., Wait, J.V. and Stuart, D.G., 1973.
    Hind limb - fore limb interactions in the cat during treadmill
    locomotion. Discussion, This Symposium.

THE FUNCTION OF LONG PROPRIOSPINAL PATHWAYS IN THE CO-ORDINATION OF QUADRUPEDAL STEPPING IN THE CAT

S. Miller and J. van der Burg

Department of Anatomy, Erasmus University
Rotterdam, The Netherlands

The functional organization and descending control of long propriospinal pathways, revealed in neurophysiological investigations in high spinal cats, were compared with the patterns of stepping and of quadrupedal co-ordination in normal and decerebrate cats. Emphasis was placed on the ascending propriospinal pathways and the coupling of hindlimb and forelimb movements.

Ascending propriospinal pathways evoke excitation mainly of reflex systems controlling physiological flexor muscles of the forelimb, while descending propriospinal pathways evoke excitation of mainly the reflex systems controlling the physiological extensors of the hindlimb. In both systems the ipsilateral projections are more effective. Transmission in the ascending pathways may be modified by at least the noradrenergic reticulospinal pathway, which has been implicated in the initiation of stepping. It is proposed that long propriospinal pathways may represent intrinsic links between the spinal 'motor centres' controlling the hindlimbs and forelimbs.

Patterns of stepping may be reduced to two basic forms of movement. (1) Alternate stepping, as in all forms of walking and trotting, where the hindlimbs step in alternation. (2) In-phase stepping, as in all forms of galloping, where the hindlimbs step more in phase, and the muscles of the back contract bilaterally to contribute to the forward thrust of the body. In both forms of

561

stepping, increase of velocity is encoded as a 'command' to
increase the force of muscle contraction. The 'routine' for
quadrupedal co-ordination is superimposed on these forms
of stepping and may be explained, at least in part, in terms
of the coupling of the first extension of the hindlimb and the
flexion of the ipsilateral forelimb. The functional organization
of ascending propriospinal pathways shows agreement with
this pattern of coupling. In the descending pathways the functional organization is at present less clear, but these pathways may serve in part to reinforce the pattern of coupling
between hindlimbs and forelimbs.

In the high spinal cat co-ordinated movements of all four limbs
resembling stepping sequences have occasionally been observed
(Guillebeau and Luchsinger, 1882; Sherrington, 1910). From
these and our own observations on spinal cats, it would appear
that the co-ordination of the four limbs in postural reactions and
in stepping is realized at least in part by reflex systems within
the spinal cord. Neuroanatomical studies (Sterling and Kuypers,
1968; Giovanelli and Kuypers, 1969) have revealed long reciprocal
connections between brachial and lumbo-sacral enlargements, and
shorter projections extending over only a few segments to terminate in the enlargements. The terminal patterns of these projections
in the gray matter of the spinal cord correspond closely with
those of the medial descending brain stem pathways (Giovanelli
and Kuypers, 1969), which are concerned with movements such
as postural adjustments and stepping (Kuypers, 1964; Lawrence
and Kuypers, 1968). Neurophysiological investigations of long
propriospinal pathways have at present shown that ascending long
projections mainly excite reflex systems controlling physiological
flexor muscles and inhibit those controlling extensors (McDonald,
1955; Miller et al., 1973a; Bergmans et al., 1973). In contrast,
descending long projections would appear mainly to excite reflex
systems controlling physiological extensors and inhibit those of
the flexors (Lloyd, 1942; Lloyd and McIntyre, 1948; Djalali, 1970),
although a more recent study would suggest a more equal distribution of excitatory effects (Jankowska et al., 1973). Transmission in the ascending pathways can be influenced by at least
two systems descending from the brain stem (Bergmans et al.,
1973). One of these is the noradrenergic reticulospinal pathway
which has been considered as one of the pathways initiating
locomotion (Grillner and Shik, 1973; Forssberg and Grillner,
1973). To obtain insight into the functional role of long proprio-

spinal systems, patterns of stepping have been studied in decerebrate cats (preparation of Shik et al., 1966) and in normal unanaesthetized cats. The neurophysiological data on ascending
propriospinal pathways show some agreement with patterns of
interlimb co-ordination (Miller et al., 1973a, b and in preparation), and this is discussed further in this paper.

NEUROPHYSIOLOGICAL STUDIES OF ASCENDING
PROPRIOSPINAL PATHWAYS

In high spinal cats (sectioned at C_1 level) propriospinal pathways ascending from lumbo-sacral segments have been shown to
exert strong excitatory and inhibitory changes in reflexes to
different groups of motoneurones supplying muscles of the forelimb (Miller et al., 1973a). In some cases the excitation was
sufficient to evoke a discharge directly in some forelimb motoneuronal cell groups, particularly those of pectoralis major and
minor (Fig. 1A-D), and this is in agreement with neuroanatomical

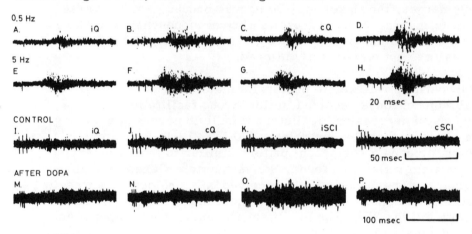

Fig. 1. Discharges recorded in the nerve to Pmaj on electrical
stimulation of hindlimb nerves. Abbreviations for Figs. 1 and 2:
c, contralateral; DC, dorsal columns; i, ipsilateral; LD, latissimus dorsi; M, median; Pmaj, pectoralis major; Q, quadriceps; SCI, sciatic; T, times threshold; U, ulnar. A-D, iQ and
cQ, 1 and 3 shocks, 20T, repetition rate 0.5 Hz. E+H, the
same, but at 5 Hz, same vertical gain. I-L, stimulation of Q
and SCI, in another experiment, 0.5 Hz. M-P, responses 15
min after i.v. injection of DOPA, 100 mg/kg, same vertical
gain as in I-L; note longer time scale.

studies showing long ascending projections to the same cell
groups (Giovanelli and Kuypers, 1969; Brinkman and Kuypers,
in preparation). On stimulation of hindlimb nerves, the latency
of the discharge (8-18 msec) depended on the repetition rate of
the stimulus. It was shortest at 3-5 Hz (Fig. 1E-H), which also
corresponds to the maximum rate of stepping in normal and
decerebrate cats (Fig. 6B). Contralateral hindlimb nerves were
always less effective and the latency of the discharge was
generally 1-2 msec longer.

Hindlimb nerve conditioning of mono- and polysynaptic forelimb reflexes revealed the excitatory changes shown in Fig. 2.
Monosynaptic reflexes to pectoralis major, biceps and deep radial
motoneurones (supplying the physiological flexor muscles) were
strongly facilitated, ipsilateral nerves being more effective than
contralateral (e.g. Fig. 2A). Conditioning of monosynaptic reflexes
to latissimus dorsi and triceps brachii (physiological extensor
muscles) showed a reciprocal pattern with depression from ipsilateral, and facilitation from contralateral hindlimb extensor
muscle nerves, the flexor muscle nerves producing the reverse
pattern (e.g. Fig. 2C). The excitability of monosynaptic reflexes
to median and ulnar motoneurones (distal physiological extensor
muscles) was not significantly altered.

Polysynaptic reflexes to pectoralis major biceps and deep
radial motoneurones received initial strong facilitation followed
by prolonged depression, ipsilateral hindlimb nerves again being
more effective than the contralateral (Fig. 2B). In latissimus
dorsi and triceps a reciprocal pattern similar to that for the
monosynaptic reflex was found. Polysynaptic reflexes to median
and ulnar motoneurones mostly received only prolonged depression,
although in one case the median motoneurones received slight
facilitation (Fig. 2D). The hindlimb afferent nerves responsible
for the discharge in forelimb motoneurones and for the facilitation
and depression of forelimb reflexes include groups II and III
muscle afferents and group II skin afferents, the nerve from quadriceps and sartorius muscles, and the sural and superficial
peroneal nerves, being especially effective. The ascending pathways are located in lower thoracic segments in the ventrolateral
funiculus (Fig. 7) and mediate effects on ipsilateral and contralateral forelimb reflex systems, the ipsilateral effects being
the stronger.

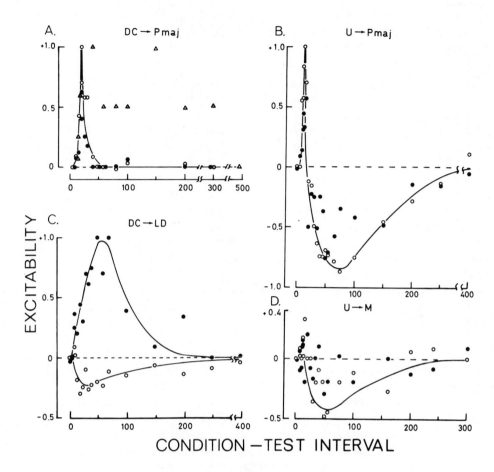

CONDITION —TEST INTERVAL

Fig. 2. Time course of excitability changes in forelimb reflexes, recorded in cut motor nerves, following electrical
conditioning stimulation of hindlimb nerves. A. Monosynaptic
reflex to Pmaj on stimulation of DC. Open circles iQ, filled
circles cQ, 3 shocks, 5T. Open triangles, excitability changes
after i.v. injection of DOPA; iQ 3 shocks 20T. B. Polysynaptic
reflex U to Pmaj at 2.4T. Open circles, iQ; filled circles cQ,
3 shocks, 10T. C. Monosynaptic reflex to LD. Open circles
iQ, filled circles cQ, 3 shocks, 7T. D. Polysynaptic reflex U
to M at 1.5 T. Open circles iSCI, filled circles cSCI, 3 shocks,
10T.

In all graphs the ordinate indicates excitability, with positive
values for facilitation and negative values for depression.
Abscissa in msec. See Miller et al. (1973a) for further
details.

DESCENDING CONTROL OF TRANSMISSION IN LONG
ASCENDING PROPRIOSPINAL PATHWAYS BY
NORADRENERGIC RETICULOSPINAL PATHWAYS

The noradrenergic terminals in the spinal cord of reticulospinal pathways may be selectively activated in low spinal cats by
intravenous injection of the catecholamine precursor DOPA
(Andén et al., 1966). This results in profound changes of reflex
excitability in lumbo-sacral segments, in particular in a depression of short latency responses in motoneurones evoked by the
flexor reflex afferents, and in an unmasking of a prolonged, long
latency reflex discharge evoked by the same afferents. The long
latency reflex responses were considered to reflect the activity
of mechanisms involved in the control of stepping (Jankowska et
al., 1967a, b), and further support for this hypothesis has been
obtained in mesencephalic (Grillner and Shik, 1973) and low
spinal (Forssberg and Grillner, 1973) cats. It has been suggested
that the noradrenergic reticulospinal pathway might represent
part of a control system for the initiation of locomotion (Grillner,
1973a).

In high spinal cats the influence of an intravenous injection of
DOPA was investigated on the transmission of long ascending
propriospinal pathways to the same groups of forelimb motoneurones as described above (Bergmans et al., 1973). The early
discharge, evoked in some preparations, in pectoralis major
motoneurones on electrical stimulation of hindlimb afferents is
enhanced after DOPA. A late discharge (30-80 msec latency)
appears after DOPA in the same forelimb motoneurones and may
often last up to 600 msec or more (Fig. 1I-O). Facilitation by
hindlimb nerves of mono- and polysynaptic segmental reflexes to
forelimb motoneurones is similarly prolonged (Fig. 2A, triangles).
Once again ipsilateral hindlimb nerves were more effective than
contralateral. Late discharges were also evoked in forelimb
motoneurones on stimulation of forelimb afferents after DOPA and
it was concluded that a broadly similar organization of late reflexes
exists in brachial segments as previously reported for lumbosacral segments by Jankowska et al. (1967a). A further system
modifying long ascending propriospinal transmission was also
disclosed (Bergmans et al., 1973). Stimulation of the ventral
quadrant just below the transection at C_1 enhanced the early discharge in forelimb motoneurones following stimulation of hindlimb
nerves without evoking a late discharge. The pathway has not yet
been identified.

BEHAVIOURAL EXPERIMENTS
ANALYSIS OF STEPPING PATTERNS

In quadruped animals, including cat, dog and horse, the sequences of contact of the four limbs with the ground have been used to characterize a wide variety of different patterns of stepping (Gray, 1968; Hildebrand, 1966; Muybridge, 1957; Roberts, 1967). Using this approach, Stuart and his collaborators (this Symposium) have made a detailed analysis of certain standard elements of the cat's gait. Before attempting to define interlimb co-ordination, we tried to answer the question: Can the different gaits observed in the cat be reduced to a few basic elements which are elaborated centrally by the deeds, for example, of balance, jumping, swimming or increased velocity?

On the basis of observations of the patterns of stepping of decerebrate and normal cats on a motor driven treadmill, and of normal cats freely moving, we have suggested that there are two fundamental types of cyclical movement (Miller et al., 1973b). (1) Alternate stepping, where the hindlimbs and also the forelimbs step alternately. This includes all forms of walking and trotting, and also swimming. (2) In-phase stepping, where the hindlimbs step more in phase with each other, and the forelimbs either alternate or step more in phase. Movements of the vertebral column can also co-operate with the combined movements of the hindlimbs to achieve greater step length and forward velocity (Hildebrand, 1959). The in-phase form of stepping includes all forms of galloping and may also serve the basic routines for such movements as jumping. This classification of locomotor movement should not detract from the value of analyses of gaits based on limb contact (Stuart et al., this Symposium), but it permits the suggestion that the same subsets of neural organization could be used with little modification in different motor behaviours, for example, walking and swimming.

The classification is based on the following observations made in both decerebrate and normal cat preparations.

1. The changeover between alternate and in-phase forms (e.g. between trotting and galloping) is always sudden and is usually completed within one step (Shik et al., 1966; Muybridge, 1957).

2. The patterns of stepping have usually been related to the patterns of contact of the four limbs on the ground (Gray, 1968;

Muybridge, 1957; Roberts, 1967) and this is shown in Fig. 3 for the commonly accepted forms of walking, trotting and galloping.

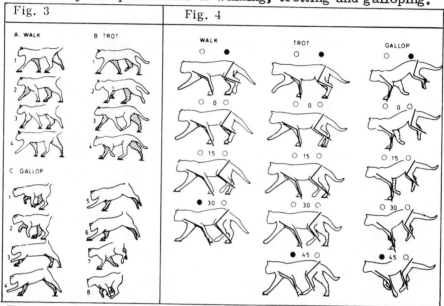

Fig. 3. Patterns of foot contact during stepping. The numbered drawings show the positions in the step cycle where the contact pattern changes. Horizontal bars indicate contact with ground. Walk 1.2 m. sec^{-1}, trot 1.7 m. sec^{-1}, gallop 3.3 m. sec^{-1}.

Fig. 4. Time coupling of first extension of hindlimb and flexion of forelimb during stepping at different velocities. The figurines in each vertical column indicate sequential frames taken every 15 msec. Solid lines show angles of knee and elbow joints. Filled circles indicate flexion, open circles extension. Figures between circles show in msec the time elapsed after the first extension of the knee joint. Walk 1.3 m. sec^{-1}, trot 1.6 m. sec^{-1}, gallop 3.1 m. sec^{-1}.

Note that in walking the time of contact of the forelimb occurs shortly after that of the ipsilateral hindlimbs (phase value of 0-0.25 on the treadmill, and about 0.20 during free movement); in trotting the hind- and forelimbs of the same side are out of phase (about 0.5 in all preparations). As its velocity increases, the cat passes progressively through walking and trotting to galloping. The interval between contact of the hindlimb and contact of the ipsilateral

forelimb follows the curve shown in Fig. 5A, open circles. In
Fig. 5B, this is replotted as phase - the interval divided by the
total step time. In all types of stepping up to approximately 2.5
m. sec^{-1}, the boundary in our data between the alternate and
in-phase forms, the curves increase smoothly. At this point the
slopes become less and there is a smaller increase during
galloping. The only change in the curve occurs at the boundary of

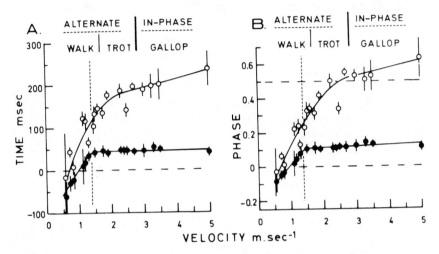

Fig. 5. Contact and coupling intervals as functions of velocity.
A. Open circles, time intervals between contact of hindlimb
and contact of ipsilateral forelimb. Filled circles, interval
between first extension of hindlimb and flexion of ipsilateral
forelimb. B. Same intervals replotted as phase: i. e. the
intervals divided by the total step time, measured from contact times of one hindlimb. Vertical bars, standard deviation.
All points from a normal cat on treadmill, except for values
at 5 m. sec^{-1}, which were taken from the same cat moving
freely.

alternate and in-phase stepping, and this and the lack of other
discontinuities is taken as further evidence that the two forms of
stepping are each homogeneous. The change in the phase of hindlimb - forelimb contact with velocity results from the fact that
increase in velocity is achieved mainly by increase in step length
(see next section), the forelimbs increasing their step by projecting
further forwards, the hindlimbs by extending further backwards.

3. During stepping certain movements of the joints of hind-
and forelimbs show a time coupling which is independent of the
form and velocity of stepping. At all velocities with freely moving
cats and at velocities greater than about 1 m. sec^{-1} with cats on
the treadmill, the first extension of the hindlimb (Philippson, 1905;
Engberg and Lundberg, 1969) is followed by flexion of the ipsilateral
forelimb (Fig. 4, figurines; Fig. 5A and B, graph, filled circles).
It is important to emphasize that the first extension of the hindlimb
has been read at the knee joint, and the forelimb flexion at the
elbow. The time interval remains remarkably constant at about
40 msec (Fig. 5A), and the phase hardly changes (Fig. 5B). At
all velocities above about 1.0 to 1.4 m. sec^{-1} the variance of the
interval is significantly less (P < 0.01) than that of the total step
time (hind- or forelimb contact to the next hind- or forelimb
contact). At present no clear coupling independent of velocity
between hindlimb and contralateral forelimb or forelimb and
hindlimb has been observed. The vertical broken line at 1.4
m. sec^{-1} (Figs. 5 and 6) represents a boundary below which the

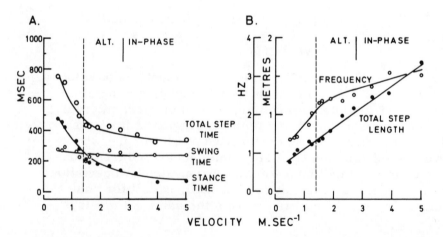

Fig. 6. Stepping parameters as a function of velocity. A.
Total step, swing and stance times. B. Frequency and total
step length. Normal cat on treadmill, same cat as Figs. 4
and 5. Values at 5.0 m. sec^{-1} from same cat freely moving.
For further discussion, see text.

step parameters are much more variable. In cats on the treadmill
this velocity has to be exceeded before the hindlimb to forelimb

coupling becomes established. This is probably in part a pecul-
iarity of the treadmill, since freely moving cats tend to have their
own preferred velocities; the phase value seldom falls below 0.2
and the hindlimb to forelimb coupling, though more variable,
is also seen at velocities below 1.0 m. sec^{-1}.

We have interpreted the coupling of hind- and forelimb movements to indicate that the central nervous system is less concerned
with precise timing of the contact of the foot with the ground, as
with the programming of the placing movements themselves. This
concept is further supported by the observation of the same
coupling of movements during swimming. The 'decision' to
initiate the first extension of the hindlimb (its placing on the
ground) enables the stance (support) phase of the forelimb to be
terminated. This 'subprogram' appears independent of the type of
stepping, except for restrictions during galloping, and it is
independent of the velocity. Whether this indicates a type of phase-
locking between segments in the neuraxis as described for the
cockroach in stepping (Pearson and Iles, 1973) or the dogfish
during swimming (Grillner, 1973b) is not at present certain,
since insufficient data has been obtained of the respective neural
and muscle activity during stepping.

THE CONTROL OF VELOCITY DURING STEPPING

From the films of the different cats measurements have been
made of the durations of the stance (support) and swing (transfer)
phases at different constant velocities of the treadmill. From
these the following quantitites have been derived: Total step time,
stance plus swing intervals; frequency of stepping, the reciprocal
of the total step time; and total length, the total step time multiplied
by velocity. These parameters, taken from a normal, unanaesthetized
cat on the treadmill, are plotted against velocity in Fig. 6. Comparable plots have been obtained in other normal cats on the
treadmill and moving freely, and also in decerebrate cats on the
treadmill. The curves in Fig. 6B demonstrate that to achieve
greater velocity the cat progressively increases the frequency of
stepping and the total step length. The frequency changes most at
velocities below 1 m. sec^{-1} and thereafter increases more slowly.
As several authors have shown the increase is largely due to a
shortening of the stance phase (Arshavsky et al., 1965; Goslow et
al., 1973). The increase of total step length is proportionately
greater than that of frequency. The transition from alternate to

in-phase stepping (e.g. trot to gallop) permits the effective total
step length to be further increased.

ROLE OF LONG PROPRIOSPINAL PATHWAYS
IN STEPPING

In the diagram of the functional connections of long propriospinal pathways (Fig. 7) it is likely to be of more relevance to

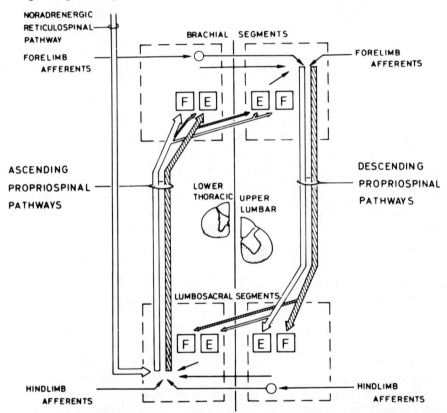

Fig. 7. Functional organization of long propriospinal pathways. Broken rectangles, segmental reflex systems controlling one limb; open arrows, excitatory effects; hatched
arrows, inhibitory effects; small arrows within broken
rectangles, interneuronal inputs to pathways; F and E, reflex
systems controlling, respectively, flexor and extensor reflex
systems; inset drawings show location of pathways in spinal
cord. All elements can indicate one or more neurones.

consider the direct or indirect connections between lumbo-sacral and brachial segments as reciprocal intrinsic links between the spinal 'motor centres' controlling respectively each hindlimb and forelimb (Miller et al., 1973a). The role of afferents may be to provide optimal regulation of the ongoing movements as they are elaborated by the central nervous system (Brown, 1911; Lundberg, 1969; for review see Grillner, 1973a). Propriospinal pathways would then serve primarily as co-ordinative links between the intrinsic activities of the segmental neuronal systems controlling the limbs (Fig. 7, broken rectangles). Transmission in the pathways would also be expected to be strongly influenced by supraspinal centres, as has been shown for segmental reflexes and various ascending pathways (Lundberg, 1971; Miller and Oscarsson, 1969; Orlovsky, 1972). It is therefore of significance that transmission in ascending propriospinal pathways may be facilitated and modified by at least two descending systems, the noradrenergic reticulospinal pathway and the descending pathway excited by ventral quadrant stimulation at C_1 (Bergmans et al., 1973). Activation of ascending propriospinal pathways by hindlimb afferents may be functionally less important than the activity of interneurones engaged in local segmental motor reflexes (Fig. 7, small arrows). This concept is further supported by the observation in decerebrate cats that the coupling of hind- and forelimb movements (Figs. 5 and 6) is not completely abolished after bilateral section of dorsal roots between L_1 and S_2 (Miller et al., in preparation).

In the long propriospinal pathways so far revealed in neurophysiological experiments it is striking that ipsilateral effects in both ascending and descending directions are more effective than contralateral (Fig. 7), and this is also supported by neuroanatomical studies (Giovanelli and Kuypers, 1969). The time coupling of the hind- and forelimb of the same side (Figs. 4 and 5) in different forms of stepping shows further similarities with the neurophysiological data. The ascending facilitation favours predominantly the flexor muscles contracting during the onset of the swing phase of the forelimb (see Miller et al., 1973a). The interval of the time-locking of about 40 msec is also compatible with the conduction delays in the ascending propriospinal pathway.

As a working hypothesis, it is suggested that the ascending propriospinal pathways contribute facilitation to the flexors of the forelimb, once the ipsilateral hindlimb has begun the first extension leading to its placing on the ground. This action might be expected to involve the ipsilateral ascending projections (Fig. 7). The postural changes in the limbs observed on hindlimb stimulation in the decerebrate cat (Pi-Suner and Fulton, 1928; Sherrington, 1898) are also consistent with this pattern, since on the side opposite to the stimulus the hindlimb assumes extension and the forelimb flexion. In in-phase stepping (i.e. as in the rotatory gallop) the onset of the first extension of the hindlimb occurs synchronously, and, depending on the laterality of the gallop, is followed after about 40 msec by flexion of one or other of the forelimbs. Here the appropriate ascending propriospinal pathway could receive bilateral activation in the lumbar cord (Fig. 7). Finally, in movements such as jumping the doubly crossed organization of ascending pathways could be brought into play securing maximal phasing of the hind- and forelimbs.

The functional organization of the descending propriospinal pathways is at present less clear than that of the ascending pathways. Attention has been largely devoted to the reflex systems controlling ankle flexors and extensors (Lloyd and McIntyre, 1948; Djalali, 1971), but it is likely that the muscles acting around the hip joint and the muscles of the back are more closely involved in long propriospinal reflexes (Sherrington, 1910; Kuypers, 1964; Grillner, 1973a). Despite this reservation it would seem that the descending pathways are also doubly crossed, and exert predominantly ipsilateral actions, while ascending pathways evoke extension of the hindlimb (Lloyd and McIntyre, 1948). Since the forelimb flexion in stepping is preceded by extension of the hindlimb the descending pathways may possibly be considered as helping to reinforce the extension and placing of the hindlimb during the flexion and swinging forwards of the forelimb. However, from preliminary observations of cats during swimming, forelimb movements would seem to 'dominate' those of the hindlimbs; in particular, that the termination of the forelimb 'stance' phase precedes the start of the 'first extension' of the ipsilateral hindlimb. It still remains to be shown if ascending and descending propriospinal projections form an integrated reflex system and how direct a role they play in actual stepping of the cat.

REFERENCES

Andén, N.E., Jukes, M.G.M., and Lundberg, A., 1966. The effect of DOPA on the spinal cord. II. Acta Physiol. Scand. 67, 387-397.

Arshavskii, Y.I., Kots, Y.M., Orlovsky, G.N., Rodionov, I.M. and
    Shik, M.L., 1965. Investigation of the biomechanics of running
    by the dog. Biofizika 10, 665-672. (Engl. Transl.)
Bergmans, J., Miller, S., and Reitsma, D.J., 1973. Influence of
    L-DOPA on transmission in long ascending propriospinal pathways
    in the cat. Brain Res. In press.
Brown, T.G., 1911. The intrinsic factors in the act of progression
    in the mammal. Proc. Roy. Soc. 84, 308-319.
Djalali, E., 1970. Relations neurophysiologiques brachio-lumbaires
    chez le chat spinal. Contribution à la connaissance de la
    physiologie de la moelle épinière. Thèse. Faculté des sciences
    de l'Université d'Aix-Marseille I. No. C.N.R.S. A.O. 4674, pp.
    150.
Engberg, I., and Lundberg, A., 1969. An electromyographic analysis
    of muscular activity in the hindlimb of the cat during unres-
    trained locomotion. Acta Physiol. Scand. 75, 614-630.
Forssberg, H., and Grillner, S., 1973. The locomotion of the acute
    spinal cat injected with clonidine i.v. Brain Res. 50, 184-186.
Giovanelli Barilari, M., and Kuypers, H.G.J.M., 1969. Proprio-
    spinal fibers interconnecting the spinal enlargements in the cat.
    Brain Res. 14, 321-330.
Goslow, G.E., Reinking, R.M., and Stuart, D.G., 1973. The cat step
    cycle: hindlimb joint angles and muscle lengths during unres-
    trained locomotion. J. Morphol. In press.
Gray, J., 1968. Animal Locomotion. Weidenfeld and Nicolson,
    London, 479 pp.
Grillner, S., 1973a. On the spinal generation of locomotion. In
    Sensory Organization of Movements. (Ed. Batuev, A.S.)
    Leningrad. In press.
Grillner, S., 1973b. Locomotion in the spinal dogfish. Acta
    Physiol. Scand. 87, 31-32A.
Grillner, S., and Shik, M.L., 1973. On the descending control of
    the lumbosacral spinal cord from the mesencephalic locomotor
    region. Acta Physiol. Scand. 87, 320-333.
Guillebeau, A., and Luchsunger, B., 1882. Fortgesetzte Studien am
    Ruckenmarke. Pflügers Arch. 28, 61-69.
Hildebrand, M., 1959. Motions of the running cheetah and horse.
    J. Mammal. 40, 481-495.
Hildebrand, M., 1966. Analysis of symmetrical gaits of tetrapods.
    Folio Biotheoret. 6, 1-22.
Jankowska, E., Jukes, M.G.M., Lund, S., and Lundberg, A., 1967a.
    The effect of DOPA on the spinal cord. 5. Reciprocal organi-
    zation of pathways transmitting excitatory action to alpha
    motoneurones of flexors and extensors. Acta Physiol. Scand.
    70, 369-388.
Jankowska, E., Jukes, M.G.M., Lund, S., and Lundberg, A., 1967b.
    The effect of DOPA on the spinal cord. 6. Half-centre organ-
    ization of interneurones transmitting effects from the flexor
    reflex afferents. Acta Physiol. Scand. 70, 389-402.

Jankowska, E., Lundberg, A., and Stuart, D., 1973. Propriospinal control of last order interneurones of spinal reflex pathways in the cat. Brain Res. 53, 227-231.

Kuypers, H.G.J.M., 1964. The descending pathways to the spinal cord, their anatomy and function. Prog. Brain Res. 11, 178-202.

Lawrence, D.G., and Kuypers, H.G.J.M., 1968. The functional organization of the motor system in the monkey. II. The effects of lesions of the descending brain-stem pathways. Brain Res. 91, 15-36.

Lloyd, D.P.C., 1942. Mediation of descending long spinal reflex activity. J. Neurophysiol. 5, 435-458.

Lloyd, D.P.C., and McIntyre, A.K., 1948. Analysis of forelimb-hindlimb reflex activity in acutely decapitate cats. J. Neurophysiol. 11, 455-470.

Lundberg, A., 1969. Reflex control of stepping. Nansen Memorial Lecture V. Universitetsforlaget, Oslo. 42 pp.

Lundberg, A., 1971. Function of the ventral spinocerebellar tract. A new hypothesis. Exp. Brain Res. 12, 317-330.

McDonald, W.I., 1955. An electrophysiological investigation of hindlimb-forelimb activity in acutely decapitate cats. B. Med. Sc. Thesis. Otago University Medical School, Dunedin, New Zealand, 117 pp.

Miller, S., and Oscarsson, O., 1969. Termination and functional organization of spino-olivocerebellar paths. In The Cerebellum in Health and Disease, pp. 172-200 (Ed. Fields, W.S. and Willis, W.D. Jr.) Warren H. Green Inc., St. Louis, Missouri, U.S.A.

Miller, S., Reitsma, D.J., and van der Meché, F.G.A., 1973a. Functional organization of long ascending propriospinal pathways linking lumbo-sacral and cervical segments in the cat. Brain Res. In press.

Miller, S., van Berkum, R., van der Burg, J., and van der Meché, F.G.A., 1973b. Interlimb co-ordination in stepping in the cat. J. Physiol. 230, 30-31P.

Muybridge, E., 1957. Animals in Motion. (Ed. Brown, L.S.) Dover Publications, Inc.: New York, 72 pp. 183 plates.

Orlovsky, G.N., 1972. The effect of different descending systems on flexor and extensor activity during locomotion. Brain Res. 40, 359-371.

Pearson, K.G., and Iles, J.F., 1973. Nervous mechanisms underlying intersegmental co-ordination of leg movements during walking in the cockroach. J. Exp. Biol. 58, 725-744.

Philippson, M., 1905. L'autonomie de la centralisation dans le système nerveux des animaux. Trav. Lab. Physiol. Inst. Solvay Bruxelles. 7, 1-208.

Pi-Suñer, J., and Fulton, J.F., 1928. The influence of the proprioceptive nerves of the hind limbs upon the posture of the fore-limbs in decerebrate cats. Amer. J. Physiol. 83, 548-553.

Roberts, T.D.M., 1967. Neurophysiology of postural mechanisms. Butterworths, London, 354 pp.

Sherrington, C.S., 1898. Decerebrate rigidity, and reflex co-ordination of movements. J. Physiol. 22, 319-332.

Sherrington, C.S., 1910. Flexion-reflex of the limb, crossed extension reflex, and reflex stepping and standing. J. Physiol. 40, 28-121.

Shik, M.L., Severin, F.V., and Orlovsky, G.N., 1966. Control of walking and running by means of electrical stimulation of the mid-brain. Biofizika 11, 659-666. (Engl. Transl.).

Sterling, P., and Kuypers, H.G.J.M., 1968. Anatomical organization of the brachial spinal cord of the cat. III. The propriospinal connections. Brain Res. 7, 419-443.

EIGHTH NERVE CONTRIBUTIONS TO THE SYNTHESIS OF LOCOMOTOR CONTROL

G. Melvill Jones, D. G. D. Watt and S. Rossignol

DRB Aviation Medical Research Unit, Department of Physiology, McGill University, Montreal

Recent experiments have demonstrated a short latency EMG response (75 msec) in human gastrocnemius on sudden un-expected initiation of a free fall. Cats were found to exhibit a similar short latency response which is permanently abol-ished by bilateral labyrinthectormy, but not by surgical in-activation of the semicircular canals. These findings point to a functionally effective vestibulo-spinal response to spec-ifically vertical linear accelerative stimulation of the vesti-bular otolith end organs. Since large cyclical changes in vertical linear acceleration of the head occur during normal human locomotion, especially running, it seems likely that this specific vestibulo-spinal influence could play an impor-tant role in the synthesis of normal locomotor control. This question has been examined in human subjects using hopping on one leg as a simplified monopedal model of cyclical loco-motor activity.

Eight subjects were found to choose very closely similar preferred frequencies of hopping (mean=2.06 Hz, S.E. 0.02). At this frequency the moment of leaving the ground (i.e. entry into zero 'g' free fall) systematically occurs close to 75 msec before commencement of the measured gastroc-nemius EMG associated with subsequent landing. Evidently the vestibulo-spinal response due to downward acceleration, implied above, would be well timed for contribution to the landing EMG. It is also shown that reversal of the vestibulo-spinal response, to be expected from the measured peak reversal of head acceleration, would be equally well timed for suppression of EMG at that moment when there is electrical muscle silence in the hopping cycle.

In view of these observations it was interesting to find that the rhythmical tempo of much traditional and contemporary dance music is based upon a fundamental cyclical frequency centred very close to the preferred hopping frequency. In this connection a formal study of audio-spinal influence on the human gastrocnemius motoneurone pool showed a sharp rise of excitability, commencing at the spinal segmental level close to 80 msec after initiation of a sudden 1 Kc auditory stimulus at the tympanum. When hopping in time to a Scottish reel played in strict tempo at 2.05 Hz (S.E. 0.002) the sharp transient sound of the "off" beat of the music was so placed that it would generate EMG potentiation at precisely the moment of actual initiation of gastrocnemius EMG. Similarly, the "on" beat would potentiate the latter part of the EMG burst responsible for projecting the body up into the "take-off" phase of the next cycle.

On the basis of other human experiments it is shown that muscle afferents due to gastrocnemius stretch after landing would also be likely to potentiate the "take-off" EMG, whilst suppression of such afferents during subsequent muscle shortening would likely contribute to the period of subsequent EMG silence.

The available data indicate that these different physiological phenomena become nicely synthesised in the common functional goal of perpetuating the on-going cycle of locomotor activity. Perhaps also we see here the elements of a physiological basis for some patterns of rhythmical organisation in music.

Recent observations on the control of stepping movements in man (Watt, 1969; Melvill Jones and Watt, 1971a) have shown that when a subject steps from a low platform to the ground, a very stereotyped pattern of electromyographic (EMG) activity occurs in the antigravity muscles of the lower leg. Fig. 1, an original record of one step down, illustrates some features of this activity. The upper trace gives the output of a strain-gauge

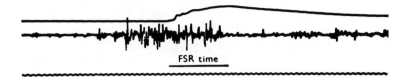

Fig. 1. Gastrocnemius EMG associated with landing from a 10" step to the ground. Upper trace - force exerted by landing platform on the foot; middle trace - surface EMG from gastrocnemius; FSR time - delay before a functionally useful EMG response to stretch would be expected to occur; bottom trace - 100 Hz sine wave (Melvill Jones and Watt, 1971a). The maximum change of force shown is approximately 2 x body weight.

measuring vertical landing force. Next is the record of gastrocnemius activity associated with one complete step down. Evidently, the muscle activity began well before landing, as must, of course, be the case for suitably timed initiation of mechanical muscle contraction. Of additional interest is the bar marked FSR, standing for Functional Stretch Response, which indicates the delay after touch-down before a functionally useful EMG response to stretch would be expected to occur on the basis of earlier experiments (Hammond et al., 1956; Melvill Jones and Watt, 1971a). The fact that this bar extends beyond the termination of 'landing' EMG suggests that electrical muscle activity was over before there could have been a functionally useful response to muscle stretch induced by the ankle dorsiflexion associated with landing. These observations led to the conclusion that in normal circumstances the whole neuromuscular sequence of activity responsible for a smooth landing is brought about by a pre-programmed sequence of neural information, accurately timed with respect to the moment of landing, but inaccessible to feedback from the mechanical event of landing itself.

This raised the question: would such a program be formulated solely on the basis of voluntary motor control in response to mixed visual and memorized knowledge, or would there be a contribution from automatic responses to the vertical accelerative stimulation which accompanies initiation of the descent?

VESTIBULO-SPINAL INFLUENCES

The results in Fig. 2 throw some light on the answer to this question (Melvill Jones and Watt, 1971b). As illustrated in this

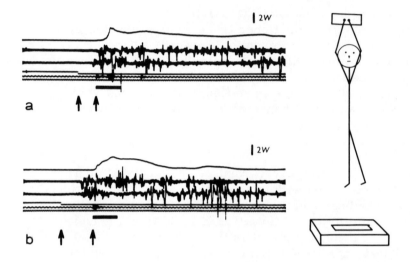

Fig. 2. Muscular activity associated with landing from unexpected falls of (a) 6.4 cm and (b) 17.8 cm. From above downwards, traces give force, gastrocnemius EMG, tibialis EMG, moment of release, sound of landing superimposed on 60 Hz and a 100 Hz sinusoidal time base. The subject is suspended by an electromagnet over the force-transducing platform. The first and second arrows of each figure give the moments of initiating fall and of contact with the ground, respectively. The solid bar beneath each set of traces gives the FSR time defined in Fig. 1. (Adapted from Melvill Jones and Watt, 1971b).

figure, the subject was suspended by an electromagnet at a variable height above a force-transducing landing platform. Each set of records in this figure shows from above downwards the landing force, gastrocnemius EMG, tibialis EMG, the moment of release (initiation of fall) and the sound of landing on the platform. The

sound trace also carries a sine wave of 60 Hz and the bottom
trace a sine wave of 100 Hz serving as a time base.

   In the context of this article, it is particularly interesting to
note that, despite differences in height of fall in the two sets of
records, the initiation of gastrocnemius EMG activity was
sharply defined in both instances at approximately 75 msec after
initiation of the fall. This is very considerably shorter than the
average voluntary response time of 163 msec measured in these
experiments in response to a light superficial touch, or by
others using different kinds of sensory stimuli (Chocholle, 1963).

   Fig. 3 plots mean values of gastrocnemius EMG latency
obtained from 8 subjects following the initiation of falls from

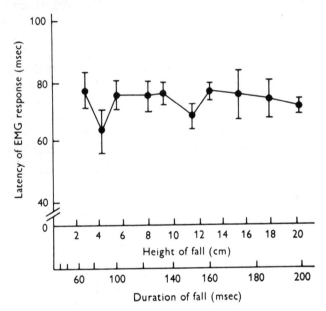

<u>Fig. 3.</u> Mean latency of gastrocnemius EMG response to
sudden falls of varying height. The overall mean of these
values is 74.2 msec (S.E. ± 1.4). (Melvill Jones and
Watt, 1971b).

different heights. Two sets of values on the abscissa give the
height of fall in cm on a linear scale and the corresponding
duration of fall, which of course is not a linear function of the
height owing to the gravitational acceleration. These results

emphasize the feature noted above, namely that the duration between initiation of fall and initiation of gastrocnemius EMG proves to be maintained constant at approximately 75 msec, independently of the height of fall. This consistency of response, together with the fact that the response time is much shorter than the voluntary response time mentioned above, is suggestive of a reflex pattern of response to the sudden transition from a normal gravitational field to the zero gravity state associated with a free-fall condition. The accelerative nature of this stimulus suggests in turn that the response might originate from vertical sensing components in the otolith organs of the vestibular system in the inner ear. Current animal experiments (Watt, 1973, unpublished data) confirm these suggestions by showing that a corresponding early response in cats is permanently (at least 14 months) abolished by bilateral labyrinthectomy, but not by selective surgical obstruction of fluid circulation in the semicircular canals.

Presumably these objective results reflect quantitatively the earlier qualitative observations of Magnus (1924) and others (Dow, 1938; Lyon, 1951; Money and Scott, 1962) who have observed sudden active extension of the limbs of animals after sudden initiation of a fall. The combined evidence points to the presence of active vestibulo-spinal modulation of the excitability of spinal motoneurone pools as a result of vertically directed head accelerations.

Against this view is the fact that, although there is clear evidence of directional polarization in the organization of the ciliated sensory epithelia of the vestibular otolith organs (Spoendlin, 1966; Loewenstein, 1967; Linderman, 1969; Flock, 1971), Malcolm (1971) has drawn attention to the fact that published illustrations indicate a rather sparse vertical projection of these polarization vectors, even in the more or less vertically oriented saccular maculae of the otolith organs. Furthermore, there has been some doubt whether the saccular component of the otolith system responds primarily to accelerative stimuli in the range of normal movement, or rather to high frequency vibrational stimuli (Ashcroft and Hallpike, 1934).

However, later neurophysiological evidence from the Ray fish (Loewenstein and Roberts, 1949) and the cat (Adrian, 1943) certainly revealed a neural component of vestibular response to vertical components of accelerative stimulation. Indeed, the more

recent work of Fernandez et al. (1972) has demonstrated heavy
representation of low frequency acceleration information in
primary afferent neurones presumed, on good experimental
evidence, to derive from the saccular end-organ of the squirrel
monkey. Again, Melvill Jones and Daunton (1973, unpublished
data) have found statistically indistinguishable intensities of
afferent neural information associated with horizontal and
vertical linear accelerative movements in vestibular components
of the cat brainstem. Fig. 4 illustrates for example the cyclical

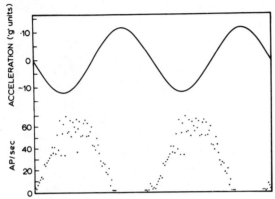

Fig. 4. Dependence of vestibular neural activity upon
vertical accelerative motion. Upper curve (0.59 Hz) gives
the sine wave of vertical accelerative stimulation (up ≈
acceleration up). Lower "spotted" curve gives correctly
phased firing frequency of single neural unit in the
inferior region of the left lateral vestibular nucleus of
cat, averaged over 60 consecutive cycles of accelerative
stimulation. Note that the activity of this cell at this
frequency of stimulation was increased by downward
acceleration and decreased by upward acceleration. The
"spontaneous" firing frequency of this unit was 23 AP/sec.

firing frequency of an otolith-dependent central vestibular neurone
averaged from 60 cycles of vertical sinusoidal acceleration of
amplitude 0.12 g and frequency 0.59 Hz. The gain of this cell's
vertical component of response was calculated as 270 action
potentials (AP) per sec per 'g', over that part of the cycle in
which it was actively firing. During the other part of the cycle
this unit was suppressed below its steady state firing frequency
of 23 AP/sec, even to the point of being silenced over a considerable segment of the cycle. The cat's head was oriented in a

stereotaxic device so that the lateral canals were in a horizontal plane. These observations make it clear that, contrary to earlier views, cyclical <u>vertical</u> linear accelerative motion of the head may be expected to feed a substantial and specific afferent input to the brainstem. Indeed, the sensitivity of such input is highlighted by the very low thresholds of unit response observed. One such unit yielded just audible modulation of AP frequency at a sinusoidal amplitude of 0.002 'g'.

Summarizing thus far, we find that (a) there is substantial representation of vertical accelerative information in both peripheral and central vestibular neural components; (b) there is a well defined short latency muscular response to sudden falls in both man and cat, and (c) permanent elimination of the cat's short latency muscular response occurs specifically after bilateral extirpation of the vestibular otolith organs. These findings encourage the view that vestibular stimulation due to vertical linear accelerative motion can bring a functionally effective influence to bear upon the postural muscles of the leg. If this is true, then since large cyclical changes in specifically vertical acceleration of the head occur during normal locomotion (Cavagna et al., 1964; Liberson et al., 1962), it would be surprising indeed if resulting vestibulo-spinal influences did not contribute in a meaningful way to cyclical events in the synthesis of locomotor control.

NEUROMUSCULAR EVENTS ASSOCIATED WITH CYCLICAL VERTICAL MOVEMENT

From an experimental point of view, it would seem reasonable to begin investigation of this question with a monopedal model of cyclical locomotor activity, to avoid the complication of reciprocal interactions between alternating limb movements. Using repetitive hopping on one leg as such a model, Watt (1969) found there was a remarkably consistent choice of "preferred" frequency of hopping among 8 subjects making 6 choices each. The resulting mean preferred frequency was 2.06 Hz (S.E. 0.02). Again, Rossignol (1973) found a remarkable consistency in the mean periodic time between successive landings in 10 subjects hopping in time to a fixed stretch of taped Scottish dance music. The mean interval between successive landings was found to be 489 msec (S.E. 1.9 msec, N = 80). For comparison with Watt's data, these results convert to a mean frequency of 2.05 Hz (S.E. 0.002).

The closeness of these two sets of data and their statistical tightness suggests greater precision than might be expected from purely voluntary control, and the following observations examine some aspects of current evidence which supports this contention.

Fig. 5 shows an extract of records obtained from a human subject hopping at his preferred frequency. The upper trace

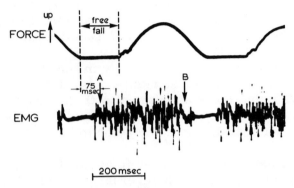

Fig. 5. Gastrocnemius EMG obtained at the preferred frequency of hopping. Upper trace - vertical force transduced from the landing platform; lower trace - gastrocnemius EMG. 'A' depicts 75 msec after the moment of leaving the ground (i. e. after entry into "free fall"); 'B' is 75 msec after the moment of maximum upward force exerted by the platform on the foot (i. e. point of maximum up acceleration).

gives the vertical force exerted by the landing platform on the subject's foot. Simultaneous records of this force profile and the output of a vertically oriented accelerometer on the head showed that such a trace of force also yields a good representation of vertical head acceleration at this frequency, despite the column of biological tissues which separates the head accelerometer from the force transducer registering at the level of the foot. This feature was again confirmed by the experiments of Rossignol (1973) in which the head accelerometer replaced the force transduction platform as an indicator of mechanical events during the hopping cycle. The lower trace in Fig. 5 shows the associated sequence of EMG activity in gastrocnemius muscle of the hopping leg. Converting upward force to upward acceleration in the top trace, it is seen that a cycle of events is established in which, during contact of the foot with the ground, the head is exposed to an upward acceleration which starts from zero, progressively increases to a peak value and then decreases again until the moment at which the body leaves the ground. At this moment, the subject suddenly enters a "free fall" or "zero 'g'" condition, as indicated in the figure. On return to the landing platform, the cycle is repeated, and so on. Bearing in mind that the moment of transition into free fall can be considered closely equivalent to the sudden fall investigated as in Fig. 2, it seems probable that approximately 75 msec later an associated moto-neurone pool excitatory input would be manifest in the EMG activity of gastrocnemius. The arrow A in Fig. 5 indicates this moment, which evidently corresponds closely in time with the initiation of EMG activity associated with landing. Presumably the time between A in the figure and contact with the ground is accounted for both by electromechanical coupling delays and the fact that there was some ankle extension prior to landing.

Since the vestibular neural response to cyclical vertical acceleration appears to reverse with reversal of the direction of acceleration (Fig. 4), it seems likely that gastrocnemius activity might be actively suppressed some 75 msec after peak upward acceleration; indeed, it has been shown that upwards acceleration of the intact cat systematically leads to suppression of extensor activity. This point in the cycle is indicated by the arrow B in Fig. 5, where it can be seen that such a suppressive effect would be entirely appropriately placed for contribution to termination of EMG activity, which, owing to electromechanical coupling delays, should also precede the moment of leaving the ground. Thus, when the evidence for vestibulo-spinal response to sudden fall is applied to the cyclical events of hopping, and presumably running, it seems plausible that a corresponding cyclical vestibulo-spinal influence may play an important role in the synthesis and precision timing of associated locomotor EMG activity.

AUDIO-SPINAL INFLUENCES

In view of the tight constraint which seems to fix the preferred frequency of hopping, it was intriguing to find that much popular dance music contains a fundamental rhythmic frequency close to this preferred frequency (Melvill Jones and Watt, 1971a). Could there be a significant audio-spinal influence on motoneurone excitability induced by the very sharp transient bursts of sound which demarcate the musical "beats", such as those seen in Fig. 7?

For these and other reasons, an experimental study has been made by Rossignol (1973) of the influence of transient auditory stimuli upon motoneurone pool excitability changes in human subjects. The method of H-reflex monosynaptic testing (Hoffman, 1922; Magladery and McDougal, 1950; Paillard, 1955) was used to quantify such changes. Briefly the method utilizes the fact that, under suitably controlled conditions, it is possible to stimulate selectively group 1 muscle afferent fibres by per-cutaneous stimulation of the posterior tibial nerve (innervating gastrocnemius) in its course through the popliteal fossa behind the knee. Such a stimulus discharges a synchronous burst of neural activity in the group 1 afferent neurones which then mono-synaptically stimulate alpha motoneurones innervating the gastrocnemius muscle of the same leg. Change in size of the resulting monosynaptic EMG reflex response, recorded from surface electrodes, has been shown to provide a reasonably valid indication of corresponding change in excitability of the relevant motoneurone pool. Thus, Paillard (1955) has successfully employed this method to measure change in motoneurone pool excitability as a result of a variety of conditioning stimuli.

In the present experiments, the conditioning stimulus chosen was a short auditory input of 1 Kc lasting 0.1 sec and a sound intensity, measured at the tympanum, of 110 dB above threshold. Taking suitable care to separate successive H-stimuli by 15 sec, found to be necessary for avoidance of interactions between successive H-stimuli, the time course of excitability changes in gastrocnemius motoneurone pool was determined in a suitable sample of human subjects (Rossignol, 1973).

Fig. 6 shows the detailed result obtained from one subject. Here the ordinate gives percentage potentiation of the H-reflex relative to a series of 10 control responses (100%) obtained before sound stimulation. The abscissa gives time, in msec, before (negative values) and after initiation of the sound stimulus, which is shown as a 100 msec block beneath the curve. Between 60 and 80 msec after sound initiation there was a sharp increase in motoneurone pool excitability, which reached in the next 30 msec or so a peak potentiation in this subject of 218%. In order to find the approximate time at which EMG activity in the peripheral

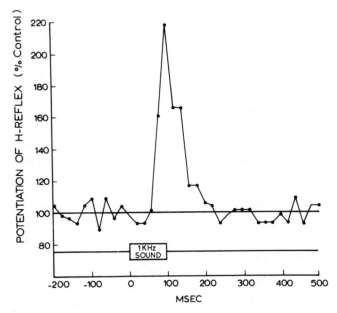

Fig. 6. Measured time course of H-reflex facilitation induced in one subject by a 100 msec tone burst of 1 Kc and 110 dB above threshold. 100% represents the mean of 10 H-reflex responses obtained prior to commencement of the sound stimulus.

muscle will be maximally potentiated, about 10 and 20 msec must be added to account for the afferent and efferent peripheral conduction times respectively. Thus on the one hand the experimental values are measured relative to the moment of H-reflex stimulation and on the other hand the effects of motoneurone excitation must travel down the efferent fibres before generating an EMG. Taking a mean measured H-reflex potentiation latency of 70 msec the corresponding EMG latency would then be about 100 msec. In the whole group of subjects examined, there was a considerable range in peak potentiation from about 150% to about 400% in the overall experiment, although the timing of both initiation and peak values of the potentiation was much more tightly constrained. Thereafter, there was a decay to the original condition over the next 200 msec or so. It is important to appreciate that these changes occurred in the absence of any overt startle reaction, as verified by continuous EMG recording during these experiments. H-reflex testing of the remote influence is, of course, only valid if that influence does not actually produce motoneurone firing, since the subsequent refractory characteristic would itself change a subsequent H-reflex response. Indeed, auditory stimuli sufficient to evoke overt startle were found to generate somewhat different patterns of response (Rossignol, 1973), although such patterns will not be further considered in this article.

From the quantitative data available in Fig. 6, we may now plot a reasonably plausible time course of motoneurone pool excitability changes likely to be associated with the transient sounds of the musical beats. Fig. 7 illustrates the outcome of

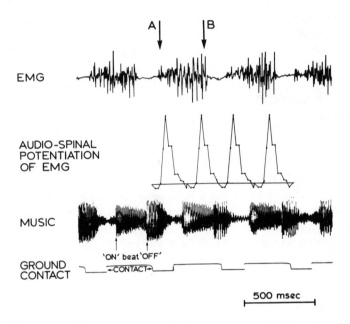

Fig. 7. EMG potentiation to be expected on the basis of Fig. 6, whilst hopping in time to a Scottish reel played in strict tempo at 2.05 Hz. From below up, traces read the cyclical shift from contact with the ground to "free fall" in the air, the sequence of sound recorded (3 dB atten at 350 Hz) from the music, the EMG potentiation to be expected from the sharp transient sounds denoted as "on" and "off" beats and actual gastrocnemius EMG. The curves of EMG potentiation are scaled replicas of the curve in Fig. 6, the initial rise of each being located 100 msec after initiation of the transient sound stimuli according to reasoning adduced in the text. A and B correspond to the similar arrows in Fig. 5.

this approach in a section of recordings obtained by Rossignol
from a subject hopping "in time" to a sequence of traditional
"reel" music played by a professional Scottish dance band.
In this figure, the musical sound is seen in the third trace from
the top. According to the written music it is easy to identify the
"on" (i. e. first beat in the bar) and "off" beats. It can be seen
that the rise time of sound intensity associated with these beats
is sharply defined and of very short duration. Moreover, in this
example the resulting auditory stimuli were comparable to the
experimental tone burst of Fig. 6, in rise time, amplitude and
duration.

    The top trace shows the recorded EMG modulation associated
with the cycle of landing and "take off", which was closely
similar to that depicted in Fig. 5. Between the EMG and sound
traces is the time course of muscle EMG potentiation which
would be expected from the motoneurone pool excitability
changes shown in Fig. 6. As will be seen each of these curves
is a scaled replica of Fig. 6, located relative to commencement
of the "on" and "off" beats according to the timing adduced above.

    Starting with the first "off" beat in the musical sound record
of Fig. 7, muscle EMG potentiation would begin about 70+.(10+20)
=100 msec later. It would then rise to a peak 30 msec beyond
that point and subsequently decline along a variable time course
according to the individual. The resulting potentiation is seen
to be most appropriately located for facilitation of the start of
the sequence of EMG activity associated with landing. Correspondingly, the following "on" beat is well placed to provide
audio-spinal potentiation for the latter part of the EMG burst
which is associated with projection of the body upwards before
take off into the short period of "free fall" depicted in Fig. 5.

    When these audio-spinal influences are integrated with the
vestibulo-spinal ones discussed above, we find that audio-spinal
potentiation due to the musical "off" beat would be nicely
synchronized with the presumed vestibulo-spinal excitatory
influence associated with the arrow A in Fig. 5; and also that
the decline of audio-spinal potentiation resulting from the "on"
beat would be nicely placed to coincide with the presumed
vestibulo-spinal suppressive influence associated with the arrow B.

RESPONSE TO MUSCLE STRETCH

Of course during landing substantial dorsiflexion of the ankle and hence lengthening of the gastrocnemius muscle occurs concurrently with the phase of deceleration of descending body velocity. It would be surprising indeed if the resulting stretch excitation in gastrocnemius did not produce a net excitatory influence contributing to the subsequent upward thrust into the next cycle. However, as indicated briefly above, a separate series of experiments (Melville Jones and Watt, 1971a) has demonstrated that in these circumstances the consequent forceful muscular response would be expected only after a considerable delay beyond the monosynaptic stretch reflex response. Fig. 8

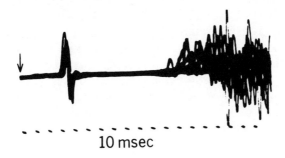

10 msec

Fig. 8. EMG response to gastrocnemius to sudden and maintained unexpected stretch. An initial synchronous monosynaptic response is always followed by a strictly silent period of about 80 msec. Only after this silent period is there a forceful maintained asynchronous EMG discharge which is therefore referred to in the text as the Functional Stretch Response (FSR). Arrow marks the moment of sudden stretch.

illustrates this feature by relating EMG activity in gastrocnemius to sudden forceful dorsiflexion of the ankle which occurred at an unexpected time marked by the arrow. The figure shows 10 superimposed responses derived from experiments of Chan (1973, unpublished data). The subject was instructed to oppose the dorsiflexion when it occurred. At the very precise monosynaptic response time there was a synchronous EMG response which corresponds closely with that due to a simple tendon tap response.

But this was followed by an extended silent period. Only after this silent period was there a prolonged strong burst of electro-myographic activity, which has been shown to be responsible for the generation of the main forceful opposition to such a stretch. For gastrocnemius in man this delayed EMG response occurred on average 120 msec after the moment of stretch, as indicated by the FSR time in Fig. 1.

Referring back to Fig. 5, and bearing in mind that stretch begins at the end of the period of free fall (i.e. on contact with the ground), it can be seen that this pattern of activity due to stretch would be located in the latter half of the EMG activity; associated, that is, with the upward thrust into the next cycle. Similarly in Fig. 7, where the cyclical frequency of hopping was on average 2.05 Hz, the delayed response to stretch would pre-sumably sum with the effects of audio-spinal facilitation in the latter half of the periods of EMG activity seen in the top trace. Furthermore, since this latter half of the EMG burst generates plantar flexion, and hence subsequent shortening of the gastroc-nemius, it seems likely there would be a subsequent phase of diminished stretch reflex afferents which in turn would be nicely placed for contribition to the postulated suppressor vestibulo-spinal influence and termination of audio-spinal influence assoc-iated with cessation of EMG.

INTEGRATION OF NEUROMUSCULAR INFLUENCES

Assembling all the information summarized above, one may postulate a reasonably plausible sequence of events as follows: assume first that a repeated cycle of hopping to a sequence of music of the kind illustrated in Fig. 7, and timed to coincide with the preferred frequency of hopping, has been in operation for several cycles. Then, in the steady state of cyclical repetition, starting at the moment of entry into "free fall" (i.e. the moment of leaving contact with the ground), a facilitatory vestibulo-spinal influence would be expected to manifest itself as an electromyographic activity close to the actual initiation of measured EMG. Meanwhile, the preceding transient auditory stimulus associated with the "off" beat of the music would be expected to raise the motoneurone pool excitability at precisely the appropriate time for the resulting peripheral EMG to summate with that due to the excitatory vestibulo-spinal influence. Thus, the vestibulo-spinal response to sudden entry into "free fall" would summate with the audio-

spinal potentiation of motoneurone pool excitability associated
with the "off" beat of the music, and both these would be suitably
timed for initiation of the EMG required for smooth arrest of the
impending landing. Then the next "on" beat of the music would
generate an excitatory influence suitably timed to summate with
the excitatory response to stretch associated with dorsiflexion
of the ankle on landing, so that the summed effect of these two
influences would be placed in the second half of the measured
EMG activity. Finally, as the potentiation due to audio-spinal
influence of the "on" beat of the music declines, reversal of
the vestibulo-spinal influence to be expected (but not yet
demonstrated) as a result of peak upward acceleration (see Fig.
4) would be suitably placed for termination of EMG activity, as
also would removal of facilitatory influence from stretch reflex
consequent upon shortening of gastrocnemius during projection
into the upward half of the cycle of body movement.

Of course, a considerable amount of conjecture is introduced
into the arguments laid out above. However, sufficient numerical
results from controlled experimental studies have been entered
into the argument to make it seem reasonably likely that we see
here the interacting influences of vestibulo-spinal, audio-spinal
and muscle afferent responses which, at a physiologically preferred
frequency, contribute one to the other in an optimal way for automatic maintenance of an on-going cyclical sequence of events.
Presumably increasing or decreasing the frequency of hopping
would substantially interfere with these nice associations. Indeed,
as demonstrated by Watt (1969), even minimal changes away from
the preferred frequency of hopping lead to an unpleasant, disorganized, sensation of movement, and also greatly increased
variability in the cyclical pattern of events. Perhaps we see here
how separate physiological entities, necessarily defined by
experiments designed to minimize all but the simple relevant
variable, become synthesized together for common purposeful
movements, to yield optimal characteristics of overall performance. Perhaps also the findings point to a physiological basis
for some patterns of rhythmical organization in music.

REFERENCES

Adrian, E.D., 1943. Discharges from vestibular receptors in the
cat. J. Physiol. 101, 389-407.

Ashcroft, D.W., and Hallpike, C.S., 1934. On the function of the
saccule. J. Laryng. Otol. 49, 450-460.

Cavagna, G.A., Saibene, F.P., and Margaria, R., 1964. Mechanical
work during running. J. Appl. Physiol. 19, 249-256.

Chocholle, R., 1963. Les temps de réaction. In Traité de
Psychologie Expérimentale. II. Sensation et Motricité. (Ed.
Fraisse, P. and Piaget, J.) Paris: Presses Universitaires de
France.

Dow, R.S., 1938. The effects of unilateral and bilateral labyrinthectomy in monkey, baboon and chimpanzee. Amer. J. Physiol.
121, 392-399.

Fernandez, G., Goldberg, J.M., and Abend, W.K., 1972. Response to
static tilts of peripheral neurones innervating otolith organs
of the squirrel monkey. J. Neurophysiol. 35, 978-997.

Flock, Å., 1971. Sensory transduction in hair cells. In Handbook
of Sensory Physiology, Vol. 1. (Ed. Loewenstein, W.R.).
Springer, N.Y., pp. 396-441.

Hammond, P.H., Merton, P.A., and Sutton, G.G., 1956. Nervous gradation of muscular control. Brit. Med. Bull. 12, 214-218.

Hoffmann, P., 1922. Untersuchung über die Eigenreflexe (Sehnen
Reflexe) menschlicher Muskeln. Berlin: Springer.

Liberson, W.T., Holmqvist, H.J., and Halls, A., 1962. Accelero-
graphic study of gait. Arch. Phys. Med. Rehabil. 43, 547-551.

Linderman, H., 1969. Studies on the morphology of the sensory
regions of the vestibular apparatus. Ergeb. Anat. Entwickl.
Gesch. 42, 1-113.

Loewenstein, O.E., 1967. Functional aspects of vestibular structure.
In Myotatic, Kinesthetic and Vestibular Mechanisms. CIBA
Foundation Symposium, London.

Loewenstein, O., and Roberts, T.D.M., 1949. The equilibrium function
of the otolith organs of the Thornback Ray. J. Physiol. 110,
392-415.

Lyon, Mary R., 1951. Hereditary absence of otoliths in the house
mouse. J. Physiol. 114, 410-418.

Magladery, J.W., and McDougal, D.B., Jr., 1950. Electrophysiological
studies of nerve and reflex activity in normal man. I: Identification of certain reflexes in the electromyogram and the conduction
velocity of peripheral nerve fibers. Bull. Johns Hopkins Hosp.
86, 265-290.

Magnus, R., 1924. Körperstellung. Springer, Berlin.

Malcolm, R., 1971. Human Response to Vestibular Stimulation. Ph.D.
Thesis, Department of Physiology, McGill University, Montreal,
Canada.

Melvill Jones, G., and Watt, D.G.D., 1971a. Observations on the
control of stepping and hopping movements in man. J. Physiol.
219, 709-727.

Melvill Jones, G., and Watt, D.G.D., 1971b. Muscular control of
    landing from unexpected falls in man. J. Physiol. 219, 729-737.
Money, K.E., and Scott, J.W., 1962. Functions of separate sensory
    receptors of non-auditory labyrinth of the cat. Amer. J. Physiol.
    202, 1211-1220.
Paillard, J., 1955. Réflexes et régulations d'origine proprioceptive
    chez l'homme. Librairie Arnette, Paris.
Rossignol, S., 1973. Auditory Influence on Motor Systems. Ph.D.
    Thesis, McGill University, Montreal, Canada.
Spoendlin, H., 1966. Ultra-structure of the vestibular sense organ.
    In The Vestibular System and Its Diseases. (Ed. Wolfson, R.J.).
    Univ. Pennsylvania Press, pp. 38-68.
Watt, D.G.D., 1969. Modes of Control in Some Anti-Gravity Muscles
    in Man. M.Sc. Thesis, Department of Physiology, McGill University,
    Montreal, Canada.

EMG OF LOCOMOTION IN GORILLA AND MAN

J. V. Basmajian and R. Tuttle

Emory University School of Medicine and Yerkes
Regional Primate Research Centre, Atlanta, Georgia
and Department of Anthropology, University of
Chicago, Chicago, Illinois

Although locomotion patterns in modern apes and man are
clearly different, the principles which control the muscular
factors are common. Specific muscles provide the motive
force when a dynamic movement occurs, but the continuance
of that activity during posture rarely is called for. Postural
mechanisms exist which allow relaxation of muscles whenever
inert mechanisms can bear the load; this state is surprisingly
prevalent in both apes and man.

Kinesiologic studies of locomotion in the gorilla inevitably
raise questions about degrees of similarity among modern man
and his ancestors. Comparisons and contrasts between two species
that have sharp differences in locomotor patterns and yet are
closely related taxonomically may illuminate and ultimately reveal
principles in both motor control mechanisms and evolution. For
the past three years we have been engaged in a systematic study
of pongid ape locomotion employing advanced electromyographic
(EMG) techniques perfected in a long series of investigations with
human subjects. Here we will emphasize our findings with gorilla
and man, leaving our work with orangutan and chimpanzee for
description elsewhere.

The predominantly quadripedal nature of gorilla locomotion
dictates a heavy emphasis in our research on the muscles of its

599

forearm and arm. Though man is bipedal, his upper limbs do
play some role in locomotion, and some notable anthropologists
believe that hominids passed through a knuckle-walking stage
quite recently in human evolution. Certain findings by our group
on the dynamics of weight bearing across joints of the upper limb
in man also illustrate important principles with broad biologic
and clinical usefulness.

EVOLUTIONARY RATIONALE

Did man evolve from relatively large-bodied "brachiators" as
various investigators have suggested? If so, did proximal des-
cendents of these "brachiators", like extant African apes, knuckle-
walk when they ventured to the ground? Or were the protohominids
virtually bipedal at the outset of their terrestrial career due to
particularities of their arboreal heritage? Can the morphological
features of the "brachiators" be explained more reasonably by the
supposition that they developed initially during a term of ground
dwelling which was followed secondarily by part-time (chimpanzee
and gorilla) and full-time (orangutan) habitation in trees (Tuttle
and Basmajian, in press)?

Detailed knowledge of the role of muscles in the hominoid forelimbs (cf. upper limbs) is imperative for resolution of the riddle
of hominoid radiation and prospectively for providing explanations
of true relationships not only among extant apes, man and their
environments, but also of fossil hominoids. This calls for inno-
vative experimentation to establish premises for the interpretation
of bone-ligament-muscle mechanics. Our electromyographic and
behavioural experiments are now in full swing and although we have
presented our early findings (Tuttle et al., 1972; Tuttle and
Basmajian, in press), final conclusions cannot be ventured in
regard to our evolutionary aims. Yet our work with apes has
provided strong support for earlier theories based on human
kinesiologic studies (described later).

Modes of Knuckle-Walking

Knuckle-walking is the characteristic hand posture employed
by gorillas and chimpanzees during quadrupedal progression and
quiescent stance. Digits II-V are flexed so that the dorsal aspect
of their middle phalangeal segments contact the ground. These

regions are covered by friction skin, forming knuckle pads similar to the skin on palms and soles. During knuckle-walking, the
metacarpus of the load bearing digital rays is nearly aligned with
the forearm. However, the wrist frequently evidences a convex
dorsal curvature or notable adduction or a combination of both
postures during progression and stance.

The proximal phalanges of digits II-V are hyperextended at the
metacarpophalangeal joints so that often a sharp angle is formed
between them and the metacarpus during load bearing activities.
The middle phalanges are flexed at the proximal interphalangeal
joints and the distal phalanges are flexed at the distal interphalangeal joints. The pulps on the distal phalanges may be apposed
against adjacent proximal segments of the hand. But frequently
the finger tips are not in contact with the palmar surface of the
hand or the substratum during knuckle-walking. The thumb does
not touch the ground (Tuttle, 1969).

KINESIOLOGIC RATIONALE

Trans-Articular Forces

Both in the compressive stages of trans-articular function and
in tension stages across the joint, EMG reveals important biological principles. In the shoulder and elbow of man and in the elbow
of gorilla we have shown that heavy tension across upper limb
joints does not recruit EMG activity except in positions where the
ligaments are relaxed - as when the shoulder joint of man is in a
partially abducted position. At least these two primates have a
ligamentous mechanism which spares the muscles and we propose
that similar mechanisms exist in other primates.

In man we have shown that human subjects suspended by their
hands from a trapeze do not show a great deal of EMG activity
nor do they let go because of muscle fatigue (Elkus and Basmajian,
1973). Slight to moderate electromyographic activity occurs in
pectoralis major and biceps muscles in the supinated position;
only the biceps activity drops in the pronated position, apparently
because that muscle is a supinator. The finger flexors and the
wrist extensors are quite active (as expected). The wrist flexors
are slightly active (with the ulnar flexor predominating) especially
with the supinated forearm.

Strapping the hands to the trapeze with a padded gauntlet (to obviate the need for the grasp) has little or no apparent effect on the EMG. It also lacks clear effect on endurance. A surprising result is the relatively short endurance of our subjects, the maximum duration being just over 3 mins (183 sec in one of the athletes, with gauntlets); most subjects last much less. The reasons given for quitting are discomfort and true pain. Most describe pain in the fingers and palm and a sense of tightness in the forearm (more on the extensor aspect). No discomfort in biceps, triceps, deltoid, or pectoralis major is cited although the last muscle is quite active. Biceps, triceps and deltoid are generally inactive. The EMG record shows no marked change in the amount of activity in those muscles that are active until the moment of quitting when any existing prior activity stops abruptly as the subject lets go. Fatigue phenomena of the EMG reported in the literature is not a significant feature. In any case, trans-articular forces appear not to require the reinforcement of muscle power, confirming earlier work.

In the gorilla, our findings for the arm muscles dovetail with these (Tuttle and Basmajian, in press). Hanging with the elbow straight permits relaxation of the brachialis and biceps.

Muscle Sparing

EMG studies in man (summarized in Basmajian, 1967) first drew closer attention to the role of ligaments. A principle emerged that stated in its simplest form is: <u>Muscles are spared where ligaments suffice.</u> This is true in both postural and dynamic situations; in the pathological situation, disturbances of ligaments lead to various secondary neuromuscular changes which again create more stir than the loss of function in the ligament.

The quiet and efficient work of ligaments allows for the operation of two laws of muscular function which MacConaill and Basmajian (1969) proposed: (i) <u>The law of minimal spurt action:</u> no more muscle fibres are brought into action than are both necessary and sufficient to stabilize or move a bone against gravity or other resistant forces, and none are used insofar as gravity can supply the motive force for movement; (ii) <u>The law of minimal shunt action:</u> only such muscle fibres are used as are necessary and sufficient to ensure that the trans-articular force directed toward a joint is equal to the weight of the stabilized or moving part together with such additional centripetal force as may be required because of the velocity of that part when it is in motion. That these two laws are valid has been demonstrated clearly by electromyography. In fact, it is the study of muscle that has revealed the role of ligaments.

Contrary to expectation, the vertically running muscles of man that cross the shoulder joint and the elbow joint are not active to prevent distraction of these joints by gravity. Much more surprising is the fact that they do not spring into action when light, moderate or even heavy loads are added unless the subject voluntarily decides to flex his shoulder or his elbow and thus to support the weight in bent positions of these joints. Quite often, he may do this intermittently or, when uninstructed, from the very onset. But it must be clear that such muscular action is a voluntary action and not a reflex one.

An analogous situation occurs in the foot where we found, some years ago, that the muscles that are usually supposed to support the arches continuously were generally inactive in standing at rest (Basmajian and Bentzon, 1954).

FORELIMB OR UPPER LIMB

Shoulder Region

While our findings in gorilla are not complete, we know that in man the muscles of the shoulder region show some activity throughout the cycle of walking. For the backward swing, even before its start, the posterior and middle parts of deltoid begin to show activity, and this continues throughout the backward swing. The upper part of latissimus dorsi and the teres major act from the onset until the arm reaches the line of the body (Basmajian, 1967). The scapular muscles and the muscles of the arm and forearm are silent.

During forward swing of the arm, activity is confined to some of the medial rotators (subscapularis, upper part of latissimus dorsi and teres major); the main flexors are strikingly silent. In some persons the rhomboids and infraspinatus are active in both swings, being most marked in persons who walk with a stoop.

Apart from brief silent periods in the extreme positions of swing, trapezius is active in both phases to maintain elevation of the shoulder. Similar activity occurs in supraspinatus; this obviously is related to the prevention of downward dislocation, noted above.

Arm and Elbow

Although notable differences exist between gorilla and man in known activity of the brachial muscles, the two species are strikingly similar in many basic features. Available evidence suggests that they share a common heritage of arboreal adaptation, including vertical climbing, hauling, hoisting, and suspensory behaviour, perhaps more recently than some authors would care to admit. Knuckle-walking probably played an inconsequential role in the protohominid career. Selection for tool use, especially involving powerful and rapid extension of the elbow joint, is the most reasonable explanation for the relatively more protruberant olecranon process in man by comparison with apes.

In the arm muscles of gorilla, our findings indicate that its elbow joint may be especially adapted for knuckle-walking and suspensory behaviour. A close packed positioning mechanism (MacConaill and Basmajian, 1969) that minimizes muscular effort during full extension of the elbow joint is indicated by remarkably low levels of EMG in the brachial muscles, particularly during knuckle-walking and suspensory behaviour on a trapeze. Extension of the elbow joint is facilitated by reduction of the upward projection of the olecranon process of the ulna, a feature that is attributable initially to aspects of an arboreal heritage in protogorilla and secondarily to selection for efficient knuckle-walking (Tuttle and Basmajian, in press).

Wrist and Hand

It is in gorilla knuckle-walking that EMG comes into its own for revealing dynamic function. Our studies on the flexor muscles in the forearm of a gorilla suggest that future comparative morphological studies on the wrists of African apes may reveal special bony features related to certain close packed positions (described below) imperative to knuckle-walking. These features may then be employed to discern evidence of knuckle-walking

heritage in the wrists of other extant hominoids and to trace the
history of knuckle-walking in available fossils.

The concept of close packing in joints is one that is fully developed in MacConaill and Basmajian (1969). In brief, it depends
on the rule that habitual motions at a joint bring it either towards
or away from its close packed position. In that position there is
maximal contact between the male and female surfaces of a
mating pair. The articular surfaces are pressed firmly together
and the bones of which they are parts cannot be separated by
traction. The ligaments are rendered taut by both the swing and
an added spin which screws the mating pair together. Thus,
muscles are spared since the ligaments produce the advantageous
situation and also maintain it until the reverse untwist and spin
movements of the mating pair are produced by muscles.

The fact that the flexor digitorum profundus muscle, which
constitutes approximately 44% of the total forearm musculature
in the gorilla, is relatively inactive during many knuckle-walking
behaviours indicates that special close packed positioning mechanisms may be operant in the metacarpophalangeal joints of digits
II-V. From studies of the distal ends and articular surfaces of
metacarpal bones II-V, we believe that special close packed
positioning mechanisms are available to safeguard against trau-
matic stressing of the hyperextended metacarpophalangeal joints,
at least during quiescent stance (Tuttle, 1969, 1970; Tuttle et al.,
1972). But these mechanisms probably are not exclusive of muscle
activity since the flexor digitorum superficialis and perhaps also
several of the lumbrical and interosseus muscles may participate
in knuckle-walking episodes.

The main wrist flexors (flexors carpi radialis et ulnaris) are
relatively inactive during quiescent quadripedal stance and progression at slow and moderate tempos. The flexor carpi ulnaris
was especially unreactive. These results suggest once more that
close packed position mechanisms safeguard the wrist joint of
knuckle-walker, relieving the muscles except during added stress.

Relative inactivity of the extensor carpi ulnaris muscle during
knuckle-walking is probably related to the fact that the same basic
posture of the wrist is maintained in the swing and stance phases
of most slow and moderately paced progressions. During swing
phase, when activity of the wrist extensors might be anticipated,
elbow flexion elevates the hand clear of the floor and shoulder

movements are probably chiefly responsible for its placement
anteriorly. No notable activities have been observed in the extensor carpi ulnaris muscle during quiescent stance, modified
palmigrade postures, or fist-walking.

LOWER OR HIND LIMB

In man, lower limb EMG studies of gait have become increasingly common. In this brief review, we cannot hope to give details
and we will omit the considerable literature on the leg and foot of
man (reviewed in Basmajian, 1967) because no similar studies
have been done on gorillas. In study after study on man, we have
noted that walking elicits very slight EMG activity in the thigh and
leg muscles compared to voluntary free movements. This has
been remarked on by others also.

Using computer analysis of EMG outputs from fine wire
electrodes in thigh and leg muscles, we found that when a subject
is permitted to walk without the imposition of a pace frequency
constraint, he selects a walking pace for the set speed in such a
manner as to allow a minimum of muscular activity (Milner et al.,
1971). During the course of such a walk, random variations in
activity seem to be more marked. This gives an indication of
some measure of ongoing adaptive control. A technique of averaging EMG records was designed primarily to eliminate the
differences between successive steps and to determine a meaningful average value. Carlsöö (1966) showed that the initiation of
walking from a stance posture consists of the body losing its
balance as a result of cessation of activity in postural muscles
(including erector spinae and certain thigh and leg muscles).
The various torques of the body weight displace the line of gravity,
first laterally and dorsally, and then ventrally, to a position in
which the propulsive muscles are able to contribute to and complete
the first step.

Hip and Thigh Muscles in Gait

The most comprehensive human study in this area is now in
the process of being written up (Greenlaw and Basmajian, unpublished). Here we will summarize the main findings, reserving
for our formal presentations the comprehensive analyses and
implications. Most impressive is the finding of relatively low

levels of activity in human lower limb muscles during ordinary gait. Human walking is an extremely economical mode of progression (its economy has presumably been carefully optimized over a long period of evolution).

The walking cycle as referred to below is based upon a normalized cycle which starts (0%) and ends (100%) at the heelstrike of the limb under consideration.

Gluteus Medius et Minimus

In the anterior fibres of gluteus medius there is moderate activity at heel contact that persists through to mid-stance. There is also a brief burst at toe-off and another just before heel contact. The posterior fibres are rather (but not exactly) similar. Gluteus minimus has only a biphasic response (at heel contact to 40% and at mid-swing).

Tensor Fasciae Latae

Its pattern is biphasic with a peak during early stance through mid-swing and another short smaller peak during toe-off.

Gluteus Maximus

Upper, middle and lower parts were all tested simultaneously. The upper part shows a clearly biphasic pattern with a small peak at heel strike and one near the end of swing phase. The middle part is more triphasic with an additional high peak just before to just after toe-off. The lower part is biphasic, rather like the upper fibres.

Hamstrings

Semitendinosus has a triphasic pattern with an initial low peak at heel contact, a second peak at 50% of the cycle, and a small third one just before the end (90% of the cycle). Semimembranosus is biphasic, lacking the peak in the middle. Biceps femoris is also biphasic, but more crisply so.

Rectus Femoris and Sartorius

Rectus femoris is generally biphasic or triphasic depending on cadence. Sartorius really shows only one peak, immediately during toe-off.

Iliopsoas

Iliacus acts continuously through the walking cycle with some rises and falls. The highest rise is during the swing phase but there is another in mid-stance. Psoas is triphasic (except with slow cadence); the main peaks correspond to those of iliacus, with a third peak at 50% of the cycle.

Adductors

Adductor Magnus is really two muscles. The upper (horizontal) part is active nearly continuously; it reaches nil only at mid-swing. The lower (vertical) part acts like a biphasic hamstring. Adductor Brevis varies with the speed of walking. At moderate speed it is biphasic with maxima at 40% and 90% of the cycle. Adductor Longus and Gracilis also have a mean peak of activity at toe-off and additional peaks at late-stance and early-swing phases.

REFERENCES

Basmajian, J.V., 1967. Muscles Alive: Their Functions Revealed by Electromyography, 2nd edition. Williams and Wilkins Co., Baltimore.

Basmajian, J.V., and Bentzon, J.W., 1954. An electromyographic study of certain muscles of the leg and foot in the standing position. Surg. Gynecol. and Obstet. 98, 662-666.

Carlsöö, S., 1966. The iniation of walking. Acta Anat. 65, 1-9.

Elkus, R., and Basmajian, J.V., 1973. Endurance: why do people hanging by their hands let go? Amer. J. Phys. Med. 52, 124-127.

MacConaill, M.A., and Basmajian, J.V., 1969. Muscles and Movements: A Basis for Human Kinesiology. Williams and Wilkins Co., Baltimore.

Milner, M., Basmajian, J.V., and Quanbury, A.O., 1971. Multi-factorial analysis of walking by electromyography and computer. Amer. J. Phys. Med. 50, 235-258.

Tuttle, R., 1969. Knuckle-walking and the problem of human origins. Science 166, 953-961.

Tuttle, R., 1970. Postural, propulsive, and prehensile capabil-
  ities in the cheiridia of chimpanzees and other great apes.
  In The Chimpanzee, Vol. 2 (Ed. Bourne, G.) Karger, Basel, pp.
  167-253.
Tuttle, R., and Basmajian, J.V., 1973. Electromyographic studies
  of brachial muscles. In Pan Gorilla and Hominoid Evolution.
  Amer. J. Phys. Anthropol. In press.
Tuttle, R., Basmajian, J.V., Regenos, E., and Shine, G., 1972.
  Electromyography of knuckle-walking: results of four experiments
  on the forearm of Pan gorilla. Amer. J. Phys. Anthropol. 37,
  255-266.

DISCUSSION SUMMARY

D. Kennedy

Stanford University, Stanford, California

The first presentation by Kennedy was followed by a general discussion of load compensation, a topic on which attention had already been focussed at earlier sessions. Melvill Jones pointed out that muscle receptors from extraocular muscles do not accomplish load compensation, but may modify patterned discharge during saccades. Houk argued against load compensation on the theoretical basis that length and force compensation are synergistic only when the compensation is for variation in the properties of the muscle itself. Referring to these and other objections to the load compensation notion, Kennedy attempted to characterize the kinds of situations in which it might be expected: locomotor or other stereotyped activities in which muscles operate against a medium that has significant and variable restoring force.

Brooks then gave an account of experiments on changes in cortical neurone discharge in response to unexpected loading. He pointed out the important distinction between load compensation carried out by spinal stretch reflexes (or tendon reflex) and other load compensating responses carried out with the help of supraspinal influences. This point was studied in his laboratory by measuring movement parameters, EMG and units in the arm area of contralateral motor cortex of three Cebus monkeys trained to turn a handle. The added procedure was the application of brief torque pulses to the handle that displaced the arm from the course of the ongoing movement. The animals compensated for the disturbance and correctly completed the voluntary movements. The protagonist EMG

611

showed three successive periods of activation, timed in relation
to the torque pulse: (1) a spinal stretch reflex starting at
approximately 12 msec and ending at 30 msec; (2) an intermediate discharge (from 30 to 60 msec); (3) a late resumption
(from 200 msec to end of movement). The cortical units displayed two successive periods of activation: (1) an "early"
burst (starting approximately at 25 msec and ending near 60
msec); (2) a "late" discharge (from near 200 msec to about
350 msec).

Brooks considers it likely that the "early" cortical burst
contributed to the intermediate muscle discharge, and that the
"late" cortical burst contributed to the late resumption of
muscle activity, which was in the range of reaction times in
voluntary movements. This experiment thus represents an
example of a load compensating response consisting of a spinal
and supraspinal component. Bizzi remarked, and Brooks agreed,
that the presence of a discharge in the cortical unit was correlated,
but not necessarily causally related, to the adaptive change in
force supplied to the muscle.

The contribution by Davis raised several questions regarding
command and phase-control in multi-membered locomotor
rhythms. In response to one of these, he re-emphasized that
there is no relationship between activity pattern in command
interneurones and those in responding motor neurones, either
as to phase or efficacy. Grillner pointed out that more complex,
ambulatory appendages (for example, the walking legs) might
have a more important role for proprioceptors. Pearson
amplified this view by citing evidence that in insect walking,
proprioceptors may influence the phase of segmental oscillators.
There was general agreement that generalizations are difficult
if not impossible in this area. Finally, the possibility of a
relationship between feedback from other moving parts and the
movement patterns of the swimmerets was cited. The experiments on swimmeret command neurones have been carried out
in isolated abdomens.

After Paul Stein's description of recent experiments on
phase co-ordination between the swimmeret oscillators, a
discussion on the general problem of phase interrelationships
was held. In response to questions by Miller and others, Stein
emphasized two points: (1) coupling between segmental oscillators
of either side can work effectively in phase co-ordination;

(2) the phase lag between two segments depends upon differences between their driven levels of excitability, that is, upon the difference between their "fundamental periods". However, the sequence of their motor outputs is independent of such differences.

Following Willows' paper, there was a discussion of the mechanisms by which periodic output bursts are generated by spiking neurones. In response to questions from Davis and Evoy, Willows clarified two points: first, that burst termination in his system involves no long-term conductance changes; and second, that the electrical junctions between bursting neurones are not rectifying except in the sense that their filtering properties which select for low-frequency events, which in this case happen to be hyperpolarizing.

Calvin then gave a discussion paper on bursting mechanisms. Davis added two further mechanisms: first, "endogenous" bursting without after-potentials as burst terminators; and second, post-inhibitory rebound, which is very marked in cells of the mollusc, Pleurobranchaea - where long-term changes in potassium conductance have also been implicated in the initiation and termination of bursts.

The papers on walking in crustaceans and insects by Evoy and Pearson produced discussion in two areas. First, Pearson's discovery of non-spiking neurones that produce reciprocally-organized motor output seemed to many to represent a direct embodiment of the "oscillator". In response to a variety of questions, Pearson emphasized that the cells are small, that their location is in a region where the dendrites of related motoneurones are clustered, and that the small synaptic potentials seen in motoneurones could be "quantal" potentials produced by a non-spiking cell via its graded membrane potential changes. Dr. W. D. Chapple (University of Connecticut, Storrs, Connecticut) inquired whether the failure to produce spikes could not be accounted for by the distance of the recording site from some local spiking region. In response, Pearson emphasized that only 6 millivolts of depolarization at the recording site is adequate to modulate the firing of post-synaptic cells, and that it is therefore unlikely that spikes in the output region of the cell would be beyond the recording range of the microelectrode. Willows continued the discussion by citing evidence that the spread of slow potentials is strongly rectified by morphological feature in some molluscan neurones,

and Pearson agreed that not all of the alternative possibilities
had yet been eliminated by experiment.

The contributions on arthropod walking also produced some
comparative treatments of other locomotor systems. Wyman
discussed the flight of flies, and Grillner the swimming of dogfish. After spinalization the head of a dogfish was fixed and the
body permitted to move freely in water. During swimming the
EMG activity was recorded in different segments along the body
in the red lateral muscle. Under resting conditions the dogfish
swims at a low steady rate around 0.5 Hz, with rostral segments
leading more caudal ones. Exteroceptive stimuli can increase
the frequency of swimming to around 2.7 Hz. The activity in
each segment was phase coupled with the adjacent segments.
Relying on the data of Lissman (1946) and von Holst (1935), the
co-ordination between the segments can be regarded as due to
a central coupling. The present results would be most simply
explained by postulating one generator in each segment producing
alternative activation of the two sides of the myotome. Each
generator (oscillator) is phase-coupled with the generator in
the adjacent segment.

In the flight of Dipteran insects, each species shows a
somewhat different motor output pattern, but generally the output
is a cyclically repeated sequence of single spikes in different
motor axons rather than bursts. This patterning is caused by
inhibitory connections among the motoneurones rather than by
premotor interneurones. A single antidromic impulse in a motor
axon activated the inhibitory cross-lines with only about a millisecond latency; a single pulse can reset the cycle timing. In
Drosophila a single gene mutation converts the normal output
to one where the various motoneurones burst together at high
frequencies for short periods, but cannot maintain activity.

Following Grillner's discussion, Miller presented evidence
that inter-limb movement in cat stepping shows a coupling which
is dependent upon the duration of the cycle period of one hindlimb.
This evidence is summarized in Fig. 1 in which cycle period
of the hindlimb (total step time) is given on the abscissa and the
ordinate gives the time interval in msec from the onset of the
first extension of the hindlimb to the onset of flexion of the ipsilateral forelimb (filled circles), and of the contact with the ground
by the hindlimb to that of the ipsilateral forelimb (open circles).
The cycle periods cover a range of stepping velocities of 0.5 to

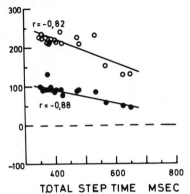

Fig. 1. Coupling Times Between Limbs

3. 3 m/sec in a normal freely-moving cat.

Increasingly, there seems to be agreement that in vertebrates as well as in invertebrates there are central pattern generators for locomotion and that separate segmental oscillators are coupled by intersegmental phase co-ordinating systems. The further question of whether these depend upon purely central neurones, or upon long proprioceptive pathways between the members, may produce different answers depending upon which system is being investigated. In cases where special central neurones are employed for phase co-ordination, there is general agreement that, although the copy of a motor message is involved, the term "efference-copy" should be avoided because of its historic use in terms of sensory comparisons.

Following Wyman's description of flight in flies, which emphasized the importance of inhibitory interconnections in generating an impulse-by-impulse phase pattern, Fourtner pointed out that in locust flight delayed excitation is used in producing part of the output pattern. The fact that for an equivalent locomotor performance there may be such substantial differences even between different species of insects emphasized the diversity of pattern generating mechanisms, which had been a recurring theme in the morning's presentations.

DISCUSSION SUMMARY

K. G. Pearson and J. B. Redford

Departments of Physiology and Rehabilitation Medicine
University of Alberta and University Hospital
Edmonton, Canada

Several major points arose in the discussion following the
three papers on cat walking (Grillner, Stuart and Miller). The
first was whether there was any evidence at the present time
for more than one oscillator controlling the rhythmic movements
of a single leg (for example, are there separate oscillators for
walking and galloping, and could different oscillators control the
rhythmic movements at different joints in a single leg?).
Grillner stated that there is evidence for at least one oscillator
for each limb but at present it is premature to speculate whether
there is more than one. The question as to whether the oscillator
was controlled by proprioceptive input was also raised. Pearson
pointed out that if in walking cockroaches or frogs the leg
extension is opposed a large extensor force develops and stepping
movements of the restrained limb cease. This suggested the
existence of an inhibitory reflex pathway onto the stepping oscillator. Grillner added that it was possible that this type of reflex
could also function in the cat, since stepping movements of the
hindlimbs of chronic, spinal kittens were inhibited if the legs
were prevented from extending.

The second major area of discussion was whether stepping
movements in spinal animals were altered after various experimental procedures. Grillner stated that holding the forelimbs of
an acute spinal kitten does not prevent the stepping of the hindlimbs. Moreover, after the foot pads have been anaesthetized
hindleg stepping movements in chronic spinal kittens are unaffected.

Following Stuart's presentation, Wetzel delivered a short
paper in which she discussed the stepping patterns of cats walking

617

on a treadmill and pointed out the differences of these stepping
patterns from those observed in freely-walking animals. Nashner
asked whether these differences could be due to the differences in
visual cues and Davis drew attention to the fact that moving
visual patterns can strongly influence the locomotor system of
lobsters and other arthropods. Wetzel agreed that visual information could be important but it was something which had not been
tested. She also suggested that the method of training cats to
walk on a treadmill could be important in determining the stepping
patterns.

Another area of discussion centred around the reliability of
measuring the phases of movement of the ipsilateral fore- and
hindlimbs. Miller's finding of a constant 40 msec latency between
the beginning of the first knee extension of the hindleg and the
beginning of the elbow flexion in the foreleg was questioned by
Stuart. When measured at the ankle, no fixed time relation
between the movements of the two limbs had been observed by
Stuart and his colleagues. Miller responded that he had observed
this fixed interval in all his preparations (intact and decerebrate)
and added that he considered Stuart's data from ankle measurements to be compatible with his own observations. Apart from
the obvious fact that before this question can be finally resolved
comparisons must be made between the same measurements,
some conference participants felt strongly that the observations
should be made at higher film speeds so as to increase the accuracy
of measurement. Both Stuart and Miller agreed.

In the discussion following the paper by Melvill Jones, the
main issue was how locomotor and other movements influenced
the transmission of information to vestibulo-spinal neurones.
Grillner commented that experiments of Orlovsky and Pavlova
(1972) indicated that there was a very poor transmission of
vestibular information during locomotion. Watt (McGill University,
Montreal) responded that Orlovsky's experiments were done with
the head held fixed and Stuart drew attention to the fact that the
inhibitory effect observed by Orlovsky was in response to lateral
tilt and not to vertical head acceleration. Stuart then stressed
the need to look closely at the effects of locomotion on the trans-
missions of vestibular activity elicited by vertical head accelerations. Bizzi (Department of Psychology, M. I. T., Cambridge,
Massachusetts) commented that in the occulomotor system there
was no suppression of vestibular input during head turning, and
that this input helps to achieve stabilization of gaze. Melvill Jones

commented that the activity in descending vestibulo-spinal neurones has not yet been studied during vertical accelerations, whereas some reticulo-spinal neurones have been found by Rossignol to be influenced by auditory inputs and it is perhaps these neurones which carry the signal to potentiate the H-reflex. In relation to the phenomenon of the potentiating effect of rhythmic auditory signals on rhythmic motor events, Redford commented that rhythmic auditory signals are often used in teaching locomotor movements to amputees and to children with cerebral palsy.

Two points of discussion arose from Basmajian's presentation. Firstly, is the pain induced when a subject hangs passively by the hands due to ischaemia, and secondly, what is the degree to which the ligaments and passive muscle properties provide mechanical stability in standing animals? Basmajian believes that ischaemia could cause some of the pain felt by hanging subjects, but considered that mechanical forces were the major factors in producing the pain. He also emphasized the economy of muscular energy in standing and walking subjects, and pointed out that many muscles are inactive during standing. Thus, he felt that mechanisms other than active muscular contractions are of major importance in stabiling posture. Kottke concurred with this point, noting that due to the remarkable balance of ligamentous structures along the vertebral column, and to the position of the centre of gravity, only a minimal action of muscles is required. Kottke also questioned whether any kind of central nervous system oscillator was needed to account for the reciprocal motion in gait. He challenged people in the audience to show more conclusively that the activity could not be all explained by reflexes that result as we change or lose our balance from a stable posture. Dr. A. Buerger (University of California, Irvine, California) presented a short paper on the plasticity of the spinal cord when shocks were delivered correlated to leg position.

REFERENCES

Orlovsky, G.N., and Pavlova, G.A., 1972. Response of Deiter's neurons to tilt during locomotion. Brain Res. 42, 212-214.

THE RELATIONSHIP OF INTERLIMB PHASE TO OSCILLATOR ACTIVITY GRADIENTS IN CRAYFISH *

P. S. G. Stein

Department of Biology, Washington University
St. Louis, Missouri

The movements of anteriad appendages lag homologous movements of more posteriad appendages during crayfish swimmeret beating. The present experiments show that the direction of metachronal movement is maintained under conditions either (1) where the anteriad oscillator has a higher intrinsic frequency than the posteriad oscillator, or (2) where the anteriad oscillator has a lower intrinsic frequency than the posteriad oscillator. The magnitude of the interlimb phase is different in the two states. These results confirm earlier predictions of experiments on the control of anteriad oscillator excitability by a single burst of co-ordinating neurone input.

Several theoretical models have been proposed which predict the magnitude and stability of interlimb phase during locomotion. It is a property of one class of these models that proper phase locking will occur only when the intrinsic frequencies of the limb oscillators monotonically change along the neuroaxis, e.g. only when a posteriad limb oscillator has a lower intrinsic frequency than a more anteriad limb oscillator (Wilson, 1966; Graham, 1972). I have recently presented data in support of a different model which predicts proper phase locking without a monotonically changing set of intrinsic oscillator frequencies

*   Suported by NSF Grant No. GB-35534 to the author.

(Stein, 1972). This latter model only requires that the set of oscillators have intrinsic frequencies within a range of each other.

A cut command neurone experimental design (Stein, 1971) has been utilized to distinguish between these two classes of models in the swimmeret system of the crayfish. This design relies on the observation that many command neurones driving the swimmeret system travel in the lateral portion of the interganglionic connectives while nearly all of the co-ordinating neurones travel in the medial portion of the interganglionic connectives. In these experiments, the lateral axons are cut   in the ipsilateral connective between two ganglia; all the axons in the contralateral connective between the same ganglia are cut. Stimulation of command half-axons in the lateral connective drives swimmeret oscillators on the same side of the cut as the stimulating electrode. Stimulation of command half-axons both above and below the cut produces phase-locking of oscillators above and below the cut.

The present experiments utilize this design with repetitive presentations of a trio of stimulating conditions. First, the posteriad half-axon of a command neurone is stimulated at Sp Hz for 10 sec and the cycle period of the posteriad oscillator is measured (Tp). Second, the anteriad half-axon of a command neurone is stimulated at Sa Hz for 10 sec and the cycle period of the anteriad oscillator (Ta) measured. Third, the anteriad half-axon is stimulated at Sa Hz and the posteriad half-axon is stimulated at Sp Hz during a 10 sec interval. If frequency equalization and phase locking of the two oscillators occur in that interval, then the cycle period of the coupled oscillators (Tc) and the interlimb phase are measured. The excitation gradient of the system is defined as the normalized difference between the intrinsic cycle periods, i.e. the excitation gradient equals (Ta -Tp)/Tc. In any one preparation Sp was kept the same and Sa was varied from trio to trio in order to alter the excitation gradient. I have examined over thirty trios in four successful preparations. The change in interlimb phase as a function of the excitation gradient from one of these preparations is shown in Fig. 1.

These data show that co-ordinated posterior to anterior metachronous crayfish swimmeret movements can occur with both negative and positive excitation gradients as well as with a zero excitation gradient. In addition, the data show the magnitude of

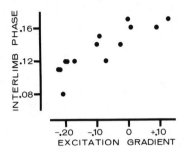

Fig. 1. Plot of interlimb phase as a function of excitation gradient. Each point represents data measured in a single trio of stimulating conditions. Ta is the intrinsic period of the anterior oscillator. Tp is the intrinsic period of the posterior oscillator. Tc is the period of the coupled system. La, p is the latency from the onset of powerstroke motor neurone discharge in the posteriad segment to the onset of homologous discharge in the next anteriad segment. Inter-limb phase equals La, p/Tc and the excitation gradient equals (Ta-Tp)/Tc.

interlimb phase is changed by alterations in the excitation grad-ient. These changes are in the direction predicted by earlier experimental data (Stein, 1972) and serve to validate the coupled oscillator model for the neuronal control of locomotion.

REFERENCES

Graham, D., 1972. A behavioural analysis of the temporal organi-zation of walking movements in the 1st instar and adult stick insect (Carausius morosus). J. Comp. Physiol. 81, 23-52.
Stein, P.S.G., 1971. Intersegmental coordination of swimmeret motoneuron activity in crayfish. J. Neurophysiol. 34, 310-318.
Stein, P.S.G., 1972. A neuronal basis for interappendage phase delay during locomotion. Soc. Neurosci. 2nd Ann. Meeting, p. 212.
Wilson, D.M., 1966. Insect walking. Ann. Rev. Entomol. 11, 103-122.

GASTROCNEMIUS MUSCLE ACTIVITY IN

HUMAN LOCOMOTION

B. R. Brandell

Department of Anatomy, University of Saskatchewan

Simultaneous and synchronized EMG and cinematographic
recordings of four male subjects were used to correlate the
intensity of medial gastrocnemius muscle activity with the
motion of lower limb segments, as they walked on a treadmill
and on the floor. For both walking media the invariable
retardation of forward shank motion, which is requisite for
mid-stance knee extension, was often associated with an early
smaller concentration of EMG, and a later more major
envelope of muscle activity was constantly synchronous with
the retardation of forward thigh motion, which necessarily
occurs at the transition from knee extension to knee flexion.
A mechanical linkage is suggested between restraint of forward
thigh motion and the initial elevation of the heel from the
ground. Plantar flexion of the ankle and upward thrust of the
shank appear to be related to residual post-activity tension of
the gastrocnemius muscle.

With reference to human locomotion, I would like to discuss
briefly the co-ordination of the gastrocnemius muscle contraction
with motions of the thigh and shank during normal human gait.
Indwelling wire electrodes and a portable tape recorder were used
to record the EMG from the medial head of the gastrocnemius
muscle of four male subjects as they walked for several minutes
on the floor and on a treadmill. Simultaneously and synchronously
a cinematographic record was made at equivalent periodic intervals

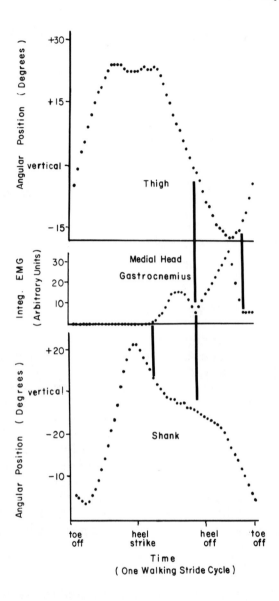

Fig. 1. Correlation of integrated EMG (arbitrary units) with
angular motion of the thigh and shank during a walking stride.
The dots represent the actual points of measurement. Note that
the early part of the Medical Head of Gastrocnemius activity
corresponds to a distinct retardation in the forward motion of
the shank, and that the most intense EMG of the Gastrocnemius
occurs at the moment when the thigh reverses its direction.

during the two walking tests. The intensity of integrated EMG and the angular position of lower limb segments were plotted against motion picture frames as units·of time (Brandell and Karger, in press; Brandell et al., 1968; Dommasch et al., 1972).

In both treadmill and floor walking the envelope of gastrocnemius activity tended to be divided into two parts. An early small part occurred in mid-stance when the knee joint was extending and appeared to be partly responsible for a marked simultaneous retardation in the forward rotation of the shank at the ankle joint (Fig. 1). The second larger part of the activity envelope occurred at the transition from knee extension to knee flexion, and apparently played a part in the simultaneous negative acceleration of the thigh.(Fig. 1). Increased tension of the gastrocnemius at this moment appears to serve two simultaneous functions: (1) it utilizes the forward rotation of the thigh to raise the heel off the ground, and (2) it promotes knee flexion by retarding forward rotation of the thigh. Plantar flexion of the ankle occurred almost entirely after gastrocnemius activity ceased and is probably related to post-activity residual tension of this muscle.

Acknowledgement: Part of a study supported by MRC Grant No. MA-4748.

REFERENCES

Brandell, B.R., and Karger, S. An analysis of muscle coordination in walking and running gaits. Med. Sport 8, Biomech. III, In press.
Brandell, B.R., Huff, G.J., and Spark, G.J., 1968. An electromyographic-cinematographic study of the thigh muscles using M.E.R.D. (Muscle Electronic Recording Device). I. Electromyography Suppl. 1, 67-76.
Dommasch, H.S., Brandell, B.R. and Murray, E.B., 1972. Investigation into techniques of gait analysis. J. Biol. Photo. Assoc. 40, 106-116.

CONTRIBUTORS

Abrahams, V.C., 191
Agarwal, G.C., 197
Atwood, H.L., 87
Baker, M.A., 187
Basmajian, J.V., 389, 599
Beck, C.H.M., 421
Blinston, G., 105
Brandell, B.R., 625
Brooks, V.B., 257
Burke, R.E., 29
Caccia, M.R., 55
Calvin, W.H., 173
Cook, T., 363
Cooke, J.D., 257
Cozzens, B., 363
Davis, W.J., 437
Emonet-Dénand, F., 119
Evoy, W.H., 477
Fetz, E.E., 187
Finocchio, D.V., 187
Fourtner, C.R., 477, 495
Freedman, W., 363
Gerlach, R.L., 179
Getting, P.A., 457
Gilman, S., 309
Goslow, G.E., Jr., 537
Gottlieb, G.L., 197
Granit, R., 3, 165
Grillner, S., 397, 515
Harris, D.A., 147
Hasan, Z., 147
Herman, R., 363
Houk, J.C., 147, 393
Kennedy, D., 429, 611
Kernell, D., 19
Künzle, H., 331
Laporte, Y., 119
Longmire, D., 55
Marshall, K.C., 425
Matthews, P.B.C., 171, 227

McComas, A.J., 55
Melvill Jones, G., 579
Miller, S., 561
Milner-Brown, H.S., 73
Monster, A.W., 347
Nashner, L.M., 291
Nichols, T.R., 407
Ovalle, W.K., 105
Padsha, S.M., 415
Pearson, K.G., 495, 617
Poppele, R.E., 127
Rack, P.M.H., 245
Rancier, F., 191
Redford, J.B., 617
Reinking, R.M., 179
Rose, P.K., 191
Rossignol, S., 579
Rymer, W.Z., 29, 411
Séguin, J.J., 331
Sica, R.E.P., 55
Smith, R.S., 105
Stein, P.S.G., 621
Stein, R.B., 73, 415
Stephens, J.A., 179
Stuart, D.G., 179, 537
Talbott, R.E., 273
Thomas, J.S., 257
Thompson, S., 457
Tuttle, R., 599
Upton, A.R.M., 55
Vallbo, Å.B., 211
Van der Burg, J., 561
Walsh, J.V., Jr., 29, 411
Watt, D.G.D., 579
Wetzel, M.C., 537
Wiesendanger, M., 331
Willows, A.O.D., 457
Withey, T.P., 537
Wong, R.K., 495
Wyman, R.J., 45

629

SUBJECT INDEX